Brain and Mind

The Ciba Foundation for the promotion of international cooperation in medical and chemical research is a scientific and educational charity established by CIBA Limited—now CIBA-GEIGY Limited—of Basle. The Foundation operates independently in London under English trust law.

Ciba Foundation Symposia are published in collaboration with Excerpta Medica in Amsterdam.

Excerpta Medica, P.O. Box 211, Amsterdam

Brain and Mind

Ciba Foundation Symposium 69 (new series)

1979

Excerpta Medica

Amsterdam · Oxford · New York

ISBN Excerpta Medica 90 219 4075 2
ISBN Elsevier/North-Holland 0 444 90095 0

Published in October 1979 by Excerpta Medica, P.O. Box 211, Amsterdam and Elsevier/North-Holland, Inc., 52 Vanderbilt Avenue, New York, N.Y. 10017.

Suggested series entry for library catalogues: Ciba Foundation Symposia.
Suggested publisher's entry for library catalogues: Excerpta Medica.

Ciba Foundation Symposium 69 (new series)
435 pages, 37 figures, 9 tables.

Library of Congress Cataloging in Publication Data

Symposium on Brain and Mind, Ciba Foundation, 1979.
    Brain and mind.

    (Ciba Foundation symposium; 69 (new ser.))
    Includes indexes.
    1. Brain–Congresses. 2. Mind and body–Congresses. 3. Neuropsychology–Congresses.
    I. Title. II. Series: Ciba Foundation. Symposium; new ser., 69.
    QP376.S878 1978   152   791–17286

ISBN 0–444–90095–0 (Elsevier/North-Holland).

Printed in The Netherlands by Casparie, Heerhugowaard

Contents

J. R. SEARLE Chairman's opening remarks 1

MARY A. B. BRAZIER Challenges from the philosophers to the neuro-scientists 5
Discussion The historical background 31

B. TOWERS Consciousness and the brain: evolutionary aspects 45

M. BUNGE The mind-body problem in an evolutionary perspective 53
Discussion Evolutionary aspects 65

D. PLOOG Phonation, emotion, cognition, with reference to the brain mechanisms involved 79

URSULA BELLUGI and E. S. KLIMA Language: perspectives from another modality 99

J. BENNETT Commentary on papers by Detlev Ploog and Ursula Bellugi 119
Discussion Language 129

C. BLAKEMORE Representation of reality in the perceptual world 139

ELIZABETH WARRINGTON Neuropsychological evidence for multiple memory systems 153

SUSAN KHIN ZAW Do philosophy and the brain sciences need each other? [Commentary] 167
Discussion Perception and memory 175

C. TREVARTHEN The tasks of consciousness: how could the brain do them? 187

O. D. CREUTZFELDT Neurophysiological mechanisms and consciousness 217

D. M. ARMSTRONG   Three types of consciousness [Commentary]   235

Discussion   Consciousness   243

I. S. COOPER   Clinical, physiological and philosophical implications of innovative brain surgery in humans   255

F. PLUM and D. E. LEVY   Outcome from severe neurological illness; should it influence medical decisions?   267

C. FRIED   Experimental surgery, and predictions of outcome from severe neurological illness: legal and ethical implications [Commentary]   279

Discussion   Experimental surgery and clinical neurology   287

P. D. WALL   Three phases of evil: the relation of injury to pain   293

C. D. MARSDEN   The emotion of pain and its chemistry   305

D. WIKLER   Pain and the senses [Commentary]   315

Discussion   Pain and mood   323

T. J. CROW   Schizophrenia: the nature of the psychological disturbance and its possible neurochemical basis   335

S. CROWN   Communication and abnormal behaviour   345

H. PUTNAM   Commentary on papers by Tim Crow and Sidney Crown   355

Discussion   Psychosis and abnormal behaviour   361

J. M. R. DELGADO   Triunism: a transmaterial brain–mind theory   369
Discussion   Triunism   395

J. Z. YOUNG   The neuroscientist's summary   397

J. R. SEARLE   Chairman's closing remarks   405

Index of contributors   415

Subject index   417

Participants

Symposium on Brain and Mind held at the Ciba Foundation, London, 5th–7th December 1978

J. R. SEARLE *(Chairman)* Department of Philosophy, University of California, Berkeley, California 94720, USA

D. M. ARMSTRONG Department of Traditional and Modern Philosophy, University of Sydney, New South Wales 2006, Australia

URSULA BELLUGI Laboratory for Language Studies, The Salk Institute, San Diego, California 92112, USA

J. BENNETT Department of Philosophy, Syracuse University, Syracuse, NY 13210, USA

C. BLAKEMORE University Laboratory of Physiology, Parks Road, Oxford OX1 3PT, UK

MARY BRAZIER Department of Anatomy, The Center for The Health Sciences, University of California, Los Angeles, California 90024, USA

M. A. BUNGE Foundations & Philosophy of Science Unit, McGill University, 3479 Peel Street, Montreal, PQ, Canada H3A 1W7

I. S. COOPER Center for Physiologic Neurosurgery, Westchester County Medical Center, Valhalla, NY 10595, USA

O. CREUTZFELDT Max-Planck-Institute for Biophysical Chemistry, PO Box 968, 3400 Göttingen, Federal Republic of Germany

T. J. CROW Division of Psychiatry, MRC Clinical Research Centre, Northwick Park Hospital, Harrow, Middlesex HA1 3UJ, UK

S. CROWN Psychiatric Department, The London Hospital, Whitechapel, London E1 1BB, UK

J. M. R. DELGADO Department of Investigation, Centro 'Ramon y Cajal', Ctra. Colmenar km. 9, Madrid 34, Spain

G. DUNSTAN Department of Moral and Social Theology, King's College, London WC2R 2LS, UK

C. FRIED Harvard Law School, Cambridge, Massachusetts 02138, USA

SUSAN KHIN ZAW Department of Philosophy, The Open University, Walton Hall, Milton Keynes, MK7 6AT, UK

C. D. MARSDEN Department of Neurology, Institute of Psychiatry, De Crespigny Park, Denmark Hill, London SE5 8AF, UK

Sir PETER MEDAWAR MRC Clinical Research Centre, Northwick Park Hospital, Harrow, Middlesex HA1 3UJ, UK

D. PLOOG Max-Planck-Institute for Psychiatry, Kraepelinstrasse 2 and 10, 8 Munich 40, Federal Republic of Germany

F. PLUM Department of Neurology, The New York Hospital–Cornell Medical Center, 525 East 68th Street, New York, NY 10021, USA

H. W. PUTNAM Department of Philosophy, Emerson Hall 207, Harvard University, Cambridge, Massachusetts 02138, USA

B. TOWERS Department of Pediatrics and Anatomy, The UCLA Program in Medicine, Law and Human Values, Center for the Health Sciences, University of California, Los Angeles, California 90024, USA

C. TREVARTHEN Department of Psychology, University of Edinburgh, 1–7 Roxburgh Street, Edinburgh EH8 9TA, UK

P. D. WALL Department of Anatomy and Embryology, University College London, Gower Street, London WC1E 6BT, UK

ELIZABETH WARRINGTON Department of Psychology, The National Hospital for Nervous Diseases, Queen Square, London WC1N 3BG, UK

D. I. WIKLER   Department of Philosophy, University of Wisconsin Center for Health Sciences, 1305 Linden Drive, Madison, Wisconsin 53706, USA

J. Z. YOUNG   The Wellcome Institute for the History of Medicine, 183 Euston Road, London NW1 2 BP, UK

Editors: Sir Gordon Wolstenholme *(Organizer)* and Maeve O'Connor

Chairman's opening remarks

JOHN R. SEARLE

Department of Philosophy, University of California, Berkeley

It was a splendid honour for me to be invited to be the Chairman of Gordon Wolstenholme's 200th and final symposium at the Ciba Foundation. My other motive for accepting the invitation was that this is a fascinating subject. I thought that the best way for me to introduce the conference would be to say why I am interested in this subject and why I think it is an important one to discuss.

When I was an undergraduate in Oxford it was commonly believed that philosophy and the sciences were hermetically sealed off from each other. There were very nice philosophical arguments designed to show that no scientific conclusion could affect any philosophical thesis. As so often happens, those arguments didn't get refuted: they just became irrelevant. One found that one's own work and the work of one's colleagues was constantly rubbing up against empirical research. Although I could give you a theoretical argument showing why philosophy and linguistics are two separate disciplines, I am constantly finding myself in discussion with my colleagues in linguistics, and they are as constantly referring to work in the philosophy of language. When it comes to the philosophy of mind the situation seems if anything even more pressing. There is an even greater need for interaction, but there have so far been rather few contacts between philosophers and what (for want of a better word) I'll continue to call neuroscientists, or brain scientists. There have been many contacts between mathematicians and philosophical logicians and between philosophers and linguists but very few contacts, as far as I know, between philosophers and neuroscientists. On the principle of grabbing whatever weaponry one needs wherever one can find it, I have dipped into some of the neuroscientific literature in a layman's sort of way, and I want to give you a few examples of why I think it is important for philosophical work.

From my point of view the two most important problems in contemporary philosophy are the relationship between language and reality, and the nature

1

of human action. The second problem is more urgent than the problem of language, because the social sciences have proved to be a disappointment. The methods of the natural sciences have not produced results in the social sciences that are at all comparable with the kinds of results that we have had in the natural sciences. There are more insistent ways of putting that second problem, such as why have the social sciences been so disappointing? Indeed, why are the social sciences such a bore? For reasons that I won't try to expound in detail I am convinced that the problem about the nature of language and the problem about the nature of human behaviour both have to do with problems in the philosophy of mind, in particular with the nature of intentionality.

As 'intentionality' is my first piece of jargon and as it may not be familiar to everybody I must say a little about it. Some of our most interesting mental states are directed at objects and states of affairs in the world: beliefs, hopes, fears, desires, motives are directed at or about objects and states of affairs. That property of being *directed at* or *about* is called intentionality by philosophers and psychologists. Not all of our mental states are like that. Pains, tickles and itches are all conscious states, and indeed in some cases more terrifyingly so than our intentional states, but they are not directed at or about objects or states of affairs. What one wants to know is what is the nature of this directedness, the nature of this intentionality? It doesn't seem possible to answer that in purely *a priori* conceptual terms. We seem constantly to be forced to take account of the empirical substructure—the physical basis or, if you like, the plumbing of intentionality.

I will give you a few examples of the sort of thing I have in mind. Consider, for example, L. Weiskrantz's experiments on blind sight (see, e.g., Ref. 1). The patients have areas of their visual fields in which they are blind, for all practical purposes, but they can nonetheless report some events and objects in that portion of their visual field. That is a good example of how empirical work can stretch our concepts. I am inclined to say that such patients have a form of intentionality. It may not be the Grade A intentionality that one gets when one actually sees objects and states of affairs but it is clear that the patients have some feelings of awareness and those feelings have truth conditions, or conditions of satisfaction, as do intentional states in general. The feelings have conditions of satisfaction characteristic of, let us say, beliefs.

That is one sort of case where I think empirical research bears on philosophical problems. There are several others. We are all familiar with the spectacular results of the split-brain operations and how they are compelling philosophers to reassess certain notions about the unity of consciousness and the identity of personhood.

Another piece of work, done some years ago by Lettvin and colleagues,[2] concerns the nervous system of the frog, on what the frog's eyes tell the frog's brain. From the philosopher's point of view their results are empirical evidence for a theory of perception that goes back to the 17th century. It is a rationalist's conception of perception according to which the mind is not a *tabula rasa*. Organisms are not, so to speak, perceptually innocent creatures that simply receive neutral data. Evidence that the structure of the nervous system structures the nature of perceptions is empirical substantiation of a long-standing philosophical hypothesis.

Several other cases are fascinating—Wilder Penfield's work for example, and the cases of *petit mal* where people are able to engage in what looks like intentional behaviour, goal-directed behaviour, though in some sense they appear to be unconscious. I think we have, in short, a large area of interaction between empirical research and philosophical investigation and analysis. The most fascinating characteristic of this research to me is that the results force a certain conceptual tension. Our ordinary ways of describing the facts often prove to be inadequate to the kinds of empirical data that have been emerging. But I must say that my epistemological hackles rise at a certain amount of this work, for the following reason. There is an anecdotal quality to some of the work that I have seen. This is to some extent inevitable because there is no way one can perform a textbook experiment. One has a patient, and one gets from one's patients the kind of information that one can get, or at least that is often what happens, as with the Weiskrantz experiments. The experiments don't all look like textbook cases of experimental design.

Finally, our other philosophical problem, the nature of language, also has important experimental implications for the nature of the localization of the linguistic capacities in the left hemisphere. Much fascinating work has been done on various forms of aphasia and in the coming years it seems to me that we can reasonably expect to learn a lot more about how language, about how our linguistic capacity, is realized in the human brain.

In short, in philosophy we have reached the point where the philosophy of mind has become central to philosophy because it has so many implications, both for traditional philosophical problems about the nature of epistemology and for the nature of language and action. We happen to have been forced into a situation where the philosophy of mind has become central at a time when, as near as I can tell, neuroscience stands on the brink of some very important discoveries. Again I must express a certain amount of caution about that. We have been told by so many sciences that they were on the threshold of spectacular discoveries that we are a little bit gun-shy. I don't want to be told again that we are going to have the solution to cancer within the next five years or that we will soon have computers that will make psychiatrists irrelevant. Nonetheless, as near as I can tell from my layman's point of view, this is a perfectly splendid time for philosophers to do what they have always done: that is, to exploit as opportunistically as they can the work of first-rate people in other fields.

References

1. WEISKRANTZ, L. (1977) Neurophysiological gaps between monkey and man. *Br. J. Psychol.* *68*, 431–445
2. LETTVIN, J. Y., MATURANA, H. R., McCULLOCH, W. S. & PITTS, W. H. (1959) What the frog's eye tells the frog's brain. *Proc. Inst. Radio Eng. 47*, 1940–1951

Challenges from the philosophers to the neuroscientists

MARY A. B. BRAZIER

Department of Anatomy and Brain Research Institute, University of California, Los Angeles

Abstract A practical science of the brain scarcely existed before the 17th century except in terms of gross anatomy. In all countries vitalistic concepts held sway, yielding only slowly to more materialistic views. These developed at a different pace in different countries, due, in each case, to the dominant philosophies of the time: the English empiricists; the French Enlightenment; the Italian and German schools of experimental neurophysiology. The last to accept the materialists' viewpoints was Russia, whose scientists imported them from their training in Western Europe in the 19th century.

A brief outline is given of how the history of brain science parallels the history of ideas in the 17th, 18th and 19th centuries.

> *Omnes homines ex anima et corpore sunt compositi*
>
> Descartes

> *I sent you lately a part of my reasonings* de intellectu humano, *which I hope came safe, for you know we are all concerned for our conceptions how idle soever.*
>
> John Locke: *Letter to a friend*

The age-old problem of Brain and Mind, coming down to us from the ancients, became a very real challenge for the brain scientist (using that denotation in its strictest sense) only when firm knowledge of the brain began to accumulate. Before then, speculation reigned alone.

The history of brain science is inevitably closely related to the history of ideas though some of these ideas have proved, to the experimentalist, to be extremely difficult to use as working hypotheses.

As we follow the outstanding thinkers through the centuries we find, hovering

between mind and brain, the ghost of the soul. This is less confusing for us
in the English language for we have a noun for 'mind', distinct from 'soul'

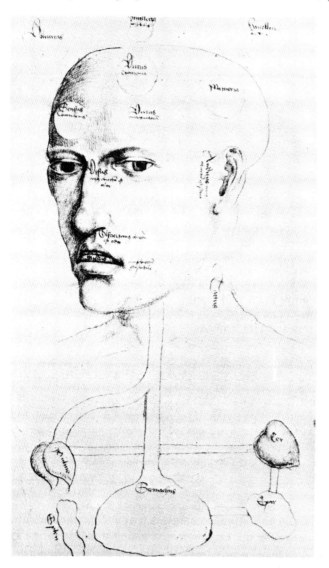

FIG. 1. From the 4th century A.D., and for several hundred years to follow, the faculties
of the mind were thought to be housed in the ventricles of the brain. This, a 15th century
illustration, was designed to illustrate the 1494 edition of Aristotle's *de Anima*. Four regions
of the brain are labelled: sensus communis, virtus cogitativa, virtus imaginativa and memoria.
(Courtesy of the Incunabula Collection at the National Library of Medicine, Bethesda,
Maryland.)

or 'spirit'. The French do not, and neither do the Russians, a difficulty which caused some of the disagreements between Sherrington and Pavlov. It is 'la vie mentale' for which the brain scientist seeks the neuronal background,

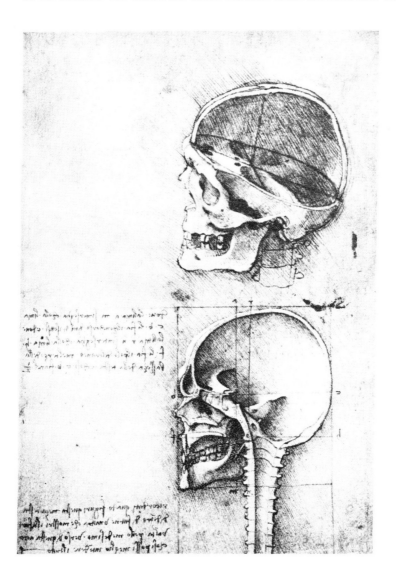

FIG. 2. Leonardo's drawing of the human skull. In the lower figure his own words state: 'Where the line a–m is intersected by the line c–b there the meeting place of all the senses (senso commune) is made . . .'
(Courtesy of the Royal Library at Windsor Castle.)

leaving aside 'l'âme' and 'l'esprit' with their overtones of the metaphysical. The later adoption by 18th century writers of the Greek 'psyche' dodged Homer's description of the psyche as a shade resembling the body.

In terms of anatomy, although for so many centuries the heart had reigned over the brain, some site in the brain for mental processes was sought even in the dark ages when, in fact, our various functions were assigned to the ventricles rather than to the solid tissue. Numerous illustrations of this idea come down to us, all devoid of scientific meaning and, all but a few, crude in execution—many being merely copies of earlier ones. What is striking, however, is that all of these depict a *sensus communis* and place it anteriorly. Fig. 1 from the 15th century, an exception for its artistic beauty, is an example of this placement of the *sensus communis* and we notice more posterior sites for 'virtus cogitativa', 'virtus imaginativa' and 'memoria'.

One great artist who, unlike the others, was also an experimentalist, gave us his exact stereotaxic coordinates for finding the sensus communis. In Fig. 2 is Leonardo's[1] drawing of the skull; in his marginal notes in mirror writing he says (in translation) 'Where the line a–m is intersected by the line c–b, there the meeting place of the senses (senso commune) is made . . .'. Elsewhere in his writings we find that he believed the *sensus communis* to be the site of the soul.

CHALLENGES FROM THE 17th CENTURY

When we reach the 17th century we find our first outstanding dualist, Descartes,[2,3,4] filling these 'holes' in the brain with a material substance carrying particles of varying sizes. These constituted his definition of les Esprits Animaux (the latter word being used in the sense of its derivation from the Latin, implying the mind). Brought to the pineal gland by the blood and directed by it to the ventricles, these spirits flowed down canals to govern all the movements of the body. Descartes, in conceiving this role for animal spirits, gave them only an efferent role. But it was imperative for his theory that the external world contribute to mental images. So he conceived the afferent influence to be effected by strings *(petits filets)*. Often presented, in secondary sources, as the original design of a reflex, this arrangement of strings coming from the sense organs to a control centre housing the soul, which then opened pores in the ventricles to release animal spirits, is far from the strict physiological concept of the reflex (as Paul Dell* has pointed out). A response controlled by the soul is far from an automatism.

---

* Footnote see p. 9.

A comment of Descartes,[4] much quoted in translation, states that 'the mind depends so much on the temperament and disposition of the bodily organs'†— but the word he himself used was 'l'esprit'. One senses that today's exponents of psychosomatic medicine would claim this as foresight. Looking back down the corridors of time one wonders whether, in this context, Descartes meant the mind or whether indeed he meant the spirit. The formulation of ideas, the intellectual life, imagination, these attributes of the mental life flourish in defiance of weakness of the body, Keats being perhaps an outstanding example among many.

Within a few years of the death of Descartes a treatise was to appear in Paris which faced up to this semantic problem. It was written by Guillaume Lamy.[5] He decided to use 'esprits animaux' for the spirits that ran through Descartes' peripheral nerve canals and 'l'âme' for the animal spirits in the brain.

The importance given to the ventricles stemmed from Galen's views that the cortex with its convolutions had no relation to mental function. This dogma ruled until the 18th century, though rare voices had been heard in dissent. The multiplicity of the cortical convolutions had fascinated the artists, but it was only when the anatomists began to trace the pathways of the cranial nerves that the possibility of sensation residing in the solid matter rather than in the ventricles began to emerge.

In the 17th century two distinguished anatomists, Sylvius[6] in Holland and Thomas Willis[7] in England, challenged the ventricles as the site of psychic spirits. Willis wrote: 'The ancients so magnified the importance of this cavity that they declared it to be the workshop where the animal spirits are created and perform the chief operations of the animal function. On the other hand the moderns consider these places as vile and assert them to be merely sewers for the carrying away of excreted matter'. And in refuting the ancient concept of the ventricles, Willis proposed the cortex as 'the part which serves for the production of animal spirits' and for their distribution 'for the various acts of imagination and memory'.

An intensely religious believer, Willis speculated that there were two souls— the corporeal soul shared with lesser animals and the rational soul of man. Willis's famous book appeared in 1664, two years after the first publication of Descartes' *De Homine* in which a similar differentiation had been made.

---

*'Descartes had a real dualistic conception ... Descartes cannot have had the concept of the reflex, since the afferent and efferent paths were so very different in constitution.'
(Dell, P. (1958) in *The Neurological Basis of Behaviour (Ciba Found. Symp.)* p. 26, Churchill, London. See also Gangueilhem, G. (1955) *La Formation du Concept de Réflexe*. Presses Universitaires, Paris.)
†'...car l'esprit depend si fort du tempérament et de la disposition des organes des cors.'

Moving mental functions from the ventricles, Willis gave the *sensus communis* a locus in tissue (the corpus striatum), placing imagination in the corpus callosum (i.e. in white matter) and memory in the cortex. Involuntary motor action he gave to the cerebellum.

This was an age dominated by great thinkers, none of them, however, an experimentalist (as Leonardo had been in the previous century). The influence of Voltaire,[8] powerful in France, spread across Europe and it is probably to him that we owe the almost immediate interest evoked by the works of Descartes (and, later, of Locke).

Another class of challenge from the 17th century for the experimentalist to meet came from the English school of Empiricism: Locke,[9,10,11] Berkeley[12] and Hume[13] with their emphasis on sense perception. Let us take only one example, John Locke.

While Locke was still a schoolboy, Descartes had died. Revolutionary as he had been in drawing 'perception' into the nervous system, Descartes nevertheless believed some ideas to be innate and that the certainty of truth could be reached by reasoning. He gave a rational soul uniquely to man.

It is essentially on these issues that Locke's concepts diverge from those of Descartes and, in doing so, usher in a new age in the theories of brain science to tease the experimentalists. As everyone knows, Locke insisted that all knowledge comes from sensory observations and from reflection on them, and that the mind is incapable of formulating ideas from any other source but the senses, and to the exclusion of all *a priori* knowledge; 'without', as he put it, 'the help of any innate impressions'. Extracts from Locke's famous Essay appeared in French[9] two years before its printing in London, and we note the translator's use of the word 'Esprit' (which was capitalized)*.

This was the period of Newton, friend and correspondent of Locke. When the movement against Locke swelled to dominance in the 19th century, Whewell,[14] the respected Master of Trinity and outstanding proponent of inductive reasoning, held that Locke's influence (which he deplored) surfaced in Newton's famous declaration of distrust in hypotheses.

The empirical method, in testing the challenge of Locke, needs neuronal evidence of a *tabula rasa* together with a storage mechanism, for Locke stated that it was 'necessary to have a repository to lay up those ideas which the senses provided' (a view he shared with St Augustine[15]).

---

*'Dans les pensées que j'ai eues, concernant notre Entendement j'ai taché d'abord de prouver que notre Esprit est au commencement ce qu'on appelle *tabula rasa* c'est à dire, sans idées & sans connoissance ... Je prétends de montrer, dans les suivants la source de laquelle nous tirons toutes les idées, qui entrent dans nos raisonnements & la manière dont elles nous viennent.'

Here are the challenges: is there neuronal evidence of development from a *tabula rasa* at birth? Is there a neuronal basis for storage?

I think today's brain scientist may perhaps say 'yes, evidence is accumulating'. Selecting single examples from experimental work in the current decade one can quote the growth of dendritic spines on cortical neurons from a paucity or complete absence in the neonate to the development of the full complement in the adult (Adinolfi,[75] Scheibel[76]), and the claims that 'usage' increases the growth of postsynaptic structures, of apical dendrites and their spines (Rutledge[77]). Neural immaturity appears to be the basis for our failure to store memories from our infant years, and there are animal experiments that show that the immature animal, although learning quickly, also forgets quickly (Rosenzweig and Bennett[78]).

The majority of early writers most often quoted on the mind–brain problem concentrated their thoughts on how the mind works in normal human beings, though the possibility existed that hints might be obtained from study of the mentally disturbed. Until the 17th century, there had been little doubt that bizarre behaviour indicated disturbance, not of the body, but of the soul. Even this opinion was considered an advance over the centuries-old belief in demons and magic as the cause of behavioural eccentricities.

One outstanding thinker from the beginning of the 17th century, Francis Bacon,[16] expressing ideas centuries before their acceptance, wrote: 'For the consideration is double; either how, and how far the humours and temperament of the body, do alter or work upon the mind; or again, how and how far, the Passions and Apprehensions of the mind do alter or work upon the Body. The former of these we see sometimes handled in the Art of Physick; but the same hath by strange ways insinuated itself into Religion. For the Physician prescribes Remedies to cure the Maladies of the mind; as in the cures of Frenzies and Melancholy; they do also administer Physick to accelerate the Mind.'

As long as mind and body were thought to be separate empires it was unusual to find a physician concerning himself with the possible neural basis for mental causes of disturbed behaviour. The great 17th century classic of psychiatry is Burton's *Anatomy of Melancholy*.[17] Burton was a Galenist, believing in humours. He believed in natural spirits, in vital spirits and in animal spirits, the first 'begotten in the liver', the second 'in the heart' and the third 'in the nerves'. A strange 'anatomy' indeed. Yet when he came to seek for 'the part affected' in melancholy Burton wrote: 'Some difference I find among writers, about the principal part affected in this disease, whether it be in the brain, or heart, or some other member. Most are of the opinion that it is the brain . . .'

CHALLENGES FROM THE 18th CENTURY

As we move to the 18th century, we find an outstanding example that posed a challenge to the neuroscientist in the works of the Abbé de Condillac.[18,19] The proposals of Locke were well known in France for they had been championed by Voltaire.[20] Condillac was aware that experiments had begun the attempt to prove or disprove the current concepts of mind and soul; outstanding among these were the ablation experiments of Claude Perrault,[21,22] the brilliant scientist, physician and architect. In attempting to test whether the brain alone was the seat of the soul (l'âme), Perrault sought to study the faculties of dogs by surgical interference with their brains. He could not accept that the control by the soul over the whole body was effected by the outflow of animal spirits from the brain. Unfortunately his animals did not survive long enough to settle this question for him. For another two centuries, however, ablation remained a chosen method for exploring brain function, until it was largely replaced by techniques that recognized that one cannot remove a part without affecting the whole. But the concept died hard and ablationists, observing postoperative functional changes in their animals, continued to consider that the piece removed and now in the bottle contained the lost function.

Well aware of this experimental approach, the Abbé Condillac had renounced his appointment as an ordained priest at the Abbey of Mureaux and before the age of 30 had become a frequenter of the salon of Madame Helvétius at Auteuil, where he met the lively group of brilliant minds that were to influence the whole of 18th century France: the Encyclopaedists. Stimulating as this company was, it was his reading of Locke in Pierre Coste's translation[9] of its rather clumsy colloquial English that provoked Condillac to write his *Essai sur l'Origine des Connaissances Humaines*[18] and, eight years later, his famous *Traité des Sensations*.[19]

Condillac introduced into his model the role of language. While agreeing with Locke that all knowledge comes from sensation and reflection,* he held that both language and symbols play a great part in the formation of ideas and that the mind itself has the active power of reflection on the ideas that (formed directly from sensations) were the result of reflection, of 'remembering, considering, reasoning . . .' Locke, however, had given no role to language other than that of communication to other minds: in man's own mind, words

---

* '. . . la refléxion n'est dans son principe que la sensation même, soit parce qu'elle est moins la source des idées que le canal par lequel elles découlent des sens.' (Extrait Raisonné 1778, Ref. 19.)

functioned only as symbols of ideas in storage. For Condillac, however, they played a part in the formation of new ideas.

For the initial sensation Condillac's model relies on the tactile sense, for actual contact, the act of touch, was held by him to be our only source of information about objects in the external world.* The other senses learnt to recognize external objects only by conjunction of their impressions with the factual evidence of touch, and in this Condillac stressed the importance of the *active movement*, not only movement of our skin but of our joints and tendons, made in touching the external object.

Condillac's fellow Idéologue, Diderot,[23] wrote of this in his *Lettres sur les Aveugles*, reporting the dying Cambridge mathematician Saunderson, who had been blind since early childhood, to have said to the priest 'If you want me to believe in God you must make me touch him'. For this and other sentiments expressed in these famous *Lettres*, Diderot was sent to prison at Vincennes.

Memory was for Condillac a *transformed* sensation, transformed in such a way that a similar sensation arriving in the present could be compared with that which arrived in the past. (This sounds like Pavlov, but I am speaking of Condillac.)

For the 20th century brain scientist with recording electrodes in the human brain, this differentiation is already becoming possible. Neuroscientists at the 1977 International Congress of Physiology heard that neuroscientists have differentiated the neuronal unit discharges evoked in single brain cells by novel stimuli from those familiar to the individual in memory.[79]

Today we readily accept the difference between seeing and gazing, between hearing and listening, between tasting and savouring, and much current work is directed towards the neuronal mechanisms involved in attention. And in fact it is Condillac who gives us the clue to what we should look for:[19] 'If a multitude of sensations operate at the same time with the same degree of vivacity, or nearly so, man is then only an animal that feels; experience suffices to convince us that then the multitude of impressions takes away all activity from the mind ... But let only one sensation subsist, or without entirely dismissing the others, let us only diminish their force; the mind is at once occupied more particularly with the sensation which preserves its vivacity, and that sensation becomes attention, without its being necessary for us to suppose anything else in the mind'.

One may note that modern neurophysiology has found the mechanisms of Condillac's 'diminished force' in the phenomenon of the inhibitory surround,

---

* 'C'est le mouvement, qui en est la cause physique et occasionelle, se reproduit dans le cerveau.'

and the mechanism of his 'sensation which preserves vivacity' in the excitatory focus.

The facet of Condillac's model that our imaginary 20th century scientist would have difficulty in testing is that he held all these faculties to be attributes not of the brain but of the soul. When an impression reaches our bodies, it is, he says, the soul which senses it: 'c'est l'âme seule qui sent'.

It was one of Condillac's most ardent followers, De Stutt de Tracy,[24] who took the lead among the Idéologues in modifying the model to bring it into the domain of the physical world. Condillac was no physiologist and had felt no urge to interpret human understanding in terms of nerves or physical events, and it is here that the Idéologues, although inspired by Condillac, parted from him.

It is perhaps of importance to note that our modern usages of the terms 'psychology' and 'ideology' have lost contact with the sense in which their French forms were used in the 18th century. The word 'psychologie' was used by Condillac to express 'science de l'âme' (knowledge of the soul). De Tracy introduced 'idéologie' to denote 'la science qui traite des idées'— knowledge of ideas.

It was, of course, essential for de Tracy's fundamentally materialistic thesis that some physiological proof be established, some action of nerves and brain. Not himself an experimentalist, he espoused the theory developed by Baglivi[25] in Rome and promoted by David Hartley[26] in England that the nerves vibrate and convey their messages by their own movements.

Baglivi, an anatomist, was a materialist ahead of his time but Hartley, a convinced dualist, would not recognize that the doctrine of vibrations was 'unfavourable to the immateriality of the soul'. He stated 'that sensations arise in the soul from motions excited in the medullary substance of the brain'.

De Tracy, a materialist, realized the difficulties inherent in the model for he recognized that the movement of nerves from the eye must be different for the perception of blue than for red; those from the ear for a dull or a sharp sound; from the nose for one odour or another; and those from touch for a prick or a burn. He hazarded that it is the same nerve that differentiates each of these sensations by carrying a different distribution of disturbance for each event, thus evoking a specific movement in the brain.*

Not himself an experimentalist, de Tracy turned to Cabanis,[27] physician

---

*One feels that de Tracy would not have been very surprised by the discoveries in the 20th century of cells in the visual cortex that differentiate the orientation of a strip of light (Hubel[80]), or of the brain cells which react differentially to the wavelength of light (DeValois[81]), or of others reacting specifically to movement (Baumgartner[82]).

Whytt was writing in the mid-18th century but the idea that some representation of the soul existed within the spinal cord was to persist to the end of the 19th century, its chief protagonist being Pflüger,[34] the founder of the famous *Pflüger's Archiv*.

This was only one of the frequent relocations the soul had had to make. We have by now seen it housed in the heart, in the ventricles, in the pineal gland, in the stomach, in the blood, in the corpus callosum and in the medulla spinalis (Aristotle, Galen, Descartes, Von Helmont, Harvey, Willis, Prochaska and Pflüger).

There was soon to develop a search for functional localization in the cortex, beginning with speculation about the convolutions. These being so obvious they had been remarked upon by almost every writer, even before Galen, but without any proposal as to their function. Galen's *Opera Omnia*[35], as given to us in translation (1822), whets our appetite by the title *De usu partium*, but in the case of the cortex we find little about its 'use'. In fact, Galen argued against there being any relationship to intelligence on the grounds that the brains of donkeys also contained so many convolutions, an opinion still extant in the 17th century (as, for example, in the writings of Bartholin[36] in 1641).

It is in the 18th century that we find the suggestion that the cerebral cortex itself initiated a control over function. We find this in the charming *Lettres d'un Médecin des Hôpitaux du Roy* written by Pourfour du Petit[37] in 1710 and published posthumously in 1788.

Pourfour, arguing from clinical observations that he (and others) had made on head injuries in soldiers, and following these up by experiments on dogs,

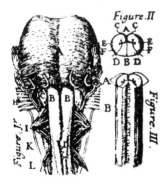

FIG. 4. Pourfour du Petit's illustration of the crossing of fibres within the cord to effect the contralateral damage he found in his experiment on dogs.
(From: Pourfour du Petit (1710) *Lettres d'un Médecin des Hôpitaux du Roy*. From the copy in the Bibliothèque Nationale. Reproduction by courtesy of the late Dr August Tournay.)

had established the crossing of the pyramids (Fig. 4). He wrote of his surprise that earlier anatomists had not come to this conclusion, especially Bonet,[38] who had reported so many examples of contracoup.

A believer in animal spirits, Pourfour argued that these must be produced unilaterally in the brain in order that they could flow to the limbs only on the opposite side of the body.* Yet when he operated to relieve these symptoms he frequently found the wounds and inflammation in the cortex rather than the ventricles ('L'inflammation n'occupoit que la partie corticale').

CHALLENGES FROM THE 19th CENTURY

It is in the 19th century that the great change came from vitalism to materialism. In the previous century, the science of the nervous system had reached different levels in the various countries of Europe. In Germany, in the first half of that century, the Thirty Years War had brought science almost to a standstill and, in the fields of chemistry and physiology, this stagnation developed into a retrogression owing to the emergence of an extremely influential figure, Georg Ernst Stahl[39] who, in opposition to the growing materialistic approach, reintroduced an immaterial *anima* which he held to be the sole activating principle of the body parts. Since the search for an immaterial agent lies outside the scope of science, this doctrine virtually extinguished experimental enquiry in his country in his times. The movement towards materialism among scientists in Germany was to come in the 19th century from leaders such as Du Bois-Reymond, Carl Ludwig and Helmholtz. They were the pupils of Johannes Müller[40,41] who had as a young man espoused the Naturphilosophie of Schelling.[42] Only later in his life was Müller to reject this vitalist philosophy, even to the extent of incinerating his early works.

In Russia, the Naturphilosophie of Schelling had a strong following among many who had been appalled by the mechanistic development of ideas in western Europe, as exemplified by the notorious treatise of La Mettrie,[43,44] *L'Homme Machine* (1748), and his earlier *L'Histoire Naturelle de l'Âme* (1745) (which, incidentally, he put in the brain).

The most influential antagonist to materialism at the turn of the century in Russia was the physiologist Vellansky[45,46] who had spent three years studying Naturphilosophie. By his prolific writings, including a textbook of physiology,

---

* 'Je vous envoie quelques remarques ... aux expériences qui prouvent, que les esprits animaux qui se filtrent dans la partie droite du Cerveau, servent pour le mouvement des parties gauches du corps; et que ceux qui se filtrent dans la partie gauche du cerveau servent pour le mouvement des parties droites du corps ...'

and by lectures in Moscow, directed not only to physiologists but to the Medical Surgical Academy, he strove to stem the tide. It was against this climate of thought that a more deterministic approach to the life sciences was to emerge in the 19th century. The change came through infiltration of ideas from the West and mainly from those of Magendie.[47,48,49]

In France the break from vitalism, with its major stronghold in Montpellier, was spearheaded by Magendie, who may be regarded as the father of experimental physiology. Until his time, the views of Bichat,[50] the brilliant French pathologist who died so young, had been dominant in France. Bichat held that the various tissues of the body, including the nervous system, had vital properties in addition to and distinct from their chemical and physical properties. This view was spread by Richerand[51] in his popular textbook of physiology and thus intensified for his period the division between physiology and the hard sciences.

Biological scientists were just beginning to free themselves from the tenet that behaviour of the human species was under command, not from an organ (the brain), but from an abstraction (the soul). But soon they were to become mired in the time-worn controversy of body versus mind.

At first accepted by Magendie, these vitalistic ideas, to which he said religion had given a 'croyance consolatrice', were gradually eroded until at last he decided to rebut them.* He did not hesitate to make his position clear. He wrote: 'Le cerveau est l'organe matériel de la pensée; une foule de faits et d'expérience le prouvent'.

But more realistic ideas about brain function had to wait for the enormous spur to the search for localization in the cortex which came from the fantastic popularity of phrenology, fathered by that master of anatomy, Franz Josef Gall.[52]

Gall's major tenet—that mental faculties must have their seat in the brain—was enormously influential in terms of cortical localization but came to final shipwreck in the form of cranioscopic mapping. His ideas did not go unchallenged. One of the most prominent men to attack Gall's doctrines was his arch-enemy, Flourens,[53] who made a sweeping rejection of all such ideas, denying the brain any discretely localized action.

More important, however, than the acrimonious wrangling between these

---

*Discussing 'intellect', Magendie wrote:[49]

'L'intelligence de l'homme se compose de phénomènes tellement différents de tout ce que présente d'ailleurs la nature, qu'on les rapporte à un être particulier que l'on regarde comme une émanation divine et dont le premier attribut est immortalité ...

Le physiologiste reçoit de la religion cette croyance consolatrice mais la sévérité de langage ou de logique que comporte maintenant la science, exige que nous traitions de l'intelligence humaine comme si elle était le résultat de l'action d'un organe.'

men was the introduction by Flourens of the experimental method into the search for cerebral localization. Like Perrault before him, he chose ablation as the means of attack. Flourens's localizations were very generalized, being divided among the medulla, the cerebellum and the cerebral hemispheres (to which he denied a role in sensation or movement).

Concerning the cerebral hemispheres, Flourens claimed that animals that survive their removal 'lose perception, judgement, memory and will . . . therefore the cerebral hemispheres are the sole site of perception and all intellectual abilities'. He did not hesitate to infer subjective qualities and faculties. In one of the more renowned of his experiments he had kept a pigeon alive after removal of its cerebral hemispheres. The bird was 'blind' and 'deaf' and appeared to be asleep, although it stirred when poked. Flourens went so far as to say that the bird lost its volition and 'even the faculty of dreaming' (Fig. 5).

Most of Flourens's observations, particularly those on the cerebellum, had been anticipated by Rolando at Sassari,[54] whose treatise of 1809 (written in Italian and illustrated by himself) was later republished in French in an abbreviated form in 1824.

Rolando did not succeed in keeping his animals alive for long and many of his conclusions were therefore incorrect, for he mistook surgical shock for paralysis. Rolando believed the cerebellum to be the source of all movement,[55]

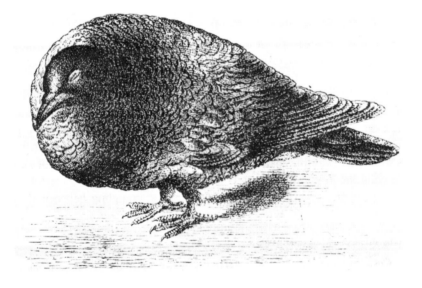

FIG. 5. A pigeon deprived of its cerebral hemispheres in the position described by Flourens. (From: Luciani, L. (1913) *Human Physiology*, English edition, Macmillan, London.)

Flourens thought it merely the regulator; Magendie disagreed, holding cerebellar function to be maintenance of equilibrium. He reached this conclusion from studying the disturbance of gait in a duck* from which he had removed the cerebellum unilaterally. The great contribution towards our modern knowledge of the cerebellum came from Luciani of Florence whose book *Il Cerveletto* (1891) is a classic.

Magendie, in the observations he made on decerebrate animals (1823), anticipated Sherrington by an accurate and detailed description of decerebrate rigidity in rabbits.

Far more successful, surgically, was Goltz,[56] the neurologist of Strasbourg; his dogs survived for long periods, his technique being to 'wash away' portions of the cerebrum, thus avoiding drastic cutting and severe impairment of the circulation (Fig. 6).

The technique thus resulted in imprecisely defined lesions and led Goltz to doubt localization of function. The brain of one of his dogs was sent to Langley[57] in Cambridge who gave it for dissection to a young colleague whose name appeared with Langley's on the resultant paper. This was in 1884, long before anyone suspected that the junior author, whose name was Sherrington, was to become one of the outstanding physiologists of his time.

But a new technique was to invade the field of brain localization. In 1870 two young doctors in Berlin, Gustav Fritsch and Eduard Hitzig[58] (apparently unaware of the work of Cabanis), demonstrated that certain regions of the cortex were excitable by electricity as evidenced by elicited movements. Less than five years later came the demonstration by Caton[59] in Liverpool that sensations evoked by visual stimuli produced a change in the ongoing electrical activity of the brain and specifically in a localized region, posterior and lateral to the midline.

In the light of history it seems strange that for over fifty years this latter discovery, though actively pursued in Poland and Russia, evoked so little attention in the West, because until that time all that experiment could reveal in animal tests was information about motor function. Until Caton's discovery, there was no direct clue to the localization of sensation in the brain, a function more clearly related to the problem of the mind. To this day, the recording of the electrical activity of the brain remains the only major non-invasive physiological technique for the assessment of cerebral function.

Fritsch and Hitzig were more fortunate than Caton,[60] for their work was

---

*Sherrington, quoting this experiment, mistranslated Magendie's word 'canard' as 'water-dog', thus making it appear to be a mammal.

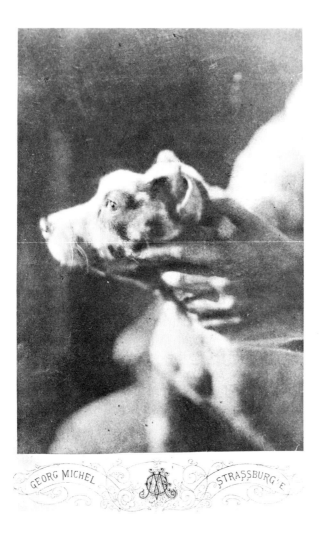

FIG. 6. Studio portrait of one of Goltz's decorticate dogs. (The gift of the late Dr Paul Dell.)

not ignored. It fell into the pattern developed so successfully by Ferrier in his popular book *The Function of the Brain*[61] and, by its restriction to motor functions, avoided controversies over sensation and how this was handled by the brain. Ferrier's experiments[62] were on monkeys but by transferring the labels to maps of the human brain, he set the stage for comparison with the cytoarchitectonic fields of Vogt[63] and of von Economo,[64] each of whom based their maps on findings from a single brain.

At approximately this same time a new proposal emerged to disturb the dualists; this was a theory of reflexes in the brain, a wholly material reflex arc. This came from Ivan Michailovich Sechenov[65] in Russia. His concept was, in fact, not completely out of keeping with developing thought. Thomas Laycock[66] twenty years earlier had published in this vein in England, using almost the same title as Sechenov's—'On the reflex function of the brain'. In 1841 Laycock wrote 'the brain, although the organ of consciousness, is subject to the laws of reflex action, and that in this respect it does not differ from the ganglia of the nervous system'. The new proposal, coming from Sechenov in St Petersburg as an essay entitled (in translation) 'Reflexes of the brain', asserted that all higher brain function is a material reflex consisting of three sectors: an afferent initiation by sensory inflow, a central process entirely subject to physical laws, and an efferent component resulting in muscular contraction.

This schema of Sechenov's is reminiscent of the three-component arc of Marshall Hall[67] and the three-component spinal reflex of Sherrington[68] but, unlike their concepts, in this schema the central component is in the brain and is purely mechanistic.

According to Sechenov, all reactions—whether described in common parlance as pleasure, fear or distress, or in other terms—were in essence muscular expressions. During the passage of the inflow through the central portion of the arc there could either be neuronal excitation which would augment the reflex motor response (as in so-called emotional states), or neuronal inhibition which would decrease the reflex movement during a thought process, the resultant being 'rational' or controlled behaviour.

Thus, according to Sechenov, all human behaviour was a balance between inhibition and excitation operating mechanically at the central link of the reflex arc.

It is intriguing that this mechanistic concept of the brain's role should have developed in Sechenov who spent so many of his years of training in the land of Kant.[69] Kant, in his moral philosophy, insisted on the role in human life of an autonomous rational will that he declared could not be comprehended within the deterministic framework of the scientific outlook.

It was the physiologists Du Bois-Reymond, Ludwig and Helmholtz whose rejection of this philosophy influenced the young Sechenov.

But in his own country, with its strong vitalistic stance, Sechenov's purely materialistic view of the mental life of our species was so disturbing that his book was at first suppressed, the Minister of the Interior stating that 'This book propagandizes in popular form the teaching of extreme materialism'. Marshall Hall, in England, in his work on reflexes had protected himself from similar onslaught by stating the movements of his decapitate animals to be 'all beautiful and demonstrative of the wisdom of Him who fashioneth all things after his own Will'.

But the influence of Sechenov's book remained and grew until, under Pavlov,[70] it became the essential foundation of conditioned reflexes. The word 'mind' ('ym' in Russian) dropped from use in Pavlov's laboratories, to be replaced by 'higher nervous activity', the term used today by all who work in that field.

What laid the foundation stone for the theory of conditioned reflexes was Sechenov's postulate that the memory trace of a past sensory experience could be evoked by the recurrence of any fraction of it, even if this fraction were quite insignificant and unrelated in its apparent meaning. This is essentially the principle underlying the formulation of the conditioned reflex theory, namely the potency of an indifferent external stimulus provided it is repeatedly time-locked to the original experience.

One should note that in Pavlov's own teaching he was describing his concepts of the processes in the brain (and specifically the cerebral cortex) without any defined neuronal foundation or any direct observations from within the brain. It was only after Pavlov's death that a younger generation of Soviet neurophysiologists began to search for (and find) in the brain supportive evidence for the conjectured neuronal mechanisms lying behind the overt behavioural responses that are the cornerstone of the original Pavlovian school.

It was largely disregard for neuronal evidence for Pavlov's concepts of conditioned reflexes that caused Sherrington, otherwise one of Pavlov's great admirers, to comment after two visits to the master himself that this would never appeal to physiologists in his own country. Pavlov must have been profoundly hurt by this for he repeated it on many occasions, even 12 years later, saying that Sherrington told him at their first meeting: 'Your conditioned reflexes will hardly be popular in England, since they have a materialistic flavour'.

Pavlov's scorn for Sherrington's dualism was worded with little restraint at several of the famous 'Wednesday' gatherings of his group. With what the late Koshtoyantz,[83] the distinguished editor of his writings, described as

Pavlov's 'spirit of militant irreconcilability', Pavlov said, in comment on Sherrington's book *The Brain and its Mechanisms*:[71]

> 'It appears that up to now he is not at all sure whether the brain bears any relation to our mind. A neurologist who has spent his whole life studying the subject is still not sure whether the brain has anything to do with the mind . . .
>
> 'How can it be that at the present time a physiologist should doubt the relation between nervous activity and the mind? This is the result of a purely dualistic concept . . . Sherrington is a dualist who resolutely divides his being in two halves: the sinful body and the eternal, immortal soul'.

One of the group protested; this was the late Kupalov, a greater scholar than Pavlov, who, while agreeing that Sherrington was a dualist, pointed out that the sense he generally imparted to certain English words, in particular the word 'mind', differed from Pavlov's interpretation. 'You', he said to Pavlov, 'interpret the concept 'mind' in your way while he regards it somewhat differently. He chiefly takes into account so to speak, the subjective emotions. He agrees that behaviour is law-governed. But he is preoccupied with what we call near sensations'. But Pavlov would not accept this and ridiculed Kupalov, saying: 'The fact that you, his advocate, despite your attempt to comprehend his viewpoint, are baffled by his phrase simply reinforces my position'.

Sherrington reserved his verbal fire until after the death of Pavlov, but his own influence on English physiology was profound. Surrounded by a group of outstanding neurophysiologists, he most surely instilled his personal views. One of his most distinguished pupils, Liddell,[84] even wrote a book in 1960 entitled *The Discovery of Reflexes*, totally ignoring conditioned reflexes and making only a single mention of Pavlov, a reference to his use of the word 'analysers'.

In Sherrington's rebuttal of Pavlov he revealed his own profound misunderstanding of Descartes, for he likened the two. 'In reflexology', he wrote, 'Descartes would find Ivan Pavlov of Petrograd his greatest successor . . .'. A strange comparison: Descartes who believed in a Deity and in a soul in man—neither of which received recognition from Pavlov.

Yet Sherrington held Pavlov in high personal esteem and, when seeking the Chair at Oxford, sought a letter of recommendation from him. The correspondence survives and provides an interesting vignette of these two men, one an experimentalist and the other, at least in his later years, essentially a conceptualist.

That Sherrington, the master of the spinal reflex, had trouble with the mind–body problem surfaces throughout his writings but becomes explicit in the more literary works of his later years *(Man on his Nature*[72] and *Goethe on Nature and Science*[73]*)*. In 1947, seizing the opportunity to write a preface to the second edition of his famous book, *The Integrative Action of the Nervous System*, Sherrington included a manifesto that stressed his dualistic outlook on the body–mind problem: 'That our being should consist of *two* fundamental elements offers I suppose no greater inherent improbability than that it should rest on one only'.

That Sherrington believed this statement deeply was revealed by yet another statement written in the first person singular, an unusual form for a scientist to use. In his Rede lecture on *The Brain and its Mechanisms*,[71] speaking of mental and physiological experiences, he wrote:

> '... to many of us a mere juxtaposition of the *two sets* of happenings proclaims their disparity... As for me, what little I know of the how of the one, does not, speaking personally, even begin to help me toward the how of the other. ... Mental experience on the one hand, and brain happenings on the other, though I cannot correlate together, I nevertheless find to coincide in time and place... But that does not help because, at least to me, neither of the two appears related to the other. As mental events I should suppose them aloof'.

This essay is not intended to cover the 20th century but these two immensely influential figures, both born at mid-19th century, were to influence profoundly the development of physiology of the brain although their viewpoints were diametrically opposite: Sherrington the dualist and Pavlov the materialist.[74]

Both lived to a great age but neither solved the brain–mind problem.

References

1. LEONARDO DA VINCI [1452–1519] *Drawings in the Royal Collection*, Windsor
2. DESCARTES, RENÉ [1596–1650] (1637) *Discours de la Méthode*, Maire, Leyden
3. DESCARTES, R. (1662) *De Homine*, Moyardus & Leffen, Leyden
4. DESCARTES, R. (1664) *L'Homme et la Formation du Foetus*, Le Gras, Paris
5. LAMY, GUILLAUME (1678) *Explication mécanique et physique des fonctions de l'âme sensitive, ou des sens, des passions et du mouvement volontaire*, Paris
6. SYLVIUS, FRANCISCUS DE LE BOË [1614–1672] (1665) *Disputationem medicarum IV. De spirituum animalium in cerebro-cerebelloque confectione per nervos distributione, atque usu vario*, Amsterdam
7. WILLIS, THOMAS [1621–1675] (1664) *Cerebri Anatome*, Martyn & Allestry, London (English translation by Samuel Pordage, London 1664)
8. VOLTAIRE, FRANÇOIS MARIE AROUET [1694–1778] (1877–83) *Oeuvres Complètes*, Garnier Frères, Paris
9. LOCKE, JOHN [1632–1704] (1688) *Extrait d'un Livre Anglais que n'est pas encore publié, intitulé ESSAI PHILOSOPHIQUE concernant L'ENTENDEMENT ou l'on montre*

quelle est l'entendue de nos connoissances certaines & la manière dont nous y pervenons, Bibliothèque Naturelle et Historique, Paris

10. LOCKE, J. (1690) *Essay Concerning Humane Understanding*, 4 books, London
11. LOCKE, J. (1977–78) *The Correspondence of John Locke*, 4 vols. (De Beer, E. S., ed.), Oxford University Press, Oxford
12. BERKELEY, GEORGE [1685–1753] (1710) *A Treatise Concerning the Principles of Human Knowledge*, Dublin
13. HUME, DAVID [1711–1776] (1739–40) *Treatise of Human Nature*, 3 vols., London
14. WHEWELL, WILLIAM [1794–1866] (1840) *The Philosophy of the Inductive Sciences Founded Upon Their History*, Parker, London (2nd enlarged edn. 1847)
15. ST AUGUSTINE [354–430] (390) *Confessions*, Book X
16. BACON, FRANCIS [1560–1626] (1605) *Of the Advancement and Proficiencie of Learning: Divine and Humane* (The quotation is taken from Wats' translation. Printed at the Golden Ball in Hosier Lane, London, 1674)
17. BURTON, ROBERT [1577–1640] (1621) *The Anatomy of Melancholy*, 3 vols., Gripps, Oxford
18. CONDILLAC, ETIENNE BONNOT [1714–1780] (1746) *Essai sur l'Origine des Connaissances Humaines. Ouvrages ou l'on Réduit à un Seul Principe tout ce que Concerne l'Entendement Humain*, Paris
19. CONDILLAC, E. B. (1754) *Traité des Sensations* (*Extrait Raisonné* added to the 2nd edn. 1778), Paris
20. VOLTAIRE, F. M. A. (1877–83) *Oeuvres Complètes*, Garnier Frères, Paris
21. PERRAULT, CLAUDE [1613–1688] (1671–76) *Mémoires pour Servir à l'Histoire des Animaux*, Académie des Sciences, Paris
22. PERRAULT, C. (1680) *Essais de Physiques*, Paris
23. DIDEROT, DENIS [1713–1784] (1749) *Lettre sur les Aveugles à l'Usage de Ceux qui Voient*, Durand, Paris
24. DE STUTT DE TRACY, ANTOINE LOUIS CLAUDE [1754–1836] (1804) *Élemens d'Idéologie*, Paris
25. BAGLIVI, GEORGIO [1668–1707] (1733) De fibra motrice et morbosa, in *Opera Omnia*, Leyden
26. HARTLEY, DAVID [1705–1757] (1749) *Observations on Man*, 3 vols, Johnson, London
27. CABANIS, PIERRE JEAN GEORGES [1757–1808] (1802) *Rapports du Physique et du Morale de l'Homme*, Paris
28. D'ALEMBERT, JEAN LE ROND [1717–1783] (1751) *Discours Préliminaire*, Paris
29. RADISHCHEV, A. N. (1941) *Complete Works*, 2 vols., Leningrad
30. STUART, ALEXANDER [1673–1742] (1739) *Croonian Lectures*, Royal Society, London
31. PROCHASKA, JIRI [1749–1820] (1779) *De Structura Nervorum*, Vindobonnae (Groeffer), Prague
32. HALLER, ALBRECHT [1708–1777] (1752) De partibus corporis humani sensibilibus et irritabilibus, *Götting. Gesell. Wiss. Acad. Sci.*, Göttingen
33. WHYTT, ROBERT [1714–1766] (1751) *An Essay on the Vital and Other Involuntary Motions of Animals*, Hamilton, Balfour & Neill, Edinburgh
34. PFLÜGER, EDUARD FRIEDRICH WILHELM [1829–1910] (1853) *Die sensorischen Functionen des Rückenmarks der Wirbelthiere nebst einer neuen Lehre über die Leitungsgesetze der Reflexionen*, Hirschwald, Berlin
35. GALEN [129–199 A.D.] (1822) *De usu partium. Opera Omnia 3 and 4* (translated by C. G. Kuhn), Leipzig
36. BARTHOLIN, CASPAR [1585–1629] (1641) *Institutiones Anatomicae ab auctoris filio Thoma Bartholino*, Hack, Leyden
37. POURFOUR DU PETIT, FRANÇOIS [1664–1741] (1788) Lettres d'un médecin des Hôpitaux du Roy, in *Recueil d'Observations d'Anatomie et de Chirurgie*, Paris
38. BONET, THEOPHILE [1620–1689] (1700) *Sepulchretum Sive Anatomia Practica* (vol. 2 Observatio VIII), Geneva

39. STAHL, GEORG ERNST [1660–1734] (1708) *Theoria Medica Vera Physiologiam et Patho-logiam, tanquam Doctrinae Medicae Partes veres Contemplativas et Naturae et Artis veris fundamentalis*, Halle

40. MÜLLER, JOHANNES [1801–1858] (1826) *Zur vergleichenden Physiologie des Gesichtsinnes des Menschen und der Thiere*

41. MÜLLER, J. (1833–38) *Handbuch der Physiologie des Menschen*, Hölscher, Coblentz

42. SCHELLING, FRIEDRICH WILHELM JOSEPH [1775–1854] (1797) Ideen zu einen Philosophie der Natur, in *Sammliche Werke*, vol. 2, Stuttgart

43. LA METTRIE, JULIEN OFFRAY DE [1709–1751] (1745) *L'Histoire Naturelle de l'Âme*, The Hague

44. LA METTRIE, J. O. DE (1748) *L'Homme Machine*, Leyden

45. VELLANSKY, DANIIL M. [1773–1848] (1805) *Dissertatio physico-medica de reformationae theoriae medicae et physicae auspicio philosophiae naturalis invente*, St Petersburg

46. VELLANSKY, D. M. (1812) *A Biological Investigation of Nature in the Form of Creator and Created, containing the Basic Outlines of General Philosophy*, St Petersburg (in Russian)

47. MAGENDIE, FRANÇOIS [1783–1855] (1809) Quelques idées générales sur les phénomènes particuliers aux corps vivants. *Bull. Sci. Méd. d'Emulation 4*, 145–170

48. MAGENDIE, F. (1823) Sur le siège du mouvement et du sentiment dans la moelle épinière. *J. Physiol. Exp. Pathol. 3*, 153–171

49. MAGENDIE, F. (1825) *Précis Élémentaire de Physiologie*, Paris

50. BICHAT, MARIE FRANÇOIS XAVIER [1771–1802] (1800) *Anatomie Générale Appliquée à la Physiologie et la Médecine*, Paris

51. RICHERAND, ANTHELINE (1807) *Nouveaux Élémens de Physiologie*, 2 vols, Crapart, Paris

52. GALL, FRANZ JOSEPH [1758–1828] (1822–5) *Sur les Fonctions du Cerveau et sur Celles de Chacune de Ses Parties*, 6 vols., Paris

53. FLOURENS, PIERRE [1794–1867] (1824) *Recherches Expérimentales sur les Propriétés et les Fonctions du Système Nerveux dans les Animaux Vertébrés*, Crevot, Paris

54. ROLANDO, LUIGI [1773–1831] (1809) *Saggio sopra la Vera Struttura del Cervello dell'Uomo degl'Animali et Sopra le Funzioni del Sistema Nervoso*, Sassari

55. ROLANDO, L. (1825) Osservazioni sul cervelletto. *Mem. Reale. Acad. Sci. Turin 29*, 163

56. GOLTZ, FRIEDRICH LEOPOLD [1834–1902] (1888) Über die Verrichtungen des Grosshirns. *Pflüger's Archiv. Gesamte Physiol. Menschen Tiere 42*, 419–487

57. LANGLEY, JOHN NEWPORT [1852–1925] & SHERRINGTON, CHARLES SCOTT [1857–1952] (1884) Secondary degeneration of nerve tracts following removal of the cortex of the cerebrum in the dog. *J. Physiol. (Lond.) 5*, 49–65

58. FRITSCH, GUSTAV [1833–1927] & HITZIG, EDUARD [1838–1907] (1870) Über die elektrische Erregbarkeit des Grosshirns. *Arch. Anat. Physiol. Wiss. Med. Leipzig, 37*, 300–332

59. CATON, RICHARD [1842–1926] (1875) The electrical currents of the brain. *Br. Med. J. 2*, 278

60. CATON, R. (1887) Researches on electrical phenomena of cerebral grey matter. *Ninth Int. Med. Congr. 3*, 846–849

61. FERRIER, DAVID [1843–1928] (1873–4) The localization of function in the brain. *Proc. R. Soc. 22*, 229–232

62, FERRIER, D. (1876) *The Function of the Brain*, Smith & Elder, London

63. VOGT, OSCAR [1870–1959] (1859–61) *Der Bau des menschlichen Gehirns durch Abbildungen mit erläuterndem Text*, Engelmann, Leipzig

64. VON ECONOMO, CONSTANTIN [1876–1931] & KOSKINAS, G. N. (1925) *Die Cytoarchitecktonik der Hirnrinde des erwachsenen Menschen*. Springer, Vienna

65. SECHENOV, IVAN MICHAILOVICH [1829–1905] (1863) *Reflexes of the Brain*, Medizinsky Vestnik (English translation in *Sechenov's Selected Works*, State Publishing House, 1935, Moscow-Leningrad)

66. LAYCOCK, THOMAS [1812–1876] (1845) On the reflex function of the brain. *Br. For. Med. Rev. 19*, 298–311

67. HALL, MARSHALL [1790–1857] (1850) *Synopsis of the Diastolic Nervous System*, Croonian Lectures of the Royal Society, London

68. SHERRINGTON, C. S. [1857–1952] (1906) *The Integrative Action of the Nervous System* (2nd edn., 1947, Yale University Press, New Haven, Conn.)

69. KANT, IMMANUEL [1724–1804] (1781) Kritik der Urteilskraft (Part 65 in *Sammliche Werke*), Leipzig

70. PAVLOV, IVAN PETROVICH [1849–1936] (1955) *Selected Works* (translated into English by S. Belsky), Foreign Language Publishing House, Moscow

71. SHERRINGTON, C. S. (1933) *The Brain and its Mechanisms*, Cambridge University Press

72. SHERRINGTON, C. S. (1941) *Man on his Nature*, Cambridge University Press

73. SHERRINGTON, C. S. (1942) *Goethe on Nature and Science*, Cambridge University Press

74. PAVLOV, I. P. (1928) *Lectures on Conditioned Reflexes*, vol. 1 (p. 60), (translated by W. H. Gantt), International Publishers, New York

References in the text to modern brain science

75. ADINOLFI, A. M. (1971) The postnatal development of synaptic contacts in the cerebral cortex, in *Brain Development and Behavior* (Sterman, M. B. *et al.*, eds.), pp. 78–89, Academic Press, New York

76. SCHEIBEL, M. E. & SCHEIBEL, A. B. (1973) Maturation of reticular dendrites: loss of spines and development of bundles. *Exp. Neurol. 38*, 301–310

77. RUTLEDGE, L. T. (1974) Synaptogenesis: effects of synaptic use, in *Neural Mechanisms of Learning and Memory* (Rosenzweig, M. R. & Bennett, E. L., eds.), pp. 329–339, MIT Press, Cambridge, Mass.

78. ROSENZWEIG, M. R. & BENNETT, E. L. (eds.) (1974) *Neural Mechanisms of Learning and Memory*, MIT Press, Cambridge, Mass.

79. BECHTEREVA, N. P. (1979) Bioelectric expression of long-term activation and its possible mechanisms, in *Brain Mechanisms in Memory and Learning* (Brazier, M. A. B., ed.) *(IBRO Monogr. Ser. vol. 4)*, pp. 311–327, Raven Press, New York

80. HUBEL, D. H. & WIESEL, T. N. (1968) Receptive fields and functional architecture of monkey striate cortex. *J. Physiol. (Lond.) 195*, 215–243

81. DEVALOIS, R. L., JACOBS, G. H. & ABRAMOV, I. (1964) Responses of single cells in visual system to shifts in the wavelength of light. *Science (Wash. D.C.) 146*, 1184–1186

82. BAUMGARTNER, G., BROWN, J. L. & SCHULZ, A. (1964) Visual motion detection in the cat. *Science (Wash. D.C.) 146*, 1070–1071

83. KOSHTOYANTZ, KH. S. (1946) *Essays on the History of Physiology in Russia*, Publishing House, Academy of Sciences, USSR

84. LIDDELL, E. G. T. (1960) *The Discovery of Reflexes*, Clarendon Press/Oxford University Press

Discussion: The historical background

Medawar: I very much regret that you hardly mentioned Kant. He is the one philosopher who, if he were alive today, would be able to look around and say 'It has all turned out just as I thought'. Immanuel Kant would surely have given an approving nod to Chomsky and to many of the neurophysiologists for demonstrating the essential soundness of his opinions.

Brazier: I agree. What interested me about Sechenov and his idea of reflexes was that he had been educated in the land of Kant, and the philosophy he heard was the philosophy of Kant.

Young: I thought you thought there was evidence in favour of a *tabula rasa* and therefore against *a priori* ideas?

Brazier: I think some neurophysiologists—such as Adinolfi, Scheibel, Rosenzweig and Rutledge—would say that there is evidence of a *tabula rasa*. As I mentioned, there is a dearth of dendritic spines on the cells of the cerebral cortex in the newborn, and experiments have shown that long-term memory traces are not laid down until the spines have developed.

Bennett: I don't think that the supposed neuronal evidence for the *tabula rasa* is evidence for anything that Locke believed. Locke says that knowledge and ideas may well exist before the time of birth. He is not talking about the state of the absolutely newborn baby but about the source of the knowledge and ideas and he says that they must all come from inner or outer perception. He could not consistently say that there are knowledge states, idea states or anything of this kind which are not present at birth, but are present shortly thereafter simply through maturational processes.

Putnam: Locke doesn't deny that there are innate propensities; learning some things is easier than learning others. If you mean by an 'innate idea' an innate *ability*, sure; but why call abilities ideas? I still don't see why that doesn't answer Chomsky.

Bunge: I am not quite sure about the innatism of either Kant or Chomsky. Kant said that an uneducated man is not human, which goes against innatism. And Chomsky doesn't distinguish between innate capabilities and inborn capabilities at all, so one might well read him as saying that man is born with certain abilities but they must develop. For instance genes must be expressed, the central nervous system must mature and so on. As he doesn't make this distinction between what is inborn and heredity, one cannot read him unambiguously as an innatist.

Ploog: I am not sure whether Chomsky's view is as you said. According to his recent lectures he seems to believe that the human nervous system is

31

made up in such a way that language is a species-specific endowed capacity which of course has to be developed by environmental forces. Each hereditary trait needs to be developed by an array of environmental stimuli. There is no one gene that expresses itself without the environment. If we view this interaction in a simplistic nature–nurture concept we get lost. Neurobiologists nowadays can say quite a bit about the development of interaction between genetically preformed structures in the brain, and what is necessary to develop the functions of seeing, of hearing and so on. I am sure we will come to that as the conference goes on.

Putnam: I recently found, looking back at Hobbes, that there is a lot of anticipation of the current computer model. One of the essential elements in the current computer model is the idea that rational thought is ultimately analysable into components which are non-significant, that the manipulation of 'meaningless signs' can constitute meaningful thought. Hobbes gives an illustration which is very charming. He reminds one that the word 'ratiocination', which is one of the more Latin words in English for rational thought, has as its etymology a word which in Latin meant reckoning, keeping accounts, *bookkeeping.* He came as close to saying that rational thought may be executing algorithms as it was possible to in his century.

Brazier: I certainly agree with you about the place of Hobbes in our thinking as neuroscientists. My only excuse for not mentioning him is that I had to choose just one person from that era. There are many to whom I have done very poor service, especially among the German school.

Bunge: You regarded Whewell as a representative of inductivism, Dr Brazier, but I think he just paid lip service to it. He was in constant polemics with J. S. Mill, the arch-inductivist, and I think that when Whewell used the word 'induction' he really meant the hypothetical deductive method.

Brazier: I really dragged him in because of his onslaught about the influence of Locke on Newton. The correspondence between Locke and Newton is, in a way, very disappointing for a scientist.

Bunge: Was Hartley really a confirmed dualist? I am not a specialist but I read him as a materialist.

Brazier: Hartley thought that the nerves vibrated, but the message that these vibrations carried went to the soul. If he isn't a dualist we have to have a more elaborate definition.

Bunge: One must always reckon that some people pay lip service in order not to be persecuted.

Brazier: Yes, like Marshall Hall.

Creutzfeldt: The history of science likes to trace the path of progress towards truth, the criterion for progress being our own presumed possession of truth.

Thus a monist may look down on those who assumed or still assume that there exist two different entities: the brain and the mind or soul. 'They' are dualists, but 'we' know better: it is all brain. But isn't there another lesson to be learned from the history of the mind/body problem—that there appears to be a 'dualistic' aspect to consciousness and to our self-understanding, which by its very nature always brings us back to a dualistic formula, in spite of our undoubted progress in factual knowledge? This 'dualistic formula' may in fact represent an essential condition of consciousness and of mind, which —if this is so—would have to be taken into account and explained by any scientific theory of the brain. It is then quite unimportant, and merely depends on the available knowledge, which mechanism is proposed for the realization of such a dualistic formula. If 'monistic materialism' or a similar position does not recognize this 'dualistic aspect' of our self-understanding (and thus of our mind), it denies the most intriguing aspect of what we include under terms such as conscious experience, mind, or self-consciousness. With such a reductionism, monistic materialism may become less scientific than straight-forward dualism, and thus a bad arbiter of progress in the brain–mind discussion.

Brazier: I agree with you but we get bogged down in our wording. We could really do with a lot more shades of meaning for words such as mind, consciousness, awareness and so on. I think we will hear later in this meeting a good deal more about this quality of consciousness or awareness.

Again, what is meant by awareness—external awareness or awareness of self? I don't believe that it helps to add 'ality' to words such as 'intention', even though this is supposed, in the country where I live now, to add some new understanding where the original word is felt to be too restrictive.

Bunge: 'Intentionality' comes from the German.

Armstrong: Descartes is a very significant but a very ambiguous figure. It is important to bring out the ambiguity. He was a dualist and all dualisms are inherently unstable, with a tendency to collapse one way or the other. Two traditions come out of Descartes. He is completely mechanistic about the body and that is very important. He gets rid of all the Aristotelian stuff, gets rid of teleology. Although Hobbes was a much more thorough materialist, it is really from Descartes that the modern materialist tradition of thought about the body springs. He is a very important nourishing source of that tradition. First we give a mechanistic account of the body, then we advance on the mind and interpret that as the workings of the brain instead of the soul. From this perspective, the Cartesian soul is just a stage in the retreat towards complete materialism.

But there is another tradition which springs from Descartes' dualism, emphasizing the soul, not the body. This was encouraged by Descartes' view that the existence of the spiritual, the existence of the mental, is much more certain than the existence of the material. He thinks he is much more certain that he thinks than that he has a body. I believe that that view is quite absurd. The certainty that I have a body and a head on my shoulders is just as great as my certainty that I am thinking now. In both cases I am rationally certain. In both cases one can think of cases where one might be wrong.

But because Descartes gave the spiritual side epistemological primacy, the philosophers, I am sorry to say, mostly grabbed hold of that side. Once you think that the special certainty is in the spiritual, you will downgrade the material, you will think that existence of the body is uncertain, and so on. Hence we get from Descartes not only the materialist tradition, which on the whole the scientists took up, but also the spiritualist tradition, the idealistic tradition. The latter led to scepticism about the external world and a lot of other nonsense. In this way Descartes led on to Berkeley, Kant and their successors, and to the general epistemological mess which philosophy, at least, has been in almost ever since.

Bunge: In support of that I would like to remind you that Descartes was called by a French philosopher 'le philosophe au masque', the masked philosopher. The Encyclopaedists paid little attention to his *Meditations* and much to his *Traité de l'Homme*—and his *Traité du Monde*. They paid attention only to two works which he didn't dare to publish in his lifetime for fear of the Inquisition. One of these was translated into English only a few years ago and the other is being translated now. These two completely materialist treatises have been totally ignored by the Anglo-Saxon philosophers.

Brazier: Only two of the illustrations in *Traité de l'Homme* are Descartes' originals. The others, which are very materialistic, were put in by la Forge and others after his death. To me Descartes is a very great figure, but those illustrations are more materialistic than the text.

Creutzfeldt: The dualistic theory that most strongly influenced German 19th century psychologists such as Wundt, and thus modern psychology as a whole, was the monadology of Leibniz. The 19th century psychologists were well aware of this tradition. The ideas of Leibniz can also be traced through the romantic psychology of the early 19th century and from then on through the often vivid and polemical brain–mind discussions up to the present time.

Plum: I think that when Gazzaniga[1] talks about more than one consciousness he is talking about a self-awareness which is fundamentally a language thing, that stands distinct from another intuitive and perhaps right-brained experience. This latter influence may or may not have self-awareness to it, or what John Searle calls intentionality. What it may possess is a kind of felt sense, a Freudian pre-language experience which influences our behaviour without our fully knowing why. When does the notion begin to creep in that we know ourselves by our words?

Brazier: You should really address that question to the philosophers. I find the introduction of language as a meaningful tool in 'la vie mentale' coming in through the French Enlightenment and the Encyclopaedists.

Searle: Your history looked like an inexorable march towards monism, but isn't there another way of seeing it? That is, it is not so much monism triumphing as a series of transformations of dualism. For example, contemporary dualist philosophers, such as Popper, have not embraced Descartes but their idea about the relationship between awareness and the brain is different from the physicalists' idea. They are not materialists in any traditional sense. Could you comment on that?

Brazier: Some of that comes in towards the end of my paper where I discuss Sherrington's kind of dualism. He doesn't write about his troubles with dualism until his old age, when he began to write *Man on his Nature* and *The Brain and its Mechanisms*, which was a Rede lecture. For that kind of lectureship he was really being asked to give a dualist lecture. Neither Sherrington nor Pavlov, both of whom lived to tremendous ages and had so much influence on brain scientists, solved the brain–mind problem.

What do others here think of the Popper/Eccles book[2]?

Armstrong: I don't think it is a very good book. The Eccles material doesn't do anything to prove dualism. His physiological material is fascinating, but seems to be absolutely compatible with the idea that the thing doing the read-out of the brain is itself something physical in the central nervous system.

The most interesting part of the book is Popper's contribution. It is very uneven and contains some very bad arguments, but it also has interesting arguments and interesting ideas for developing a dualist view. But I must say that, as a materialist, I wish that the dualist case had been presented more strongly.

Brazier: I was very disappointed in the book. Jack Eccles had told us about it for some years and I really expected them to present their cases very well. I didn't even think Popper presented his case as well as he does in his other books.

Armstrong: The great dualist counter-attack has still to be launched. If only for the health of materialism, it is desirable that it should be launched.

Medawar: I thought the most interesting part of that book was the agreed statement at the beginning by Popper and Eccles that the problem of the relationship between brain and mind might well be insoluble. There are good reasons for thinking they are right. Certainly nothing occurs during the course of the book to challenge that statement.

Bunge: I was very disappointed in the book too. Eccles doesn't say anything he hasn't said in other books and I find several faults with Popper's part. First he builds a straw man, which he calls materialism, but which is really 18th century mechanism. He doesn't take into account emergent materialism such as Diderot's. Second, he totally ignores contemporary physiological psychology. Both Popper and Eccles think that they can jump from neuroscience to the philosophy of mind without passing through psychology, which is a methodological mistake. Third, I found no arguments at all for dualism. Fourth, Popper oscillates between two very different dualistic positions. One is animism in the style of Plato, namely the idea that the soul controls the body; he recalls several times Plato's simile of the helmsman and the ship. Then in the subtitle and in other parts of the book Popper contends that what he is defending is interactionism, which is a totally different theory. Finally the so-called World 3 is not a world at all. A world is supposed to be a system, something self-contained and homogeneous. Popper's World 3 is composed on the one hand of ideas, programmes, theories and so on, and on the other hand of material objects such as pencils, books and so on. How can a world be made up with these heterogeneous objects? One must say at least what the composition operation is in order to get a world proper, i.e. a system.

On these five counts I felt the whole book was very weak and thus an argument for materialism, not for dualism.

Brazier: Yes, I agree.

Armstrong: The interactionism seems to me to be the good part. I can't see how there can be any evolutionary explanation of consciousness otherwise. To the extent that Popper emphasizes interactionism, I think that is excellent. The only point is, why does the interaction have to be between something material and something spiritual? Why should it not be interaction inside the physical system?

Bunge: They don't define 'interaction'. In science interaction is a relation among things or among events.

Creutzfeldt: My comment is only indirectly related to the Popper/Eccles book[2] but I should like to try to prevent our discussions from getting too involved in a dispute between materialistic and dualistic beliefs. In the true sense of the word, dualistic theories may well be materialistic if they attribute to the mind a material nature of some sort (a force, a state, or even a real substance). In this sense even Eccles' dualistic hypothesis may still be considered materialistic as it presupposes some 'mechanism' which interacts with the brain. However, what appears more important is that Eccles comes to the conclusion that our present-day models of brain mechanisms are not sufficient to explain the working of the mind as we experience and understand it. Many prominent neuroscientists have arrived at this conclusion. What is not answered by dualism or monism is the nature of the mechanism which may be in the brain or connected with it and which forces us to understand ourselves in dualistic terms. And in that sense, one wonders whether the relevant question is being asked in the monism/dualism controversy.

Putnam: The expression 'the mind–body problem' brings in a host of pre-suppositions, most of which are false.

Medawar: Contrary to what Mario Bunge says, I believe that the World 3 concept[2] is defensible and rather useful.

Blakemore: One problem here is that we are trying to trace continuity between Cartesian dualism and some forms of modern dualism. For Descartes, dualism was fundamentally tied up with religion and the concept of continuity of spirit beyond death: 'l'âme' had a quality quite different from any known material substance. Some modern dualists believe, rather, that so-called 'emergent' properties of the mind cannot be accounted for, in a reductionist fashion, in terms of the properties of the individual components of the brain. Two levels of description are needed, they say.

Creutzfeldt: The problem here, as you rightly point out, is the religious context of classical dualism. But I think that we shouldn't discuss religion here: the question of the soul and eternal life has nothing to do directly with our problem but is a matter of belief for the individual. On the other hand, a relevant question may be why religion is part of human nature and whether we can define brain mechanisms which make religion a necessary condition of the human being.

Blakemore: If we don't bring religion, in the broadest sense, into our discussion we shall have nothing to discuss.

Young: Believing is a property of the human brain and we are here to discuss the brain.

Trevarthen: I am struck by what seems to me a restriction of the history of the mind–brain problem, as this was presented by Dr Brazier, to problems of *awareness;* that is to experiences of the outside world. All questions about the control of action appeared to relate to responses reflecting outside events.

This does not cover the phenomena of intention. Behind intention are motives; these too were not included in the history in an explicit way. Another feature of consciousness is the ability of people to transmit and understand intentions with other people, and to share or conjoin them in cooperative activity.

Language plays a leading part in that ability, but I do not see language as causing or creating that cooperation. I think that the question of religion must concern itself with any conceptions we might have about how human beings perceive their existence together. It is no good thinking of just one individual. Dr Brazier, were you pushed by the history of western European ideas to make an account of the relationship of the mind to the brain in terms of solitary awareness?

Brazier: I think history had the effect of pushing things in that direction, but one could develop it from another point of view. And I don't see how we can cut out the religious attitudes in dualism. It would be a false break to me if you say we can leave out religion when we are going to talk about monism and dualism.

Fried: There is a lot to be said for dualism but it is important to see that it has not got anything necessarily to do with religion, though it clearly has been tied up with religion in the past. We are sure we can discuss logic, mathematics, language, even psychological phenomena, emotions and so on, as though they were a sort of autonomous field, without any feeling that we must know the physiological substrates of our knowledge of these matters. At the same time, in a way which I think is rather Cartesian, we assume that there are physiological processes correlated with our knowledge of all the things we are discussing. And we admit that we do not know what the connection is between these domains of substantive discussion and the physiological domain. We don't think that the connection runs through the pineal gland, as did Descartes. Nor do we feel any necessity to assume religious truth or the absence of religious truth in order to speak in this dualistic fashion. So the issue is very much there. Ordinary people, some of them with and others without religious beliefs, talk about psychology, for example, as if it were a domain which it is perfectly possible to discuss, even though one has little idea what its physiological mechanisms are.

To show how totally irrelevant religion is to this kind of dualism, Hilary Putnam gives the example of computer science. Computer scientists can discuss all kinds of problems about programming without having the first notion about the wiring and electrical mechanisms of the computer. Very competent computer scientists may not even know whether the computer is working electronically, whether it has transistors or vacuum tubes or hydraulic gates. All of those kinds of mechanical substrates might be consistent with the same kind of logic. Religion doesn't enter into it at all.

Bunge: The discussion of dualism is essential: it is the whole point of this conference. The difficulty is great because it is not only a philosophical problem but also a scientific and ideological one. We are all motivated more or less by ideological ideas. It is not futile to discuss the problem provided we do it clearly. One of the first things to realize is that when we speak of dualism we may not be very clear on it because there are several kinds of dualism. There is a substance dualism and property dualism. Substance dualism says there are two kinds of substance, such as Descartes' *res extensa* (matter) and *res cogitans* (mind). This kind of dualism was rejected by Spinoza, who on the other hand maintained that there is a plurality of properties. Modern materialists need not say that the properties of the brain are exactly the same as those of the computer or those of an atom. They recognize that the nervous tissue has emergent properties that other things don't have—for instance the ability to program computers or to write poems and so on. Although they are substance monists they may be property pluralists.

Medawar: Dr Searle, you referred to your Oxford upbringing and the attitude of linguistic philosophers to the problems we are discussing. Isn't it true to say that the attitude of linguistic philosophers to physiologists is mainly a defence against what the philosophers suspect is another attempted usurpation of their subject matter by those pesky scientists? Gilbert Ryle's book, *The Concept of Mind*,[3] would annul our meeting if everyone believed in it without qualification. I believe that the argument in that book is mistaken but I would very much like to hear your views.

Searle: There was a theory behind the thesis that philosophy is not continuous with the empirical disciplines. Any theory may have motivations of a non-intellectual kind and it may have been that the usual territorial imperative was operative in philosophy, as it is in other academic disciplines, but that was not the reason advanced. The reasons advanced for the idea that philosophy is not continuous with empirical disciplines were not totally bogus but were quite interesting reasons. The theory, which goes back to Wittgenstein and in some ways to Socrates, says that philosophy is essentially conceptual analysis: we inherit a series of concepts, most of them non-technical and most of them part of the heritage of natural languages, and the task of the philosopher is to analyse the relations between these concepts and the way the concepts relate to reality. If that is the task then it looks as if there is no direct impact on this task from scientific results.

I myself think that this theory was not refuted but just became irrelevant by the march of events. Philosophy is much more interesting today than it was twenty years ago, simply because we no longer want to make a distinction between philosophical questions and other kinds. If that means that the empirical researchers are marching in on our territory, so much the better, because if they look behind them they will see that we are marching in on their territory too.

I shall resist the temptation to launch into an answer to the question about Gilbert Ryle, because it would have to be very long.

Medawar: What about all his category arguments? I don't think Gilbert Ryle really knew what Husserl* meant by a 'semantic category mistake'.

Searle: The idea of a category mistake has, I think, a legitimate but rather limited place in the armoury of philosophical investigation.

Bennett: In Ryle's famous recantation of the concept of the category mistake he says that this concept is needed, not for the usual reason that there is an exact professional way of using it, in which like a skeleton key it will undo locks for us, but rather for the unusual reason that there is a rough amateurish way of using it in which it will make a satisfactory thumping noise upon doors which we want opened.

Putnam: The Concept of Mind is a great book but I don't think it proves any of the things that Chapter 1 says it is going to prove, although Chapter 1 is excellent advertising. What the book really shows could be put this way: if the traditional philosophical view is right, that the fact that we could be mistaken about whether there is a rostrum in this room shows that we don't directly observe rostra, then the universality of the phenomenon of self-deception shows that we don't directly observe our own volitions, thoughts, beliefs or 90% of what has been called the mental. That is a very powerful argument and I wish that the book hadn't been written in such a way that everybody got to talking about category mistakes or whether it is all dispositions.

Searle: I don't think it is a great book. I think we will find it embarrassing in twenty years' time to read the reviews that say it is a great classic in English philosophy. The real weakness of the book is precisely that it leaves out the most interesting property of the mind, namely its capacity to direct itself at objects and states of affairs by means of intentionality. The behaviourism running through that book tries to reduce intentionality to dispositions to behaviour, and that seems to me its fatal weakness.

Putnam: I couldn't agree less.

Young: Dr Searle, would you redefine intentionality?

Searle: I don't think there is a philosopher's definition of intentionality in terms of simpler notions that don't themselves contain any intentionalistic notions. The intuitive idea is this. Some mental states are essentially directed at objects and states of affairs other than themselves. It is not true of all mental states that they are intentional and it is not true of all intentional states that they are conscious, but there is obviously a close connection between

---

* Edmund Husserl (1859–1938), author of *Phenomenology* and founder of the discipline so described.

intentionality and consciousness. Wherever we have an intentional state, it appears to be the case that we are at least in principle able to bring it to consciousness. That is the assumption on which Freudian psychology rests, namely that we can bring repressed intentional states to some sort of consciousness.

If one wanted a formal definition or formal criteria for intentionality there are certain syntactical clues. The intentional concepts such as hope, fear, belief, desire, wish, want and so on have a syntactical feature in the Indo-European languages that is not shared by pains, tickles and itches. That is, the verbs require certain kinds of direct objects, usually sentential direct objects. That is a clue that certain kinds of semantics are operating. Namely, there is a sense in which the intentional states that we are interested in—beliefs, fears, hopes, desire, loves, hates and so on—are about objects and states of affairs, and the sorts of direct objects that the corresponding verbs require are representations of those objects and states of affairs. Thus, the syntax is a clue to the fact that the key to understanding intentionality is representation. The mind represents objects and states of affairs by way of its intentional states; and the key to understanding representation is the conditions of satisfaction of the representations: what it is that makes your belief true, what makes your fear be realized, what makes your desire satisfied. In these cases we find the clue to understanding what fears, beliefs, hopes and desires are, because it is their essential characteristic that they represent their conditions of satisfaction.

Bunge: Don't you think that the word 'intentionality', which was introduced by Franz Brentano in order to differentiate between psychic and physical objects, is ambiguous? It designates two different concepts, namely that of purposive action on the one hand, which is a psychological notion, and the concept of external reference, which is a semantic notion. By conflating the two, Brentano introduced enormous confusion into the literature. One might say that every purposive action is referential but the converse is certainly not true.

Searle: My own view about this is that the intention behind intentional action is no more and no less referential than the intentionality of, say, belief. The difference is that when I have an intention to do something, my mental state is a representation of my subsequent behaviour and also figures in the causation of that behaviour. The fascinating question for this conference is, how are these intentional states realized in the brain? In answer to your question, I want to say that in the sense of 'representation' in which my intention represents my subsequent behaviour, my belief that it is raining represents the state of the weather, and the form of intentionality in both cases is the same.

Bunge: But if you want to define a mathematical function or some other abstract object, where is the external reference and where is the intention regarding your future behaviour?

Searle: If it is my intention to define a mathematical function, then the future behaviour is that I should produce a satisfactory definition.

Bunge: Yes, but where is the external reference?

Searle: The 'external reference' will be in the definition that I have produced.

Bunge: That is not external.

Searle: The conditions of satisfaction of an intentional state need not be in that sense 'external'. My intentions could be, for example, to have thoughts. I could have an intention to think about Kansas City and the condition of satisfaction of that intention would be that I think about Kansas City.

Bunge: Kansas City is out there but a function is not out there.

Searle: That is a problem about the nature of mathematics, not about the nature of intentionality. To get the conditions of satisfaction of beliefs about mathematics, plug in your favourite theory of mathematics.

Bunge: But you have to distinguish between intention and external reference.

Searle: I can have beliefs about mathematics and their conditions of satisfaction are about mathematics.

Young: But you said that belief is one of the characteristics of intentionality.

Searle: No; intentionality is one of the characteristics of belief. I should explain that the verb 'intend' is only accidentally connected with the notion of intentionality. It is an unfortunate term but we are stuck with it.

Brazier: I am not a philosopher so I have been very pleased to hear the philosophers speaking. We have had more discussions from the philosophers than from the neuroscientists. Of course I was speaking from the historical point of view and historically the division between the mind and the soul was very flimsy indeed. I think that is why in the historical development the religious tinge to duality appears very strongly. Religion is there in its development. All of us have commented on the language, the metaphysical terms, used in many countries, including the country of Descartes. I can't divide those concepts into purely materialistic terms, however much I try, and I find no evidence that Descartes intended us to. I doubt if many of the people who have written since then intended that either. This is where I part company from Otto Creutzfeldt. I don't think that you can divide dualism and religious belief with a sharp line. This is obviously a point of interest to everybody. We could also talk a great deal more than we have so far on the part that language plays in our thoughts, in our minds, in our brains.

References

1. GAZZANIGA, M. S. & LEDOUX, J. E. (1978) *The Integrated Mind*, Plenum, New York
2. POPPER, K. R. & ECCLES, J. C. (1977) *The Self and its Brain*, Springer International, Berlin
3. RYLE, G. (1962) *The Concept of Mind*, Barnes & Noble/Harper & Row, Scranton, PA. (Reprint of 1949 edn., Hutchinson, London)

Consciousness and the brain: evolutionary aspects

BERNARD TOWERS

School of Medicine, University of California, Los Angeles

Abstract Self-reflective consciousness is distinguished from 'simple' awareness and from conscious awareness. Awareness is a fundamental property of living matter as it reacts to environmental stimuli. A hypothesis is advanced to account for the general phenomenon of decussation of nerve fibres in the central nervous system of vertebrates. This feature, the crossing over of nerve fibres to the opposite side of the brain, is interpreted as exemplifying the inherent caution of living forms. The evolution of increasing complexity of structure in spinal cord and brain is a prerequisite for increasing awareness of the environment and for increasing freedom from its constraints. Conscious awareness is manifested in living forms primarily when they are learning to respond either to new stimuli or to internal demands such as breathing and walking. The relegation of learnt activities to the realm of unconscious reflex allows for concentration on new and more complex responses, which leads to further freedom of action. The seeming simplicity of human thinking rests on the increasing complexity of the evolving brain and of appropriate responses learnt during phylogenetic development. The human brain and its thinking functions are basically trustworthy because they are rooted in biological evolution.

Some of the philosophers I have spoken to about this symposium on *Brain and Mind* have said 'but surely it ought to be the other way round?' For philosophers Mind must come first. The ability to reason and to engage in self-reflective conscious awareness is of the essence of their trade. 'One not only knows', it has been said, 'but one knows that one knows. Other species do not'. This is the hallmark of the human species, and the joy of the philosophical mind.

I respond to the objection as an anatomist and developmental biologist must: 'But no, in order to think as a philosopher thinks it is not only important, but absolutely essential, that one first has a human *brain*, and a well functioning one at that. The brain is unquestionably a product of the evolutionary process. So the title for the symposium is absolutely right: *Brain and Mind*'.

The philosopher's mind, with its powers of reflecting or turning in on itself, does not represent the only kind of consciousness or conscious awareness that exists in nature. It is the end-result (to date) of a *capacity* in biological evolution that has become actualized over a period of three-and-a-half-thousand million years. Mind is as much a product of the evolutionary process as is the brain. Therefore we must consider the concept of 'Emergence and the mind', to use the title itself of a stimulating contribution by my philosopher-respondent, Mario Bunge.[1] In that paper Bunge develops a powerful theory of 'emergentist materialism'. I accept his phrase, and find myself in sympathy with the position he takes. But now I want to develop, as an evolutionary biologist, a theory of what I will call, by analogy, 'emergentist psychism', and wait to see what responses it attracts.

My own paper reverses the order of words again, being entitled, as you see, 'Consciousness and the Brain: Evolutionary Aspects'. I shall argue that there is no contradiction between this title and what I have said about the correctness of the order of words in the overall title of the symposium, *Brain and Mind*.

Self-reflective consciousness, as a manifestation of the human mind, requires simpler forms of consciousness or conscious awareness as a substratum for its functioning. The reverse is clearly not the case. In the Cartesian heyday animal experiments were performed without regard to the yelps of pain they produced; these were regarded as no more significant than the squeaking of metal parts in a badly-oiled machine. Animals were machines, and machines were clearly not 'conscious' or 'aware'. So the squeals of pain were tolerated by possessors of the Cartesian 'mind'. They inflicted the pain apparently without loss of composure. It sounds not only cruel but absurd. The reason it sounds absurd is, in my opinion, because we are all of us now, to some degree or other, affected by knowledge of the evolutionary process, of our own emergence. I refer to the emergence of the genus *Homo*, whether *H. sapiens*, or *H. faber* or *H. ludens* (as our own species is better named, in my view) or *H. habilis*—I am mixing them up in evolutionary time simply to illustrate that there *is* a unity to the genus despite the different forms within it, just as there *is* a unity to the species *Homo sapiens* despite the variety of races that comprise it.

Let us grant, then, in this post-Cartesian evolutionary age, that animals *are* aware. They are conscious of their environment, and aware enough to do something about it if they don't like it. It might be argued that this is 'simple' awareness only, with response by simple reflex. That takes us back to the machine model, and to the need for a ghost in the human machine to account for the human mind and its more profound form of consciousness. That way leads to biological nonsense. Real awareness of the environment is obvious in higher mammals. When the cat is on the mat and the fire gets too hot, the cat gets up, looks around, and goes and finds a cooler mat. That represents a highly developed form of conscious awareness. I don't want to say that other mammals are *just* like us. But I do want to say they are conscious in some quite elaborate sense.

Let us now move away from comparisons of higher mammals with human beings. Such comparisons are intriguing (especially in higher primates, some of which today seem to know how to *talk*, using sign language), but they are apt to deflect us from consideration of consciousness in other biological forms. The real fact is, as every student of biology knows, that it is characteristic of living matter at whatever level one observes it (multicellular, unicellular, subcellular, microbiological) that amongst its many intriguing properties are those of awareness of and reaction to environmental stimuli. It might be said that I am diluting the concept of consciousness too much. Not, I think, if I stick with living matter. I propose to do that here, although living matter itself must have arisen from reactive non-living material, at least for anyone who doesn't want to give up on evolution.[2] But for this occasion I will stick with the living.

Let us take what we refer to as a simple living organism, like *Amoeba*. Simple, we say. Yet it is already unbelievably more complex than bacteria or viruses—which themselves are so complex as to stretch the mind and sophisticated techniques of the modern scientist, as he or she attempts to understand them. Amoeba has its nucleus, cytoplasm and complex cell membrane. It has all the complexities of organelles and mitochondria, and a nucleus with its double-helix strands of DNA. What a chemical (biochemical) laboratory it is! Moreover, it *does* things. It acts and reacts in astonishingly complicated ways. Incidentally, we ourselves have cells in our bodies that behave in many ways just like amoeba—the macrophages, for instance. Watch them in tissue culture: they act and react, they do things and they respond to stimuli. Are they aware, or conscious in any meaningful sense? Where, one might ask, is the brain, the so-called 'seat of consciousness'? Well, there is no brain, of course, nor was there in evolution, for a very, very long time. There was, however, a potential, a capacity, for the development of brain. First there had to develop the metazoan (many-celled) organisms. Then the cells of metazoa had to start to specialize. All the cells carry the same genetic material and have identical potential, but they cannot help but start to differentiate and specialize, initially simply as surface cells and internal cells. It is the surface cells that are the receptors of information from the external environment. It is no surprise that in all vertebrate forms, including ourselves as embryos, it is the surface cells which give rise to the nervous system, including the brain. Nerves are, first and foremost, receivers of information, and then transmitters of that information to some kind of effector mechanism. Plants never developed nerves, and they remain forever locked into their physical environment through inability to *do anything* either to it or for themselves. The recent book by Paul Shepard[3] arrived too late on my desk for incorporation into this paper. But I commend his interpretation of the immense contribution of plants and insects to the emergence of mind. They literally 'prepared the soil' without which animals would not have been possible. Their presence has always been, and continues to be, essential for the development of powers of thought and imagination.

So now I return to animal forms and the development of a nervous system that is capable of freeing its possessor, in part, from the constraints of the environment. I want to hypothesize about the extraordinary, and hitherto unexplained, phenomenon that all the information that we ourselves receive (and the same is true of all vertebrates) from one or other side of our individual environments, is carried to and is organized by the opposite side of the brain. This is what is known as the great decussation of nerve tracts in the central nervous system. It is a puzzle how that feature ever got started in evolution. Why *should* almost all nerve fibres cross from one side of the central nervous system to the other in order to transmit signals from and to the functioning body and its environment? A solution to that puzzle might prove significant for understanding the more fundamental features of reactivity of biological organisms and of their capacity for conscious awareness.

Take amoeba again. Stimulated on one side its first reaction is to retreat. Subsequently it may learn by experience that the stimulus is not noxious but may in fact be something worth pursuing, like food, and then its response changes. The initial retreat is produced by cytoplasmic flow into a pseudopodium that goes out on the side of the cell opposite to that of the unknown stimulus. Living matter is basically cautious. Now imagine a primitive metazoan that has a few receptor nerves derived from its surface, and a few contractile elements within its body. My hypothesis is that stimulation of a nerve on one side would induce a flow of information to a contractile cell on the opposite side, and thereby cause the organism to retreat from the possible danger. When the system had become sufficiently complex, and there was exchange of information between cells in a primitive central nervous system, the creature could learn, as amoeba does, not simply to retreat from possibly noxious stimuli but also to pursue desirable ones. The original decussation of fibres, once initiated, would be permanent, because new nerves grow along established pathways.

From such small beginnings, as I see it, has come the immense complexity of the modern decussating vertebrate nervous system, with the human type the most sophisticated. Special sense organs developed for the most part at the forwardly-moving end of primitive creatures, as they still do in us. Special senses convey more information, through larger nerve bundles, than do ordinary surface receptors. The front end of the central nervous system expanded, and we call that expanded part the brain. When an individual human brain ceases to function, while other tissues of the body continue to live, we are tempted, and in some jurisdictions urged, to equate brain death with death itself. There is peculiar tragedy in the sight of the severely brain-damaged neonate who we know will never communicate except at a very basic, so-called vegetative level. Why is this tragic when vegetables themselves are not? The tragedy, I suggest, lies in the loss or non-development of an expected capacity or potential. Things that make us laugh, make us feel happy, joyful or 'fulfilled' are what make life worth living—for us. I agree with Jacob[4] that living forms, in evolution, show more of this 'fun' side of living than they do of the tragic.[2]

The fun seems to come from the efforts we exert in concentrating on doing something new, and especially from learning how to do it successfully. In his Tarner Lectures of 1956 Erwin Schrödinger[5] developed a fascinating theory of the function of conscious awareness, in both ontogeny and phylogeny, as the expression of this impulse in living organisms to learn how to respond either to new environmental stimuli or to self-imposed tasks that require some effort of concentration. He refers to the attempts of the infant to stand, to maintain balance, and eventually (with many mishaps and setbacks) actually to walk. The effort of concentration is obvious to the observer. It is experienced by adults, too, if they ever have to learn to walk again after a debilitating illness or accident. The gratification achieved by both infant and adult, on learning how to do it, is one of the joys of living. Once one's neuromuscular apparatus has learnt the task of simple walking, one can go on to other things, like jumping or running, or, as Schrödinger points out, one can leave the learnt task to the body itself, and simply *walk* while talking, or reading a book, or thinking a poem or a piece of music. This is liberation. Increasing freedom from the constraints of the environment is the hallmark of an evolutionary process that leads both towards the complexity of the human brain and to the seeming simplicity of human freedom to think. The experienced simplicity of mind is built upon, or allowed only by, the complexity of brain structure.

Schrödinger[5] took his argument about learning, achieving and then relegating the learnt tasks to the realm of the autonomic or unconscious activity of the central nervous system, back through the evolution of increasing complexity of the central nervous system. He argued that the activities that modern complex mammals can take for granted, such as breathing, or keeping the heart pumping, were once activities that had to be *learnt* by their progenitors. It was during that learning period, he suggests, that they too manifested conscious awareness of what they were about. We may be inclined, looking down from our own lofty heights, to disparage those efforts as menial, non-rational, unworthy of the attention of philosophers. And yet, if those progenitors of ours, hundreds of millions of years ago, had not exercised their 'minds' or their 'efforts of will' on achieving them, we would not be here to think about it or talk about it at all.

The same kind of thing is true in ontogeny. For instance, babies seem sometimes simply to 'forget to breathe'. Apnoeic spells are common enough in nurseries for the newborn, especially in intensive-care units where premature babies are cared for until they are mature enough to 'care for themselves'—though none of us ever really reaches quite that stage, not even if, or especially if, one lives to be a hundred. The organism, operating through the complex pathways of its central nervous system—and let us remember that *any* nervous system, no matter how simple it looks, is very complex in form and function compared to any other organ system that has evolved—constantly learns its tasks and goes on to new ones. This is what eventually made it possible for us, with the brain now at a level of prodigious complexity, not only to learn and to know, but to know that we know, and to discuss the nature of that knowledge.

If 'awareness' in some rudimentary form is an inherent property of living matter, then conscious awareness was always a possibility as an effect of increasing specialization and complexity in the organization of a nervous system in which a 'central' exchange-component evolved. This in turn allowed, in evolution, for development of self-conscious awareness or 'reflection'.

As I have said, I am attracted by Schrödinger's[5] thesis that every vertebrate organism in its ontogeny, and every group of vertebrates in phylogeny, engages in activities that deserve to be called 'conscious'. Those vertebrates have tasks to learn. The structure must be present to allow such learning, at whatever level of sophistication is appropriate to the individual or the group. If they had not learnt their appropriate tasks, and had not learnt how to embed them in their brains so that they became routine or automatic, then the vertebrate phylum would never have got to the point of examining itself, through us. The phylum is now capable of turning in on itself and on the world, in the way that the modern scientific mind, and the modern imagination, make possible.

In his *Autobiography* Charles Darwin[6] wrote, in 1876, of the 'impossibility of conceiving this immense and wonderful universe . . . as the result of blind chance and necessity. When thus reflecting I feel compelled to look to a First Cause having an intelligent mind in some degree analogous to that of man'. And then he wrote, 'but then arises the doubt—can the mind of man, which has, as I fully believe, been developed from a mind as low as that possessed by the lowest animal, be trusted when it draws such grand conclusions?' The answer, I think, is 'yes—with reservations'. Increased freedom implies freedom to be wrong as well as to be right. Drawing correct conclusions about nature and the evolutionary process is the peculiar task of our species for today. We should give that task (both scientific and philosophical) our full attention, our full concentration. And then we shall become free to attempt other tasks, just as our more recent ancestors, having learnt to walk on two legs and to manipulate things with their hands, gave themselves freedom to concentrate on thinking *something*. They themselves were dependent on the success of biological ancestors which learnt how to breathe, and made it automatic—and they in turn on progenitors which learnt how to keep the heart pumping. Conscious awareness, and concentration of effort, have been vital at all stages. On the whole the process has worked pretty well. At least it has reached the point now where we can examine it and talk about it. So I think we should trust it, and trust ourselves. The emergent mind is to be trusted precisely because it is bound up inextricably with evolutionary biology. Darwin had his doubts a hundred years ago. Today we can afford to be more sanguine, in the light of our more sophisticated insights. When Margaret Fuller announced that she was prepared to 'accept the universe' Thomas Carlyle is reputed to have said, 'Gad! She'd better!' In similar spirit, I think we had better accept the brain, and have faith in the general trustworthiness of its workings. If we don't, we shall end up, as so many have done in the last half-century, in meaninglessness and absurdity, the antithesis of worthwhile philosophy.

ACKNOWLEDGEMENTS

My debts to my pupils across the decades, and to my teachers across the centuries, are too numerous to list. In recent years I have profited greatly from the contacts resulting from invitations to take part in: a series of US Symposia on Philosophy and Medicine; meetings of the Hastings Center, NY; Concern for Dying (an educational council), NY; The Kennedy Institute for the Study of Human Reproduction and Bioethics, Washington, DC; The Society for Health and Human Values, Philadelphia, Pa; The Society for the Study of Medical Ethics, London, UK; and, most of all, the UCLA Medicine and Society Forum and the UCLA Program in Medicine, Law and Human Values. In particular, I would like to acknowledge my debt to participants in that Program, especially to its co-director (with me), William J. Winslade, Ph D, J D, for many stimulating discussions. The Administration and Faculty at UCLA have done much to encourage this Program in its early years, not least by giving me relative freedom to develop it. The President of the University of California has been particularly supportive.

References

1. BUNGE, M. (1977) Emergence and the mind. *Neuroscience 2*, 501–509
2. TOWERS, B. (1978) The origin and development of living forms. *J. Med. Philos. 3*, 88–106
3. SHEPARD, P. (1978) *Thinking Animals: Animals and the Development of Human Intelligence*, Viking Press, New York
4. JACOB, F. (1977) Evolution and tinkering. *Science (Wash. D.C.) 196*, 1161–1166
5. SCHRÖDINGER, E. (1958) *Mind and Matter*, pp. 3–9, Cambridge University Press, London
6. DARWIN, C. (1958) *The Autobiography of Charles Darwin, 1809–1882. The First Complete Version* (Barlow, N., ed.), pp. 92–93, Collins, London

The mind–body problem in an evolutionary perspective

MARIO BUNGE

Foundations and Philosophy of Science Unit, McGill University, Montreal

Abstract Charles Darwin realized that his theory of evolution, jointly with the psychoneural identity hypothesis, implies the conjecture that behaviour and ideation evolve alongside anatomical and physiological traits. He was therefore the founder of evolutionary psychology. However, this science has not been pursued with vigour: not even its name has attained currency. In fact most psychologists still think in a pre-evolutionary fashion and seldom ask questions about the adaptive value and possible evolution of behavioural and mental traits.

One reason for the underdevelopment of evolutionary psychology is that, on the whole, psychology is still separate from biology. In turn, one reason for this estrangement between close relatives is that psychology is still to some extent in the grip of psychoneural dualism, or the prehistoric belief that mind and body are separate entities. This doctrine is bound to block the advance of evolutionary psychology because a dualist must either deny mental evolution or speculate that it proceeds by some mechanism other than genic variation and natural (and social) selection.

On the other hand the psychoneural identity hypothesis fits in with biology and, in particular, with evolutionary biology. Moreover, by construing ideation as a brain process, psychoneural monism explains how ideas (via behaviour) can become a motor of evolution as well as an outcome of it. So, it is in the interest of evolutionary psychologists to pay closer attention to the mind–body problem and to adopt the psychoneural identity hypothesis and turn it into a full-fledged scientific theory.

ONE CENTURY OF EVOLUTIONARY PSYCHOLOGY

Until recently the mind was generally regarded as a human prerogative as well as immaterial, unchanging, and often also as supernatural. Charles Darwin changed all this, if not *de facto* at least *de jure*. In fact he conjectured that subhuman animals too can have a mental life, that ideation is a bodily process, and that it is subject to natural selection just like any other biofunction. Indeed Darwin adopted a materialist and evolutionist view of mind as early as 1838, as revealed by his recently published M and N Notebooks, which he edited himself the same year (1856) as he began writing *Natural Selection*, the unfinished ancestor of the *Origin of Species*.[1] In the M Notebook we read: 'Origin of man now proved.—Metaphysics must flourish.—He who understands baboon would do more toward metaphysics than Locke' (M84). And in the N Notebook he draws the methodological consequence of the hypothesis that mind is a bodily function: 'To study Metaphysics, as they have always been studied appears to me to be like puzzling at astronomy without mechanics.— Experience shows the problem of the mind cannot be solved by attacking the citadel itself.—the mind is function of body.—we must bring some *stable* foundation to argue from.—' (N5).

Darwin of course did more than confide his thoughts on the nature and evolution of behaviour and ideation to his notebooks. He wrote *The Descent of Man* (1871) and *The Expression of the Emotions in Animals and Men* (1872), the founding stones of evolutionary psychology and ethology—not to speak of anthropology and prehistory. The first book, in particular, exerted a tremendous influence—on all but psychologists and philosophers of mind. True, George Romanes wrote several books on animal intelligence and mental development (which he misleadingly called 'evolution'). However, those works fell short of scientific rigour. Besides, Romanes rejected mental evolution on religious grounds. Likewise Alfred Russel Wallace, the cofounder of evolutionary biology (though not an enthusiast for natural selection), resisted Darwin's generalization of evolution to mental abilities.

The field lay fallow until C. Lloyd Morgan published his *Introduction to Comparative Psychology* (1894). From then on psychologists have taken it for granted that the study of pigeons, rats, dogs and monkeys is relevant to the understanding of the human species. But, unlike the behaviourists who followed (in particular Watson and Skinner), Morgan believed not only in the continuity of the evolutionary process but also in the emergence of new properties and laws during it: he wrote *The Emergence of Novelty* (1933) to emphasize that point. And the distinguished animal psychologist Theodore Schneirla emphasized the qualitative differences among evolutionary stages in his long essay 'Levels in the psychological capacities of animals'.[2]

Like most other evolutionists, the eminent geneticist Theodosius Dobzhansky thought that evolution has been punctuated by qualitative novelties. In particular he stated that man is 'a possessor of mental abilities which occur in other animals only in most rudimentary forms, if at all.'[3] This acknowledgement of qualitative difference drew the irate reaction of a distinguished primatologist, who stated that 'There is no evidence of an intellectual gulf [between man and subhuman animals] at any point'. And yet, despite all the astonishing accomplishments of apes—particularly in artificial environments—none of them has designed a machine, or written a song, or proposed a social reform. So, abyss there is, though it was formed only recently and in one and the same mountain range.

Evolutionary psychologists will then stress the discontinuities (through emergence) as well as the continuity (through descent) of the evolutionary process. Hence, although they will regard rat psychology as highly relevant to human psychology, they will also investigate the peculiarities of human behaviour and ideation. But how many behavioural scientists actually think in evolutionary terms? A perusal of scientific publications will exhibit but few works on the evolution of the nervous system aside from the monumental volume on the evolution of the cerebellum edited by Llinas in 1969.[5] Only a handful of books on the evolution of behaviour and mentation appeared after the volume edited by Roe and Simpson in 1958:[4] Munn,[6] Jerison,[7] and Masterton and colleagues.[8,9] And although there are hundreds of journals of psychology, with a few papers on evolutionary psychology scattered among them, none seems exclusively devoted to evolutionary psychology—a term that is not even in current usage.

It seems then that most psychologists are not used to thinking in evolutionary terms or, indeed, in biological terms. For the most part they have received no biological training and they seldom mix with biologists. (Neuroscientists retaliate by ignoring psychology.) I know of only one Department of Psychobiology (University of California at Irvine), one of Biobehavioral Sciences (University of Connecticut) and one of Psychiatry and Biobehavioral Sciences (University of California at Los Angeles), and one Laboratory of Neuropsychology (National Institute of Mental Health, Bethesda). Moreover it is only recently that courses in physiological psychology have become standard components of psychology curricula. Even so, few textbooks in the field adopt an explicit evolutionary viewpoint (an exception is Thompson[10]).

The disregard for evolutionary biology is particularly notable among the practitioners of artificial intelligence (AI). Intent as they are on designing machines imitating human behaviour or ideation, they often take simulation for identity and claim that human beings are machines. By thus skipping the biological and social levels they gloss over three billion years of evolution. And by so doing they fall into the dualist trap: indeed the AI people are fond of likening the mind–body distinction to the software–hardware distinction. They also forget that, unlike self-assembled (or self-organizing) systems, all machines have been designed and none of them is free in any sense, for every one of them acts by proxy. A pinch of evolutionary thought would have spared them these mistakes—and deprived the dualist of the joy of receiving comfort from the mechanist.

If psychologists on the whole ignore evolution, it is little wonder that philosophers of mind pay hardly any attention to it. A well-known Wittgensteinian philosopher of mind noted for his attacks on the psychoneural identity hypothesis has gone so far as to hold that 'it is really senseless to conjecture that animals *may* have thoughts' (Malcolm[11]). Yet we have known for some years now, particularly thanks to the work of the Gardners and the Premacks, that apes can learn to express their thoughts by means of certain artificial languages such as that of the deaf-mutes.

There is no justification for a philosopher to continue to talk of mind as a human prerogative as well as immaterial and unchanging, let alone as supernatural. There is even less justification for a neuroscientist to continue to hold such prescientific views on mind. However this is exactly what the eminent neurophysiologist Sir John Eccles has been saying for the past three decades: that mind is immaterial yet can act on neurons;[12] and that the existence of consciousness and that of the cosmos 'require a supernatural explanation to be admitted by we scientists in all humility'.[13] Not surprisingly, Eccles claims that *Homo sapiens* has not been subject to evolution. In fact, since the brain of man (seems to have) ceased to grow over the past 250 000 years, 'our human inheritance of brains averaging about 1400 cc in size is the end of the evolutionary story. And now, in any case, biological evolution for man is at an end because selection pressure has been eliminated by the welfare state'.[14]

This startling conclusion rests on the following false presuppositions: (a) that genic variation (by mutation and recombination) stopped long ago in human beings; (b) that behaviour and ideation, though possibly dependent upon brain size, do not depend upon the organization and plasticity of the neurons; (c) that behaviour and ideation play no active role in adaptation, hence in human evolution; (d) that hominids and humans have never faced new challenges (such as glaciations and droughts) calling for new abilities; (e) that the Welfare State, by alleviating poverty, raising the health level and assuring education for all, does not set a premium on any skills. In sum Eccles has managed to do violence to genetics, evolutionary biology, history and sociology in one breath. (For further criticism see Dimond[15].) This is not a coincidence but an unavoidable consequence of the dualistic and supernaturalistic philosophy of mind according to which mental evolution either does not exist or, if it does, then it is not an aspect of biological (and social) evolution. Evolutionary neuroscientists think otherwise: to them 'The relation between brain and mind evolves in association with a physiological substratum, and hence there is no dualism'.[16] (See details in Refs. 8 and 9).

RESEARCH PROBLEMS SPARKED OFF BY PSYCHONEURAL MONISM

It would seem that we are back in square one, in the pre-Darwin days, when biologists and philosophers of mind held a palaeolithic view of mind. But this is not quite true, for psychoneural monism has now a growing number of adepts, and evolutionary thinking is making important inroads in psychology, particularly among primatologists, developmental psychologists and socio-biologists. These scientists are at least beginning to pose problems that make no sense in a dualistic and pre-evolutionary context, and that are spawning some interesting hypotheses and experiments. Here is a random sample:

(1) How new is the neocortex and, in particular, the associative 'area'?

(2) How new is synaptic plasticity—or, equivalently, when did Hebb's mechanism of use and disuse[17] emerge? (Hebb's principle is 'Neurons that fire together tend to stay together'.)

(3) What is the origin of brain lateralization? Is there any adaptive advantage in it? (See, for example, Levy.[18])

(4) Why does parental behaviour occur at all, given that it is energy- and time-consuming and that it renders parents easy targets for predators (Barash[19])?

(5) What has been the evolution of parental behaviour in the higher vertebrates and how is it affected by ideation?

(6) Is altruism genetically programmed or learnt? (Prior question: is it legitimate to treat inheritance and experience as additive factors and consequently ask what the contribution of each is?)

(7) Is aggression genetically programmed? (Prior questions: the one in point (6), and whether aggression can be equated with defence and making a living.)

(8) When and how did empathy and solidarity emerge?

(9) What are the origins of goodness and of cruelty?

(10) How did smiling and laughter evolve from grimacing, and what if any are their adaptive advantages?

(11) At what evolutionary level did imagination, ideation, foresight (or foresmell), goal-seeking behaviour and self-consciousness start?

(12) How did human language originate and evolve? (See Jaynes.[20])

(13) Is acquisitiveness instinctive or learnt, and how did it evolve?

(14) Is there an inherited moral sense, and in any case at what point in evolution did morality emerge? (Recall Darwin's *Notebook M* (144): 'What is the Philosophy of Shame & Blushing? Does Elephant know shame—dog knows triumph.—' For recent work on the development of morality see Goslan.[21])

(15) What if any, are the biological roots of managerial, political and military behaviour patterns?

The above are just a few of the many questions that are currently being investigated, or are likely to be tackled soon, by evolutionary psychologists, ethologists, sociobiologists, anthropologists and social scientists. No such questions arise in the framework of psychophysical dualism even if dualists occasionally pay lip service to evolutionary biology (e.g. Popper & Eccles[22]). The reason is transparent: according to the neo-Darwinian theory, evolution proceeds by genic variation (a material event) and natural selection (another material event). That theory leaves no room for immaterial agencies such as non-embodied souls, ideas in themselves, and other Platonic inmates of Popper's World 3. Dualists do not accept materialistic (biological) explanations in the matter of mind: they cannot admit that molecular changes and environmental factors can act on minds. So, they must either deny mental evolution altogether or speculate that it proceeds by some mechanism other than genic variation and natural (and social) selection. In either case they come into conflict with evolutionary biology and psychology, regardless of the frequency with which they use the term 'evolution'. And, to the extent that their views are influential, dualists slow down the advance of both sciences.

Psychoneural identity theorists, on the other hand, are in harmony with evolutionary biology and psychology. In fact to them mental functions are brain functions, so mental evolution is an aspect of the evolution of animals possessing brains capable of 'minding'—i.e. the higher vertebrates. (For a half-way formalization of the identity theory see Bunge.[23]) To be sure, for social animals, in particular human beings, we must add social (economic, political and cultural) evolution to biological evolution. But, since societies are concrete or material (though not just physical) systems, biosocial evolution is a material process—albeit one exhibiting properties unknown to physics or even biology. This is not to deny the influence of behaviour and ideation on adaptation, and hence on evolution. On the contrary, the efficacy of behaviour and ideation is assured by construing them as bodily functions, whereas if detached from matter they are deprived of testable power.

In sum, psychoneural monism is the philosophy of mind behind evolutionary (and physiological) psychology. And, while the latter has yet to make its mark, at least it has made a good start by asking some of the proper questions—questions whose investigation does not call for the postulating of immaterial or supernatural agencies.

OBSTACLES: GENUINE AND SPURIOUS

Several objections have been raised against the neo-Darwinian approach to behaviour and evolution. One of them is that, because behaviour is not only a result of evolution but also a factor in it, the theory must be corrected with a dose of Lamarckism (Piaget[24]). This claim seems to be mistaken: behavioural (and mental) adaptation can be explained by (natural or artificial) selection acting on genic variation. The environment selects behaving organisms, not naked genes or disembodied behaviour repertoires. To be sure, the higher vertebrates can learn new behaviour patterns in response to environmental changes or mental processes, so they are not at the mercy of their genomes—or, rather, they can make full use of their genetic potentialities. Still, such potentialities are inherited and, when actualized, they work on a par with other biological traits. If successful, a new behaviour pattern—whether acquired by genic change or by learning—is bound to have some genetic effect because it favours certain genotypes over others.

Example 1: A mutant synthesizes certain enzymes, allowing it to eat certain plants that the normal variety cannot digest. This allows the mutant to occupy a different (perhaps larger) ecological niche, which confers some advantage upon it though at the same time setting it in competition with other species. If successful, the mutation will tend to spread. *Example 2:* An animal learns a new advantageous behaviour pattern, i.e. one that eases its way of making a living. As a consequence it reproduces earlier or more abundantly than its conspecifics, so that its peculiar genes have better chances of spreading and becoming entrenched In either case the rate of change of the new population depends upon the difference between the birth and death rates —as is the case with all organisms—but now these rates depend partly on behavioural traits, some of which are phenotypic rather than genotypic.

So, while behaviour can make the difference between radiation and extinction, it fits within the neo-Darwinian schema. What is true is not that the latter is grossly in error but that behaviour, in particular social behaviour, enriches the modes of adaptation and quickens considerably the pace of evolution. (Methodological consequence: genetics is necessary but insufficient to explain behavioural evolution.) This applies particularly to the plastic behaviour of the higher vertebrates, which is partly controlled by ideation. The overall advantage (and occasional disadvantage) of possessing mental abilities is quite obvious in an evolutionary psychobiological perspective. If on the other hand mind were immaterial, evolutionary theory would have nothing to say about it.

Another popular idea is that human history transcends biological history (true) to the point that the latter is irrelevant to the former (false). This is like saying that, because biology deals with emergent properties and laws ignored by physics, the latter is irrelevant to the former. Surely human history is more than biological evolution: it encompasses the latter, in the sense that human history is artificial rather than natural evolution, for history is largely shaped (though not fully controlled) by human beings themselves. But this history is concrete and thus a far cry from the mythical history of independently evolving ideas imagined by Hegel and other idealist philosophers. Human history is concrete because it is the evolution of human populations, i.e. of systems of human beings interacting amongst themselves and with their natural and social environments.

What is undoubtedly true is that the weight of intelligence in human affairs has increased dramatically over the past fifty millennia and even more so since the beginning of agriculture about 10 000 years ago. However, intelligence is a property of the brain—and one extremely sensitive to social stimuli— not of an immaterial mind. And in any case let us not forget that, with the increasingly important role of intelligence in the process of artificial selection that we call 'human history', the roles of human stupidity, greed and cruelty have also become more important. Side by side with the inventor, the scientist and the social reformer, human societies have created the dogmatist, the mystic and the military butcher. While more and more individuals have become enlightened during certain exceptional periods, greater and greater masses have been driven to disaster, and now a couple of individuals have the technical ability to extinguish all life on earth—several times over. There is no room for such monstrous stupidity in the idealistic philosophy of history.

A third popular objection to evolutionary psychology is that it is untestable, for a collection of fossil bones can tell us nothing about the behaviour and mentation of their departed owners. This objection is quite natural if behaviour and ideation are taken to be immaterial, but it is no more than a challenge if the psychobiological standpoint is adopted. Moreover the challenge is being met by the usual methods elaborated by palaeontologists, anthropologists and prehistorians. There are three such methods and, while all three involve admirable efforts of imagination, neither surpasses the imagination invested by physicists in conjecturing the structure of the atom or by biochemists in guessing the structure of the DNA molecule.

There is, first, the direct approach of studying fossils and their associated natural and artificial remains, and trying to reconstruct not only their anatomy but also the physiology and the behaviour of their owners (in particular posture, locomotion and feeding habits). *Example:* the hypothetical reconstructions of the ways of life of hominids living two million years ago in East Africa. (For a beautiful semipopular account see Leakey and Lewin.[25])

Then there is the comparative approach, which is both indirect and empirical, as it consists of studying specimens of modern taxa conjectured to be close relatives of extinct ones. (Not all comparative studies are relevant to evolutionary psychology even when they focus on behaviour; only those are relevant which compare the behavioural repertoires and mental abilities of species belonging to the same phyletic line. See Hodos and Campbell.[26]) *Example:* Primatologists have been shedding considerable light on the possible life styles and behavioural repertoires of our prehuman ancestors. Finally there is the armchair approach of asking how, on the basis of our general neurobiological knowledge, certain neuronal systems and their functions could have evolved, or how such and such behaviour or thought patterns might have arisen or evolved. All three approaches are necessary and should be better integrated, particularly in the case of behaviour and ideation, for they throw light on complementary sides and control each other. (Cf. Jerison.[7])

In sum, although evolutionary psychology is a tough subject, it may not be tougher than cosmology and, in any case, it is just as interesting if not more so.

SUMMARY AND CONCLUSIONS

Our first conclusion is that evolutionary psychology, created by Darwin one century ago, is a going concern, admittedly still a rather weak one though one that deserves strong support.

Secondly, the underdeveloped state of evolutionary psychology may be explained by (a) the youth of evolutionary thinking in general, (b) the neglect of the theory of evolution (and in general of biology) by most psychologists, (c) the difficulty of generating reasonable hypotheses about the evolution of behaviour and ideation—particularly given the strong prejudice against framing hypotheses and theories in the behavioural sciences, (d) the difficulty of obtaining and interpreting empirical data relevant to such hypotheses, and (e) last, but not least, the dualistic philosophy of mind that has dominated for thousands of years.

Thirdly, evolutionary biology has done more than trace the ancestry of some contemporary biospecies: it has reoriented biological thought. Thus where pre-Darwinians saw design in adaptation, contemporary biologists see the outcome of natural or artificial selection on the products of random genic variation. The impact of the new outlook on the sciences of man has been just as dramatic. Thus while the pre-Darwinians often saw man as a spiritual being (Plato's model), we see ourselves as animals, albeit exceptional ones (Aristotle's model). While the pre-Darwinians (in particular the believers in the arcane) believed man to have paranormal abilities independent of the brain (such as telepathy and psychokinesis), we believe all our mental functions to be lawful (though not always normal) brain functions. And while the pre-Darwinians (in particular the psychoanalysts) sought a purpose or 'meaning' in every bit of human behaviour and mentation, we regard purposeful behaviour as exceptional and moreover as something to be explained rather than as having explanatory force. (*Example*: 'She did X in order to attain Y' is explained as either 'She has been conditioned to do X every time she wanted Y', or 'Knowing (or suspecting) that X causes Y, and valuing Y, she did X'.)

Fourthly, when scientists underrate philosophical issues they risk falling victims to unscientific philosophies likely to slow down or even derail the train of their research. The mind–body problem is a case in point: as an eminent psychologist wrote three decades ago 'The study of mental evolution has been handicapped by a metaphysical [mind–body] dualism', for it denies the evolutionary hypothesis that 'The evolution of mind is the evolution of nervous mechanisms' (Lashley[27]). Indeed (a) instead of suggesting promising questions that may be investigated with the means at the disposal of biologists, anthropologists and prehistorians, dualism diverts the attention of these investigators to an inscrutable entity—the proverbial immaterial soul; (b) because it contends that mind is immaterial, dualism must either deny that it has evolved or assert that its evolutionary mechanism is non-Darwinian: in either case it is anti-evolutionary.

Fifthly, in contrast to psychoneural dualism, the psychoneural identity theory suggests a host of interesting research problems, such as those of the forms 'What neural systems are required by such and such behaviour patterns or mental functions?', and 'How may such and such behaviour patterns or mental capacities have evolved?' Yet, the psychoneural identity theory is so far a skeleton waiting to be fleshed out, and evolutionary psychology little more than an incipient science that can boast of far more problems than solutions. But at least these problems are interesting and can be investigated by the scientific method, and those few solutions that we do have are not ready-made ideological slogans but scientific hypotheses that can be perfected or even rejected altogether.

ACKNOWLEDGEMENT

I thank Victor H. Denenberg (Department of Biobehavioral Sciences, University of Connecticut) for instructive exchanges.

References

1. GRUBER, H. E. & BARRETT, P. H. (1974) *Darwin on Man. Together with Darwin's Early and Unpublished Notebooks*, Dutton, New York
2. SCHNEIRLA, T. C. (1949) Levels in the psychological capacities of animals, in *Philosophy for the Future* (Sellars, R. W. *et al.*, eds.), pp. 243–286, Macmillan, New York
3. DOBZHANSKY, TH. (1955) *Evolution, Genetics and Man*, p. 338, Wiley, New York
4. HARLOW, H. F. (1958) The evolution of learning, in *Behavior and Evolution* (Roe, A. & Simpson, G. G., eds.), pp. 269–290, Yale University Press, New Haven
5. LLINÁS, R. (ed) (1969) *Neurobiology of Cerebellar Evolution and Development*, American Medical Association, Chicago
6. MUNN, N. L. (1971) *The Evolution of the Human Mind*, Houghton & Mifflin, Boston
7. JERISON, H. J. (1973) *Evolution of the Brain and Intelligence*, Academic Press, New York
8. MASTERTON, R. B., CAMPBELL, C. B. G., BITTERMAN, M. E. & HOTTON, N. (eds.) (1976) *Evolution of Brain and Behavior in Vertebrates*, Erlbaum, Hillsdale, N.J.
9. MASTERTON, R. B., HODOS, W. & JERISON, H. J. (eds.) (1976) *Evolution, Brain and Behavior. Persistent Problems*, Erlbaum, Hillsdale, N. J.
10. THOMPSON, R. F. (1975) *Introduction to Physiological Psychology*, Harper & Row, New York
11. MALCOLM, N. (1973) Thoughtless brutes. *Proc. Addresses Am. Philos. Assoc. 46*, 5–20
12. ECCLES, J. C. (1951) Hypotheses relating to the mind-body problem. *Nature (Lond.) 168*, 53–64
13. ECCLES, J. C. (1978) Keynote address to the 1975 ICUS Congress, in *What ICUS is*, International Cultural Foundation [Rev. Myung Moon, Chairman], New York
14. ECCLES, J. C. (1977) Evolution of the brain in relation to the development of the self-conscious mind. *Ann. N. Y. Acad. Sci. 299*, 161–179
15. DIMOND, S. J. (1977) Evolution and lateralization of the brain: concluding remarks. *Ann. N. Y. Acad. Sci. 299*, 477–501
16. BULLOCK, T. H. (1958) Evolution and neurophysiological mechanisms, in *Behavior and Evolution* (Roe, A. & Simpson, G. G., eds.), pp. 165–177, Yale University Press, New Haven
17. HEBB, D. O. (1949) *The Organization of Behavior*, Wiley, New York
18. LEVY, J. (1977) The mammalian brain and the adaptive advantage of cerebral asymmetry. *Ann. N. Y. Acad. Sci. 299*, 264–272
19. BARASH, D. P. (1976) Some evolutionary aspects of parental behavior in animals and man. *Am. J. Psychol. 89*, 195–217
20. JAYNES, J. (1976) The evolution of language in the late Pleistocene. *Ann. N. Y. Acad. Sci. 280*, 312–325
21. GOSLAN, D. A. (ed.) (1969) *Handbook of Socialization Theory and Research*, Rand McNally, Chicago
22. POPPER, K. R. & ECCLES, J. C. (1977) *The Self and Its Brain*, Springer International, New York
23. BUNGE, M. (1979) *Treatise on Basic Philosophy*, vol. 4: *A World of Systems*, Reidel, Dordrecht
24. PIAGET, J. (1976) *Le Comportement, Moteur de l'Evolution*, Gallimard, Paris
25. LEAKEY, R. & LEWIN, R. (1977) *Origins*, Dutton, New York
26. HODOS, W. & CAMPBELL, C. B. G. (1969) *Scala naturae*: why there is no theory in comparative psychology. *Psychol. Rev. 76*, 337–350
27. LASHLEY, K. S. (1949) Persistent problems in the evolution of mind. *Q. Rev. Biol. 24*, 28–42

Discussion: Evolutionary aspects

Bennett: I can see how being a dualist is going to lead to problems about the evolution of the mind, but I wasn't clear about how Eccles' dualism is involved in his statement that in human beings selection pressures have been eliminated by the welfare state. I didn't see why that was clearly wrong.

Bunge: Eccles says explicitly that since the brain-case has stopped growing over the past 250 000 years we must infer that the evolution of the human species is at an end. That is wrong because it rests on the false presuppositions that I listed (p. 56) and that Eccles doesn't examine.

Medawar: If that is a true representation of what Jack Eccles said, I am very sorry.

Bunge: I am simply saying that his statement presupposes those propositions. I am not quoting him.

Brazier: The seeds of that are to be found in what Eccles[1] said at the meeting at the Vatican.

Medawar: Darwin made a remark which is always held up to young philosophers as an example of the deep philosophical illiteracy of scientists. In one of his Notebooks he asked 'Why is thought being a secretion of brain more wonderful than gravity, a property of matter?' (cited by Gould[2]). That is a straight question. Let's have a straight answer from someone, without talking about categories.

Putnam: I have great sympathy with that question of Darwin's. But a lot of philosophers now want the theory of evolution to do too much work in epistemology and psychology. The tide if anything is that way, and I am sceptical about the claim that evolution can be much help in epistemology. I want to share my problem with you.

People say that we can explain by evolution why our beliefs tend to be true. The general idea is to try to solve the old problems of epistemology by rehabilitating the move that most English philosophers have been making anyway since Hume, even if they haven't admitted it. That is, 'Hume was right—we can't *justify* any of this stuff, but thank goodness enough of our basic beliefs are true!' Then, of course, other people come out with the old objection, which I think is right, that that is saying there is no difference between reason and animal faith. Now the first people say, 'instead of talking about *justification* let's talk about *reliability*. The problem is to show that our belief-making mechanism is a *reliable* one, that is, one that has a tendency to produce true beliefs. All we can ask is empirical support for the claim that our belief-making mechanism is a reliable one, proof that that claim is coherent with total science'. And lo and behold there is this wonderful theory of evolution which talks about adaptation, and we have a truth-producing belief mechanism which is obviously adaptive, so everything is fine.

The trouble with this story is that it would fit better with dualism. It was suggested that the dualist would be in trouble with the theory of evolution, but if intelligence is a *faculty for perceiving truths* that would have great adaptive advantage and the evolutionary story would be wonderful. But intelligence *isn't* a faculty for perceiving truths; it is a faculty for producing beliefs that meet certain operational and theoretical constraints.

Young: What is a faculty?

Putnam: It is a program, to use computer language, for churning out propositions which satisfy certain operational and methodological constraints.

Young: Is it a brain program or a soul program?

Putnam: I think it is a brain program. On a materialist view it is a program for producing beliefs which agree with your experiences and which meet certain simplicity constraints. There is nothing there that logically guarantees that these beliefs would be *true*. Worse than that, even if the world is such that the beliefs which agree with your operational constraints and are simplest tend to be true in one part of the world, it is perfectly possible that they be false in another area. People talk about 'causal theories of knowledge' these days. In a causal theory of knowledge you do not have to *justify* a belief for it to count as knowledge; you just have to be situated so that you wouldn't have had that belief if it hadn't been true. The evolutionary story works fine, it seems to me, for knowledge about tables and chairs. We have evolved in such a way that in general we wouldn't believe there is a chair in this room if there were no chairs here. I wouldn't believe that John Searle was in front of me if John Searle wasn't in front of me. When we come to our most general beliefs, such as that the laws of nature are the same at the micro level as at the macro level, the evolutionary explanation of the origin of the propensity to believe them doesn't connect with their being true. The evolutionary explanation of why I believe that there are infinitely many natural numbers will not connect with its being true.

Plum: The discussion seems not to be focusing on what the questions are. Are you talking about consciousness as equivalent to wakefulness? Are you talking about awareness of the environment as the same thing as awareness of self? In the evolutionary tree, isn't self-awareness apparently limited to the higher primates and especially to those that possess language?

To what do the philosophers refer when they talk about truth? What is the independent evidence for truth, and how do you verify it? How can truth be susceptible to evolution? Are you talking about controlled experiments to verify truth, are you talking about statistical validation, or have you a set of philosophical principles which amount to a Codex? We biologists need you to inform us on these matters.

Towers: There is a good deal of misunderstanding about the nature of evolution and what it leads to. Hilary Putnam was propounding the idea that what some philosophers understand by evolution is that somehow or other it will lead us to truth. This is to misinterpret biological evolution, which is not some kind of programme which leads in a direct line towards some predetermined end. Evolution is essentially opportunistic; it is a tinker system that picks up anything that happens to be around, and manipulates and incorporates it. Whether whatever is produced by a tinker is beneficial and adaptive is a matter of luck. The things that are not beneficial and adaptive will go under. The rest will be incorporated into the next stages but there is nothing that guarantees that you are going in a specific direction. It is like oil on water. It goes here, there and everywhere, eventually ending up in the place where it is best fitted to end up. There are many such places for many different organisms.

Young: Will you also tell us about the awareness of arthropods?

Searle: One of the things that was worrying Dr Plum was your use of the term 'awareness', Dr Towers, and I was a little puzzled by it myself.

Towers: There are various levels of conscious awareness. There is the simple response to environmental stimuli. When we observe animals we see that they are aware of the environment in that they respond to it, do something to it. I don't want to say that that is self-conscious awareness and I certainly don't want to say that it is reflective conscious awareness. But for *Homo sapiens* to have developed the capacity of reflective conscious awareness, all of these other stages of awareness had to be developed earlier in evolutionary history.

Searle: You used the term in connection with amoebae, but do you also want to say that during photosynthesis plants are aware of the sun?

Towers: I remember once discussing Fred Hoyle's book *The Black Cloud* with an astronomer. To what extent is the black cloud, because it responds, aware of its environment? There are astronomers who would want to say that the physical principles that make one material body respond to another material body represent a primitive form of awareness, that this is inherent and built into the structure of matter.

Searle: The question was, do *you* want to say that?

Towers: Yes, ultimately I would.

Creutzfeldt: Aren't we now getting close to panpsychism? Is that a position that we really want to defend when we talk about the evolution of the human species?

Towers: No. I said I wanted, in my paper, to stick to biological forms and not go into the prebiological. But somewhere, of course, you have to incorporate prebiological if you want to be an evolutionary theorist all the way through. I would say that the propensity of inorganic matter to respond to other inorganic matter in the environment by forming molecules, super-molecules and so on simply indicates the nature of the material universe in which we live. This is how matter behaves. If it behaves that way for a long enough period, we are involved in an evolutionary process which eventually provides us with the opportunity of reflecting back on it and trying to analyse what it is all about. I am not postulating anything supernatural, such as a universal soul.

Wikler: Perhaps you can hold the evolutionary view about the validity of our belief about tables and chairs without having to postulate a direction for evolution, or having to say that somehow evolution is pushing us to a realization of the truth. It is enough to hold that even if evolution does proceed in a tinkering way, the kinds of animals that had brains that led them to constantly false beliefs about tables and chairs wouldn't be with us any more. So, we can assume that evolution has provided us with a mechanism for generating true beliefs. At least this would seem likely in the case of ordinary, mundane beliefs.

It is another thing to use evolution as evidence for the truth of global beliefs about the nature of time and so on; perhaps this would require your other premises.

Marsden: In a conversation like this the biologists amongst us become uncomfortable, as Dr Plum did. My discomfort arises from hearing that if an organism responds to the environment, that indicates some awareness and perhaps a primitive consciousness. A man who has lost his brain completely will still respond to a pinprick if his spinal cord is intact, but can you call that awareness? In human terms it is not consciousness at all.

Towers: The pithed frog will respond to stimuli. Presumably that animal without its head and brain is not aware of what is going on. One reason why it is not aware is that the simple reflex functions which it is now exhibiting as a pithed animal had earlier been taken over by the development of brain at some previous stage of evolution. So now when you remove its brain, you remove its consciousness. This is not to say that a much more primitive organism than a frog, one which did not yet have a brain, would not respond with its own level of conscious awareness.

Young: That is wholly specious, if I may say so. For example, I have never seen a newly born squid which couldn't breathe. You mentioned some babies who don't breathe much and we all know that there are many such cases, but every animal is born with these capacities. To say that they have to learn them painfully is wholly misleading.

Towers: I don't think the individual has to learn them but they had to be learnt at some stage in evolution. The diaphragm, for example, is a voluntary muscle, with its nerve supply from the spinal cord. That must have been under conscious control, just as other voluntary muscles are, and now for the most part we simply let it do its own job, whether we are awake or asleep. Of course, we can always reassert voluntary control in this instance if the situation calls for it, as in holding one's breath or taking deep breaths.

Plum: That is a different interpretation from the one most of us would place on ontogeny. Most of us would see ontogeny as consisting of a whole series of automatic developments, none of which had to be learnt. If the development led to enhanced chances of individual or species survival, it persisted; if it was detrimental to survival, it failed. It is hard to envision learning or a sense of struggle entering into the almost limitless biological trials and errors which lie behind the making of the human species.

Towers: I am thinking of phylogenetic development, not ontogenetic development.

Searle: I think what Dr Plum is getting at is how far does the thesis go? For example, do you want to say that at one time it is likely that human beings had to digest as a conscious activity, or secrete bile or adrenaline?

Towers: Not human beings.

Searle: Our predecessors, then?

Towers: This is Schrödinger's hypothesis.

Young: He was a physicist, not a biologist.

Medawar: I had some correspondence with Schrödinger in which he withdrew these particular views when I introduced him to the idea of antibody formation. He had to agree that this wouldn't fall within his theory. He was a very great man, a very nice man, and he admitted that he was wrong!

Crow: Surely what Dr Towers is suggesting is a form of Lamarckism: that what is acquired is then incorporated into the genome.

Cooper: A very profound question that Dr Towers raised which didn't at first seem to be related to the conference was: why is the sight of a vegetative baby tragic? First, not everyone thinks that that is tragic, and many who do, particularly the parents, eventually adopt a different view. It is a cultural preconception but it is not necessarily universally accepted when people are put to the test. I personally think it is tragic, and I have to admit that the reason is partially aesthetic, though there are many other reasons. The parents of these vegetative babies, although they always try to upgrade them, care for them and enjoy them. Above all they love them and in return they get very visible signs of loving symbolism, which to me represents a level of awareness, if that is what we are talking about. In this tragic group, infanticide is virtually non-existent, in contrast to what happens to normal but unwanted infants. In addition, a very high level of non-verbal communication develops between these babies and all of those who spend a lot of time with them. This includes what we would accept as signs of joy, which you said was one of the criteria of consciousness and life. This struck a very responsive chord in me.

There are people who insist that their plants thrive when they speak to them and do very poorly when they don't. On the other hand I am going to consider the possibility that plants may be affected by sound vibrations produced by speech, as well as Dr Towers' suggestions of amoeba awareness.

Young: Darwin played the trumpet to flowers.

Trevarthen: One of my students recently gave me the privilege of reading an unpublished diary written by Darwin and his wife Emma about their children. It is full of accurate psychological insights into the development of human consciousness in babies. But Darwin was in a moral dilemma about acknowledging the materialistic mentalism to which evolutionary theory led him.[3] When he wrote *The Descent of Man* and *The Expression of the Emotions in Animals and Men* he was very much concerned to not fully acknowledge his beliefs publicly. The scholars suggest that, after all the terrible troubles he had had in gaining acceptance for his theory of evolution, and being sensitive to public criticism, Darwin feared he would lose the battle if he said he thought that the highest mental and spiritual attributes of our species were materialistic. He certainly felt that if he did so he would hurt his family and their sensibilities.

Darwin was a courageous thinker and he was deliberately concerned about the highest moral questions when he wrote about human evolution. That preoccupation of his has perhaps been betrayed by psychology in a rather cowardly way in this century. I agree with you about that, Dr Towers.

I am interested in your suggestion that you understand the special kind of awareness of human beings to be expressed in play: you said you preferred *Homo ludens* to *Homo sapiens.* Surely we have *Felix ludens?* Cats play?

Towers: I think we have suffered so much from our Puritan inheritance that enjoying life is regarded as rather reprehensible.

Trevarthen: Yes, animals do not have a Puritan inheritance and they enjoy life, or they don't worry about it. But there must be some other special feature of human play. I have been trying hard to work out what it is.[4] Babies seem to illustrate an important difference very early in their behaviour. We find them spontaneously doing things that are not done by any chimpanzee. The formula that I have reached to explain this difference is related to the understanding of shared tasks. Young infants, about one year of age, exhibit unique forms of cooperative understanding when playing with their mothers. So play seems to have a *social* function.

Young: There is a danger in looking for the whole range of human faculties in babies.

Trevarthen: But there are very complex psychological events happening by the age of one year, some of which are not seen in any other species. Surely these are a clue to the nature of human consciousness. Darwin believed so. Dr Towers, what motivates your preference for the name *Homo ludens?*

Towers: Playing represents, in sum, the nature of the evolutionary process. That is François Jacob's 'tinkering'. That is what living is all about.

Trevarthen: But you agree that the human species is not the only one that plays. It just plays better than any of the others?

Towers: Yes; the development of the capacity for self-reflective consciousness ought to provide further freedom from the constraints of the environment and allow further advances in the evolutionary process. What I said was that this gives human beings the freedom both to be right and to be wrong.

Trevarthen: Some ideas are thought wrong because other people do not believe in them. They do not meet tests of the collective consciousness. When you were talking about the reality of tables and chairs I realized that there are lots of things that I believe for which I have never had any real evidence. I believe them because other people believe them. There must be some important link between reflective consciousness and the ability to communicate either knowledge or disbelief to other people. You talked about an activity which tests consequences, but what about beliefs which we have no chance of testing?

Fried: The question of evolution has probably been too simple-mindedly pushed off into the domain of physical genes, but we must all realize that there is a form of evolution which is cultural. People get upset about that because they think that a new dualism is being introduced. Needless to say, the culture has its substratum in capacities which have their basis in physical capacities. Nevertheless, human learning is transmitted in a way that is rather analogous to gene transmission and that has an adaptive significance. We talk about cultures being subject to adaptive pressures when the mechanism of adaptation is not the mechanism of DNA and RNA but another kind. If you were playing the game of discovering what was unique about human beings, you might say that human beings may be the only species where cultural evolution has become particularly important. In other species it is the evolution of physical structures which is distinctive.

Searle: Do the evolutionists here accept the extension of the idea of Darwinian evolution to cover cultural evolution?

Trevarthen: Yes. I would say we are now in a phase of 'psychosocial cultural evolution'.

Searle: Is it Darwinian? Do you think the same mechanisms are operating?

Trevarthen: Formally, yes, because there is transmission of learnt behaviour patterns between generations and a natural selection process. Of course, the mechanisms are not the same.

Medawar: It is Lamarckian. What is transmitted is Popper's World 3. What pass from one generation to the next are ideas, theories, arguments, hypotheses, and the physical institutions that embody them. This aspect has been extensively written about by people who shall be nameless, such as me!

Searle: In response to Mario Bunge's paper one could say that evolutionary thinking, as a pattern of analysis, is neutral between monism and dualism. Dogmatic monism can be just as much an obstacle to evolutionary thinking as dogmatic dualism. It may be useful to point out some examples of that. One striking thing about Wilson's book on sociobiology[5] is his dogmatic assumption of epiphenomenalism—the idea that the mental doesn't really make any difference. His account of communication, which I think is the weakest thing in the book, is very crude. He doesn't see that it is intrinsically intentional—that it involves intentionality at a rather sophisticated level. The sociobiologists' explanation of the incest taboo also leaves out intentionality. I want to suggest that the facts of mental development are among the things that require evolutionary explanation. That is, if the mind doesn't really matter, then why did it evolve? That seems to me a question that is neutral as between dogmatic monism and dualism.

I want to tie this in with the problem about awareness. The neuroscientists are right to be worried about the definition of this word: there is a phenomenon that we want to identify. There is a phenomenon of awareness which is somehow a property of human beings and I don't think it is a property of galaxies, billiard balls or plants in the sunshine. If we use the word generally, so that it covers all these things, we lose something essential in the characterization of what we are trying to explain.

Bunge: I don't think that biology is sufficient to solve any epistemological problems. I am not a reductionist and I think it would be foolish to try and do that. But I don't think epistemology ought to forget about biology, in particular about the theory of evolution. This theory, however, is too general to explain any specific processes. In order to predict any specific evolutionary process, you have to add a number of special assumptions concerning the genetic constitution of the animals, the environment, and so forth. I have made this point in a mathematical model of evolution.[6]

Secondly, not everything that we do, feel, think, etc., has an adaptive value. Although many people in psychology hold a Panglossian view of biology —everything that happens is for the best, in the best of all possible worlds— this is of course nonsense.

I am not acquainted with the causal theory of knowledge but if it is similar to the causal theory of perception then I am against it. For general reasons, I don't think that causality is the only mode of becoming. We must reckon with randomness and, in the particular case of higher vertebrates, we must reckon also with purposive action. Although it can perhaps be explained in causal terms, I don't think that we can dispense with those other modes.

Concerning the puzzle of how to define human beings, I don't think that a single property will do. A whole conglomerate, a whole cluster of properties, may do. A human being is not just *Homo ludens* but many other things as well, among them *faber, culturifex,* and *politicus.* Among other things we can build and destroy social institutions.

I don't think that the mechanisms of social evolution are the same as those of biological evolution. For one thing, cultural evolution is artificial. For another, most of it is not adaptive. Just think of the fifty thousand nuclear bombs that we have accumulated in order to kill ourselves several times over.

Concerning Professor Searle's doubts, I don't think that the theory of evolution is neutral between materialism and dualism. The mechanisms of biological evolution are variations of material processes. Natural selection is a thoroughly material process. There is no room there for anything disembodied or immaterial. You are interested in saving the mind, but so am I and so was Darwin. You don't have to be a physicalist or a reductionist of some kind! You can recognize the mental as being a function of the brain, yet a function that individual neurons don't have and one that took millions of years to evolve from more primitive brain functions.

Searle: I take it that by dualism you mean straight Cartesianism, two independent substances with no interaction?

Bunge: Yes.

Searle: Are there any such dualists any more?

Bunge: Yes, we are surrounded by them.

Creutzfeldt: In case you are referring to me, I should like to point out again that I am not interested in the problem of substantive dualism. The problem we are discussing here is the very weak and soft evolutionary theory of consciousness. What does an evolutionary theory of consciousness teach us about consciousness except that it may be useful for survival?

Bunge: If you think of the *mind* as looking at itself then of course you are being a dualist. When we say that the *brain* can think about itself, about its past brain states, that is a different thing.

Creutzfeldt: But this is the phenomenon that we want to learn about and explain. The evolutionary story hasn't yet taught us anything about this property of the brain, i.e. how it becomes conscious of itself.

Towers: The suggestion that I am a panpsychic (p. 67) is not true. Nor is it true that I am a kind of crypto-Lamarckian (p. 69)—at least I am no more Lamarckian than Darwin was.[7] In so far as I am a philosopher at all, I am fundamentally Aristotelian, but with modern process philosophy overcoming the static Aristotelianism of Aristotle. Philosophy today *has* to move into process philosophy if it is to make any kind of sense of what we know now about the evolutionary history of this planet. This knowledge is very new. It is only in the last hundred years that people have been able to articulate anything worthwhile about our past history—not only our own past history (other than the recent past), but the past history of the universe. All that I am saying is that the universe as we see it today, which we know has evolved in various stages that we do know something about, must have had the capacity to develop, ultimately, the power to reflect back in a self-conscious awareness incorporated into its structure from the beginning.

Plum: That is teleological.

Towers: No, it is not.

Plum: The human species is an accident of fate, from repeated throwing of the genetic dice. The way we have ended up has nothing directly to do with what the universe was like in the beginning, although it is quite true that our species has had to adapt to the universe that surrounded our evolution. But dualism is unthinkable in the sense that there was a guiding hand that said what we should evolve to at this particular time.

Towers: I agree absolutely with that. I am not saying anything more than that.

Searle: I didn't take it that you were denying that point. The way that one is taught to think of mentation, as some people have been calling it, or intentionality or the mind or what have you, is that from an evolutionary point of view it is the result of a series of causal processes of a fairly specific type, which probably had something to do with certain kinds of nervous systems. The way I hear you talk about it, Dr Towers, is completely counter to that, and I wonder if I am understanding you correctly. The picture you have seems to be that there are all kinds of things that at one time had mental processes involved, such as digestion or photosynthesis. All sorts of things may have been a matter of conscious effort. Somehow the mental part then went away and was reserved for a smaller area. Is that your picture?

Towers: No; what I am saying is that once organisms have learnt the things they have to do in order to survive, they can then allow those learnt processes to be incorporated into the autonomic nervous system and proceed with increasing complexity to other levels of awareness.

Searle: But aren't there all sorts of things that organisms do in order to survive, such as photosynthesis and digestion, that don't require any mental process at all?

Towers: Yes.

Bennett: You were challenged several times about whether you are really a crypto-panpsychist ('There is a mental aspect to everything'); and this certainly was the label that occurred to me when I was listening to you on the subject of amoebae. At any rate you seemed to hold that there is a mental side to anything that has any degree of organic organization. But then you appeared to retreat into saying merely that the capacity for the whole story was there from the beginning, and my question is: could this be true in any sense in which it is not trivial? What does it mean to say that the capacity was there from the beginning, except that it was always true that what did happen could happen? I could imagine people saying that it wasn't there from the beginning if they positively believed in a cataclysmic divine intervention at the level of natural law. There is that much content in it—you are saying that nothing of that sort occurred—but is there any more in it than that? What I detect behind your words is the idea of the capacity being there in the form of a foreshadowing of it, so that even in the simplest physical systems you do in fact think that, if not mentality, then there is something analogous to mentality but a bit simpler. That is what I think of as panpsychism, and I don't use that as a term of abuse. I am not sure that panpsychism is false. It seems no worse than any of the other theories kicking around. How do you stand on that?

Towers: I would just say that we ought to reflect on whether or not, in this universe about which we are beginning to discover a few realities, there is the possibility that on other planets processes similar to those on this planet have taken place. There are many people who would say that, given the immensity of the universe, it is inevitable that similar processes should have taken place and that there should be intelligent beings of some kind—maybe looking very different but who have developed a capacity to know, and to know that they know, and to understand.

Young: That is quite different from anything you said earlier.

Blakemore: I don't like the idea of inorganic panpsychism. One is only reduced to that kind of argument if one believes that mentational behaviour in humans is a *property* of the system rather than a *function* of it. A physical property, such as mass or electrical charge, can be rightly ascribed to a physical object. Mental behaviour is not such a property. It is a function of nervous systems, and the human brain has it in an exaggerated form, just as we have more sophisticated mechanisms of homeostatic regulation than are possessed by primitive organisms. Would one want to argue that the ability to regulate one's environment is a *property* that already exists in inorganic molecules?

Putnam: We are not recognizing how terribly conflicting our intuitions are on this question of consciousness. For example, most of us think that dogs and cats are conscious.

Plum: That is only because we haven't defined consciousness today!

Putnam: The definitions come at the end, when you have solved the philosophical problem, not at the beginning.

If you drop a lobster in a pot of boiling water there is a momentary screech. At that moment it is not ridiculous to worry about whether a lobster feels pain. If we come to construct robots that have something like our range of abilities and can conduct conversations, the question of whether we are dealing with a mere machine or something that is really conscious will really bother us. With a split brain, the question of whether there are two distinct loci of sense data, two distinct centres of consciousness, only one of which has access to speech, or whether there is one locus of consciousness and something else which is simulating consciousness, bothers most of us. Why not solve this conflict of intuitions by definition? It is of course because we are worried about whether the definition is right. By definition robots aren't conscious. Part of the definition of consciousness is that you have to have DNA, so never mind about that robot. But that is not going to satisfy anyone. The argument will simply reappear as an argument over the correctness of the definition, which is why you can't solve any philosophical question by first defining your terms. All philosophers will define their terms so that they win!

I am sympathetic to identity theory. As Colin Blakemore was saying, we may be dealing here with properties which are ultimately functional properties, but the trouble is that there exist *operationally indiscernible identity theories*. By that I mean that there are formally incompatible identity theories which lead to the same predictions with respect to the experiences of all normal observers. For example the theory that the lobster is really not conscious and the theory that it is lead to the same predictions with respect to the experiences of all objects other than lobsters. The theory that there are two loci of consciousness in the split brain and the theory that only one lobe is conscious lead to the same predictions about the experiences of all unsplit brains. Similar things occur in other branches of science. There are for example observationally indistinguishable topologies for space–time, but the problem seems really acute in our subject. Dr Plum's suggestion that the notion of truth itself may be implicated may be right. I have thought along those directions myself but again one couldn't start by just defining the right notion of truth. That would have to be the outcome of a philosophical investigation.

We have been talking as if somewhat strange or funny questions had been raised by Dr Towers. I don't think they are strange or funny. I think all of us in different moods worry about the same things as he worries about.

Towers: I am very glad to discover at this meeting that the philosophers, perhaps even more than some of the scientific members, are prepared to take the theory of evolution seriously. I have had some brushes with philosophers quite recently who were prepared to dismiss it as irrelevant.[8] I speak as a developmental biologist who tries to interpret for first-year medical students something of the complexities of the anatomical organization of the human body, which they find mind-boggling. It is a great relief to some of them to learn, after struggling with all those extraordinary facts about the structure of the human body, some of the features I try to explain to them in terms of development. Once they understand that first this and then that structure is laid down, and why it must be so, it begins to make sense to them, and that is a great relief. I think that the nature of the human species and our ratiocination will only make sense if we treat it developmentally. I am glad to see that several members of this symposium are prepared to do that.

Bunge: Some of this discussion illustrates the perennial dilemma of all evolutionary biologists—namely, should we stress continuity through the genes, or discontinuity through the emergence of new properties, functions and so on? I think that a balanced view will recognize both continuity and discontinuity.

References

1. ECCLES, J. C. (1966) *Brain and Conscious Experience (Pontificia Academia Scientarum, Study Week, Sept. 1964)*, vol. 30, Springer, New York
2. GOULD, S. J. (1977) *Ever Since Darwin: Reflections in Natural History*, Norton, New York
3. GRUBER, H. E. & BARRETT, P. H. (1974) *Darwin on Man*, Wildwood House, London
4. TREVARTHEN, C. (1979) Instincts for human understanding and for cultural cooperation: their development in infancy, in *Human Ethology* (von Cranach, M. & Aschoff, J. eds.), Cambridge University Press, Cambridge, in press
5, WILSON, E. O. (1975) *Sociobiology: The New Synthesis*, Harvard University Press, Cambridge, Mass,
6. BUNGE, M. (1978) A model of evolution. *Appl. Math. Mod. 2*, 201 204
7. TOWERS, B. (1968) The impact of Darwin's 'Origin of Species' on medicine and biology, in *Medicine and Science in the 1860's (Proc. Sixth Br. Congr. History of Medicine, 1967)* (Poynter, F. N. L., ed.), Wellcome Institute of the History of Medicine, London
8. TOWERS, B. (1978) The origin and development of living forms. *J. Med. Philos. 3*, 88–106 (see especially p. 90)

Phonation, emotion, cognition, with reference to the brain mechanisms involved

DETLEV PLOOG

Max-Planck-Institut für Psychiatrie, Munich

Abstract Phylogenetic steps in the evolution of vocal communication have a bearing on the brain mechanisms involved in the emergence of human language and speech. A schema of the neuronal organization of voicing in a hierarchical manner is presented. At the lowest mesencephalic level the movements of the vocal apparatus are coordinated and integrated into species-specific vocal gestures. At the middle level these signals are controlled by the anterior limbic cortex, which serves this function in primates only, and only in the human species is the highest level around the cortical larynx and facial area actively involved in the vocal signalling process. This functional schema is used to explain the sequential stages in the ontogenetic process of phonemicization in the human infant, and special emphasis is placed on vocal–auditory feedback mechanisms which come into play from the lowest to the highest level of the central nervous system during maturation. Even feedback loops of the lowest level enable the distinction to be made between self-produced vocalizations and those produced by others. These mechanisms are thought to be an early means for the development of self-awareness. If one grants that the human infant possesses self-awareness, one must concede that such stages of the mind were developed before the emergence of the human species.

'Dead matter seems to have more potentialities than merely to produce dead matter. In particular, it has produced minds—no doubt in slow stages—and in the end the human brain and the human mind, the human consciousness of self, and the human awareness of the universe'. Karl Popper (Ref. 1, p. 11) continues in the same paragraph: 'One of the first products of the human mind is human language. In fact, I conjecture', he says, 'that it was the very first of these products, and that the human brain and the human mind evolved in interaction with language'. Was language really the first product of the human mind? And what were the products of other minds which preceded the human mind in slow stages?

Throughout my presentation I shall have these two questions at the back of my mind and shall be considering facts and hypotheses from the perspective of organic evolution and the ontogenetic development of the human brain and the human mind.

As I see it, communication among conspecifics was one of the first products in evolution which made interactions between individuals possible. From ethology we know that social signalling has two facets: the signal carries the message to the recipient and simultaneously expresses the sender's emotional state. In human beings, the voice is the predominant means of social signalling, and many stages in the evolution of vocal communication made contributions to the brain mechanisms involved in the emergence of human speech and language.

What is known about the role of the cerebral system in the production of vocal signals? As has been shown, in monkeys vocalization can be elicited by electrical brain stimulation of a great number of subcortical structures[2,3] and specific vocal patterns in the repertoire can be assigned to specific brain structures.[4,5]

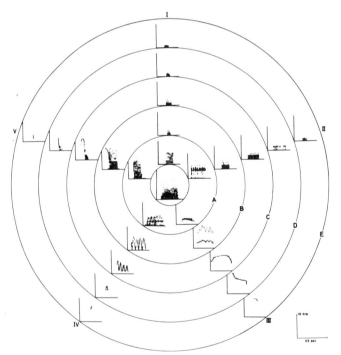

FIG. 1. Vocal repertoire of the squirrel monkey. The calls are represented as frequency-time diagrams.[63]

Fig. 1 shows a schematic representation of the squirrel monkey's vocal repertoire. The sounds can be heard under electrical brain stimulation as well as under natural conditions. The individual sounds are depicted in frequency/ time diagrams, with shrieking close to white noise in the centre of the circle. Five groups of calls, first described in 1966,[6] are shown as graded signals from the centre towards the periphery. Each group (and most probably each graded signal) is assigned a certain function. Group II calls, for example, are heard in the context of directed aggression; Group III calls, among them the one known as the isolation peep (IIIc), serve a number of cohesive functions; and so on.

Fig. 2 indicates the brain structures from which the above-mentioned groups of vocalizations can be elicited electrically. The great extent of these structures, reaching from orbito-frontal and temporal through thalamic and hypothalamic structures into midbrain and pons and their intimate connections with the limbic system, is shown. The extent of the system and the observation that the elicited calls are often accompanied by other motor and autonomic reactions, as well as the relatively long latencies to onset of the calls, suggest rather strongly that not all of the structures are directly involved in the generation of the calls. Rather, it is likely that stimulation of these systems causes a motivational change in the animal which is then expressed by the call. This hypothesis was tested by means of self-stimulation experiments in which the animal could switch the electrical stimulation of vocalization-producing brain structures on and off. In this way, it could be determined whether stimulation of a given vocalization point was aversive, pleasurable or neutral. In two areas only—shown as stippled areas in Fig. 3—there was no correlation between self-stimulation behaviour and vocalization type elicited. One area extends from the so-called supplementary motor area of the neocortex and the anterior cingulate gyrus to the gyrus rectus and along the ventromedial border of the capsula interna. The second area consists of the posterior central grey matter of the dorsal midbrain with the latero-caudally adjacent pontine tegmentum. Our interpretation is that we are dealing here with primary vocalization areas.[7] This dorsal midbrain–pons area yields vocalizations in other mammals such as cats and dogs[8,9] and also in amphibians and reptiles.[10,11] Destruction of this area causes mutism in frogs, cats and humans.[10,12,13] This area appears to be controlled, however, at least in primates, by the above-mentioned cingulate area of the forebrain, which is part of the limbic mesocortex. Sutton et al.[14] have demonstrated that rhesus monkeys can control their vocal behaviour contingent upon conditional stimuli and rewards. The monkeys were required to produce a 'coo' of a certain duration and intensity. After bilateral ablation of the cingulate area this

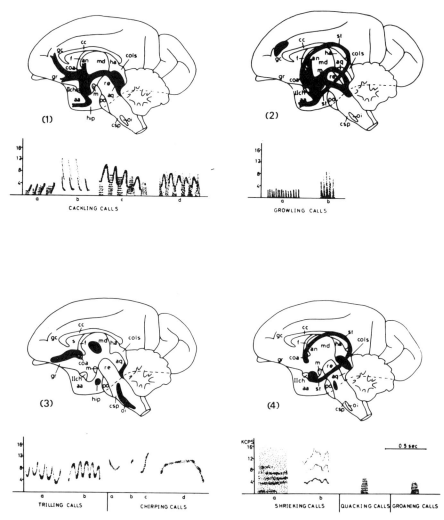

Fig. 2. Vocalization elicited by electrical stimulation of the squirrel monkey's brain. General view of the cerebral system (in black) yielding cackling calls (1), growling calls (2), chirping calls (3) and shrieking calls (4). The calls are represented as frequency-time diagrams. Abbreviations: aa = area anterior amygdalae; an = nucleus anterior; aq = substantia grisea centralis; cc = corpus callosum; coa = commissura anterior; cols = colliculus superior; csp = tractus corticospinalis; f = fornix; gc = gyrus cinguli; gr = gyrus rectus; ha = nucleus habenularis; hip = hippocampus; m = corpus mammillare; md = nucleus medialis dorsalis thalami; oi = nucleus olivaris inferior; po = griseum pontis; re = formatio reticularis tegmenti; st = stria terminalis; IIch = chiasma nervorum opticorum. Compiled from Jürgens [64] and Jürgens & Ploog.[5]

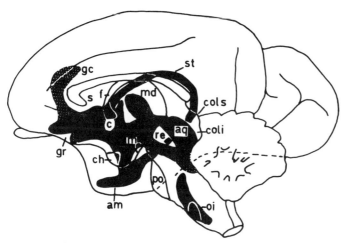

FIG. 3. Vocalization-producing brain areas in the squirrel monkey.[63] The stippled regions represent vocalization areas in which the electrically elicited calls are independent of concomitant motivational effects. For abbreviations see Fig. 2.

instrumental response was abolished, although the monkeys were still able to vocalize adequately in response to fear-eliciting stimuli. After bilateral ablation of the frontal neocortex, including the homologue of Broca's area and the cortical face area, neither the instrumental response nor spontaneous vocalization was affected. From these experiments it can be concluded that in monkeys the cortical face area does not play an appreciable role in the vocalization process, whereas the cingulate area seems to control the instrumental use of the voice, depending on external conditions. The published clinical work[13,15] reveals that lesions of the cingulate area and the adjacent supplementary motor cortex result in disturbances of the vocalization process, ranging from slight dysarthria to akinetic mutism. Rubens[16] found that patients with lesions in these areas have only slight difficulties in repeating sentences but may often lose spontaneous speech completely. When they repeat sentences the melody is lost and the voice sounds monotonous.

Neither in the squirrel monkey nor in the rhesus monkey, and hardly ever in the chimpanzee, was it possible to elicit vocalizations from the cortical area where the face, the tongue and the larynx are represented. In human beings, however, it is possible to elicit non-verbal vocalizations bilaterally from these zones; furthermore, ablation of these zones, especially in the dominant hemisphere, is followed by a severe disturbance of articulation. Ablation within the supplementary motor area causes transient articulatory difficulties; impulsive utterances and word repetitions can be elicited by

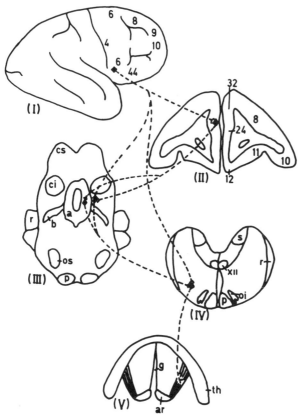

FIG. 4. Neural pathways from the cortical larynx area and cingular vocalization area to the larynx in higher primates.[63]

electrical stimulation. Broca's field, however, is not essential for proper articulation.

For further clarification of the neuronal pathways and brain structures which mediate vocalization the autoradiographic tracing technique was used, with the squirrel monkey as the experimental animal.[17,58] The results of these extensive studies are shown in Fig. 4. In Section I of this schematic representation the cortical larynx area is depicted, the stimulation of which results in movements of the monkey's vocal cords but not in vocalization.[18]

Injection of labelled material in this area reveals projections to the cingulate area, as shown in Section II of Fig. 4. From here the pathway leads to the dorsal midbrain–pons area which was mentioned before (see Section III). There is also a direct connection from the cortical larynx area to this lower centre. The connection from the midbrain–pons area to the nucleus ambiguus, the final relay station for the peripheral phonatory apparatus (shown in Section IV), has recently been demonstrated.[19] In the chimpanzee and in the human there seems to be a pathway running directly from the cortical larynx area to the nucleus ambiguus.[20, 21]

In a more recent study[22] the functions of the anatomical projections of the cingular vocalization area (see Section II) were investigated. The effects of various brain lesions on vocalizations elicited from the precallosal cingulate gyrus were studied. Lesions which abolish these vocalizations completely can be traced continuously from the stimulation site down to the laryngeal motor neurons in the nucleus ambiguus. The pathway thus determined follows the corticospinal tract down to the caudal diencephalon. Here, the effective lesions leave this tract and ascend dorsally into the periaqueductal grey matter. The pathway follows this structure to its end, where it sweeps laterally through the parabrachial area and then descends through the lateral pons and ventro-lateral medulla to the nucleus ambiguus. Our diagram thus demonstrates the neuronal organization of voicing in a hierarchical manner. At the lowest level, the ponto-mesencephalic area, the vocal cords, the respiratory movements and the movements of the supralaryngeal apparatus are coordinated and integrated into species-specific vocal gestures. At the middle level these signals are controlled and modulated by the anterior limbic cortex, which serves this function in primates only. It is assumed that the structures involved here control the readiness to react vocally. Only in humans is the highest level around the cortical larynx and facial area actively involved in the vocal signalling process. It is assumed that these structures play a role in the process of vocal learning and mediate learnt articulatory movements.

Our model helps to explain clinical speech disorders of many kinds, especially the intrinsic involvement of emotion in speech, such as the profane utterances of vestigial speech in motor aphasia and the various forms of language behaviour in psychotic states.[23] In fact, emotion is involved in everyday verbal communication, in songs without words, and in the cooing and babbling of small infants.[24]

Although Ernst Haeckel's view that the stages of evolution are recapitulated in ontogeny has received more criticism than acceptance, such a comparison does seem relevant to the development of phonation. Lower vertebrates such as toads and lizards can produce only a few innate species-specific vocalizations. In land mammals, with increasing levels of organization, such as in cats and dogs, the repertoire of sounds is increasingly varied, and it is at its largest in both number and variety in the subhuman primates. As shown in Fig. 4, among the primates not only the ponto-mesencephalic functions but also the limbic functions play a role in phonation. Phonation in turn is embedded in the increasingly complex organization of social behaviour, which is reflected in the increasingly complex forms of communication.[25]

At birth the human being is equipped with only one form of vocalization—crying. But this crying becomes differentiated almost immediately, and soon there is a wide range of cries reflecting different moods and having distinguishable signalling functions.[26] The second kind of vocalization, which appears simultaneously with social smiling, is cooing. This kind of vocalization, consisting of various palatal, velar and labial sounds, has a definite social function, and mother and infant enjoy cooing at each other. This pattern of alternative cooing and waiting can be observed in children between four and eight weeks of age. Pitch, volume, frequency and pattern of vocalization are sometimes already modulated at this age. The infant seeks opportunities for such vocal dialogues and takes pleasure in these interactions.[27] Lenneberg[28] reports that cooing is just as frequent in infants whose parents are deaf-mutes as in those with normal parents.

At about eight weeks of age, after social smiling is well developed, a new and more variable kind of vocalization appears—babbling. It consists of series of consonant–vowel combinations, is not as dependent on 'dialogue' as cooing, and often occurs even when the baby is alone. Otto Koehler[29] was the first to recognize the universality of these monologues. At this age babies all over the world produce the same sounds and combinations of sounds.[30,31] At this stage of development the endogenous generation of sounds is apparently preprogrammed in such a way that imitation of a model is not necessary. The vocal gestures have the character of fixed action patterns which are produced even in the absence of releasing stimuli, i.e. they are 'vacuum activities'.[32] The number of consonants and vowels used increases at a steady pace. When an adult talks directly to a baby, or even when the baby merely overhears the adult's voice, this stimulates vocalization in the baby, but it does not influence the pattern of development of vocalizations.[33]

At about nine months of age there is a turning point. Babbling decreases or even stops completely for a time. The baby begins to address familiar faces with simple sounds (/ae/, /ba/, etc.). 'The phonetic richness of the babbling period thus gives way to phonological limitation'.[34] It is as if vocalization reorganizes itself and begins again with what appear to be simple sounds.[35] At about 10 months the baby begins to imitate speech sounds emitted by adults. Thus towards the end of the first year another process begins which lasts roughly one year: gradually the child gains command of words, i.e. learns to articulate. Again, the development of articulation follows a pattern, i.e. the order in which certain phonemes first appear is independent of which language the child will learn later. The sequence of stages is based on 'the principle of maximum contrast' and 'development proceeds from the simple and undifferentiated to the stratified and differentiated'.[36]

In this discussion of phonological development in humans three points should have become clear: (1) Phonological development in humans is different from that in subhuman primates from the very beginning. Whereas the latter are born with a repertoire of sounds which undergoes hardly any subsequent changes,[37] and are unable to imitate sounds or learn any new kinds of vocalizations, in the human species the range of vocalizations expands and changes in a process that begins in the first few weeks of life and proceeds through a number of genetically predetermined stages before the development of actual speech. (2) Although the development of vocalization in humans is unique, *during the first year of life* there are similarities with phonation in subhuman primates: the great variety of vocalizations and the innumerable variations within them; the resulting possibility of finely differentiated expression of emotional state, with a multitude of different meanings expressible through vocalization; the inability to imitate sounds in spite of a superior ability to recognize species-specific vocalizations.[38,39,40] (3) The fixed pattern of phonological development in humans, which is independent of the language spoken by the baby's caretakers, indicates that maturational processes in the central nervous system determine the stages of this development. Our hypothesis is that vocalization in the human infant during the first few weeks of life is controlled by the ponto-mesencephalic region (see lower stippled area in Fig. 3 and Section III in Fig. 4).

Crying has an automatic character and a simple signalling function. When the cooing stage begins, the limbic cingulate area begins to function. Now the vocalizations allow more variety of expression and are related to the baby's social environment. Several investigators have shown that at the age of about three months operant conditioning of infant babbling can be established. During the conditioning phase, each vocalization by the baby was followed, after a 1.5-second delay, by 5 seconds of tape-recorded auditory reinforcement, which consisted of an adult female voice slowly repeating phrases such as 'hello baby'.[33] But response-independent social stimulation, with the adult looking into the eyes of the baby as the releasing stimulus for infant vocal sounds, produces equivalent increases from baseline level in the vocalization rate of infants.[41] Towards the end of the first year of age, when the baby starts to imitate sounds and when the reorganization of vocalization mentioned earlier begins, the neocortical functions begin to play a role in phonation which will become increasingly important. The patterns of movement present at birth are gradually transformed into articulatory gestures of the caretaker's language. In the middle of the second year there is a marked increase in the number of phonemes the child is able to articulate and in the number of words used. The increase in the number of phonemes goes hand in hand with an increase in the symbolic use of vocalizations (words). At the same pace the child's utterances become differentiated gradually, though not completely, from the bodily expression of emotion. It takes several more years of maturation before the partial uncoupling of propositional speech and the expression of emotions becomes routine. Parallel to this development the child gains control over facial expressions. The growing fluency of vocal gestures (articulated sounds) is clearly a function of the differentiation of localized cortical activity states. The child speaks with the accent of the parents' dialect, though articulation is not completely correct as yet. At the end of the fourth year most children can master all phonemes. The phonemicization process is complete.[35]

According to Lenneberg,[28] language is a central, maturationally defined mental function and the manifestation of species-specific cognitive propensities. In his last publication Lenneberg[42] says, 'If we want to understand the relationship between language and the brain, we must look for neurological processes, their nature and their function'. One way of looking at maturational processes in the brain and related functions is to compare the myelogenesis of structures involved in such functions and the behaviour observable at subsequent stages of development. Lecours[43] has provided this comparison. At the time babbling begins to appear, the motor roots of the cranial nerves related to the production of sounds have completed their myelogenetic cycles[44] and myelogenesis of several brain-stem structures, including the pre-thalamic pathways for all sensory modalities, is not far from completion; but the corticobulbar pathway, the association fibres and the thalamocortical projections (with the exception of the visual system, in which myelination is completed quite early) are only beginning their myelogenetic cycles. Thus babbling is essentially governed from lower subcortical levels, where a certain degree of anatomical maturation has already been achieved.

At the time when imitation of adult speech sounds becomes the child's predominant phonological activity, the pathways presumably involved in speech production have all, according to the findings of Lecours, reached a certain degree of myelogenetic maturation, but not all of them have completed their cycle. Myelogenesis of the post-thalamic component of the acoustic pathway, through which the specific inputs for phonemic imitation reach the auditory cortex, is not yet complete. The cycles of longer association fibres such as the fasciculus arcuatus, through which auditory information is presumably transmitted to motor areas, are quite advanced yet still incomplete. Myelogenesis is nearly terminated in the pyramidal and extrapyramidal systems, which govern and modulate the production of speech sounds, and in the pre-thalamic and post-thalamic exteroceptive and proprioceptive pathways that bring proprioceptive feedback to the precentral gyrus. Lecours states that if this circuit is indeed the one subserving imitation of phonemes, this activity begins when maturation of its anatomical substratum is not quite complete, and imitation becomes progressively more perfect as anatomical maturation gets closer to its conclusion.

Auditory–vocal feedback mechanisms are often assumed to be a major factor in language acquisition without there being any clear idea of how they might work. On the one hand the articulatory movements of the phonatory apparatus are so rapid that what is known about the physiology of proprioceptive feedback mechanisms in the lower brain-stem does not provide an adequate explanation; on the other hand, especially with reference to language acquisition, the assumption must be made that feedback signals from the individual's own speech movements travel over a number of synapses into the buccopharyngeal area of the motor cortex. Without doubt a number of feedback mechanisms are involved which are quite different anatomically and physiologically and which function on different organizational levels within the central nervous system. Here again a comparison of humans and monkeys can be of help.

For example, we deafened adult squirrel monkeys[45] and found that even after several years there were no changes in vocal patterns; however the monkeys' voices became louder and the number of vocalizations decreased. Thus, if they are to control the volume of their own voices monkeys, too, need acoustic feedback, but this is not necessary for controlling the vocal patterns themselves. The decrease in the total number of vocalizations can be considered as resulting from the social isolation due to lack of auditory-vocal interaction. Thus exteroceptive input stimulates the animal's own production of vocalizations. This view is supported by the observation that a monkey kept in isolation will stop vocalizing after a few days. To find out what a squirrel monkey must learn from an external model, infants were raised from birth by muted mothers, i.e. mothers whose vocal cords were cut during pregnancy. In spite of this complete deprivation of species-specific vocal experience, the infants vocalized immediately after birth and produced all types of adult calls (see Fig. 1). They did not have to learn either their species-specific vocal patterns or the appropriate situation in which a vocalization normally occurs. Even an infant which was deafened on the fourth day of life produced the regular vocal behaviour of the species.[37] From this we can conclude that the vocalizations of this primate are genetically preprogrammed, fixed-action patterns which do not have to be learned by imitation. In this regard, then, the monkey's vocal behaviour is comparable to the human infant's during the first stages of vocal development, i.e. both vocalize regardless of exteroceptive input or deafness. There are, however, profound differences between the monkey and the human infant. While the monkey's vocal repertoire remains more or less invariant, the human infant's vocal production undergoes preprogrammed changes. The monkey's vocal utterances seem to depend either on certain internal states —for example, even as an isolate raised with a dummy mother the animal utters a typical purr to get milk[46,47]—or on external events, predominantly on social cues, especially vocalizations of other monkeys. The human infant, although producing vocalizations depending on internal states and social cues such as the human voice, also produces whole 'monologues' over long stretches of time, sometimes up to 30 minutes, in the absence of a social partner and obviously independent of internal needs. All observers of infant babbling agree that this behaviour resembles play with the buccopharyngeal muscles, occurs in a relaxed mood and is obviously an exercise of the phonatory apparatus. It is very likely that the feedback mechanisms which operate in this audio–vocal play are of a different nature from the invariant, goal–oriented and response-dependent vocalization of the infant monkey. In contrast to the human infant, the infant monkey will continue to utter vocal fixed-action patterns when deafened, while the deaf human infant or the infant with mute parents and without exposure to spoken language will not move on from the babbling stages to the first imitated words and will not learn to speak.

In our examination of similarities and differences between the development of vocal behaviour in monkeys and humans it might be worth looking at a specific aspect of motor development in general, i.e. at the effect of the individual's actions on the environment and the consequences of these actions for the individual. It is well established that if the rhesus monkey and several other species are raised completely alone or with motionless surrogate mothers from immediately after birth, their social behaviour develops abnormally. The infants also exhibit deviant self-directed motor behaviour such as clasping, rocking or biting themselves. There is clinical and circumstantial evidence that isolation of human children leads to comparable self-directed deviant behaviour. Mason and coworkers[48] have quite convincingly shown that the behavioural development of an infant monkey will take an almost normal course if the surrogate mother makes simple movements and can be manipulated by the infant to a certain degree. Thus, if infant monkeys experience the consequences of their own actions, their behaviour develops normally and motor stereotypes do not occur. For human neonates it has been demonstrated that operant conditioning reactions can be established as early as the end of the first postnatal week.[49] In their third month of life human infants express pleasure by facial expressions and vocal utterances if they have mastered an operant conditioning task, for example switching lights on by rule-governed head-turning movements, and they continue to perform the task without further nutritional reward as if they were addicted to their task.[50] It is obvious that it is their own actions in causing the changes in the environment which attract the attention of the infants and reinforce their activities. This has also been demonstrated nicely by Watson,[51] who found that three-month-old babies paid attention for only a short while to a mobile over their heads. However, if this object was connected with the baby's leg by a thread the baby quickly discovered that movements of the leg set the mobile in motion. Under this condition the infant remained attracted and kept the object moving for long periods of time. When the mobile was disconnected, interest was rapidly lost and leg movements ceased to occur.

The point I want to make here is that the orderly development of monkey and human infants depends on feedback behaviour of the above-mentioned kind. While this is certainly true for other higher mammals too, as first demonstrated by Held & Hein[52] in cats, primates especially tend to manipulate their environment, including their social environment, thereby being rewarded by their own actions which bring about these changes. In contrast to the monkey, human infants are comparatively immobile for the better part of the first year of life. Movements by which they can manipulate their environment are few and relatively ineffective. However, this is altogether different for vocal activity. From the first day of life human infants receive exteroceptive and proprioceptive feedback from their own voices. By crying and early modifications of crying they bring their caretakers close and thereby manipulate the environment through their own activity. Through their propensity to modify their voices at a very early stage of development they receive a varying proprioceptive input from the proprioceptors of the vocal apparatus, whose activity is then perceived by auditory perception. The infants thereby experience the consequences of their own actions, i.e. the varying patterning of movements of the vocal apparatus, through audio–vocal feedback. As indicated, this control of the effects of one's own activity has a strongly reinforcing quality. It is therefore very likely that the relatively large amount of vocal production (as compared with other primates) during the cooing and babbling phase, although genetically preprogrammed, is reinforced by the rewarding effects of control over one's own movements.

The question arises, at what point in the vocal development towards speech do we want to call the vocal movements initiated by the infant in social or non-social situations voluntary movements? Are the beginning and end of a cooing episode in a dialogue between child and caretaker voluntary acts? Is the termination of a babbling period when the caretaker appears voluntary? When the child begins to imitate and to make the first attempts to articulate words, I assume that these motor acts will unanimously be called voluntary movements. I am raising these questions to show that there is a certain arbitrariness in whether a motor act or at least a vocal gesture is regarded as voluntary or automatic, and there are certainly transitions between these extremes. A clearly willed imitative articulatory movement can become completely automatic some time later. And just this gradual shift from automatic production of fixed action patterns to voluntary acts and then to automatic articulatory movements is an important part of language acquisition.

In the discussion on brain and mind, however, voluntary movements play an important role in regard to the emergence of consciousness. Popper (Ref. 1, p. 29) suggests that we have reason to accept the view that there are lower and higher stages of consciousness. 'If the fact', he says, 'that animals cannot speak is a sufficient reason to deny consciousness to them, it would also be a sufficient reason to deny it to babies at an age before they learn to speak'. But it is obvious that babies do have consciousness before they learn to speak. They have a concept of social interactions consisting of a donor and a recipient, of an object and its transmission, and so on. There is a pre-speech grammar before the first words have emerged.[53,54] And babies have, no doubt, self-awareness, i.e. they distinguish themselves from others.

My conjecture is that auditory–vocal feedback is the earliest and most effective mechanism in human ontogeny for the development of self-awareness and thereby of consciousness of the self. For auditory–vocal feedback is the first experience of the ability to control one's own actions and is therefore highly suitable for the development of the concept of one's own identity. One way of searching for brain mechanisms which mediate 'lower and higher stages of consciousness' is therefore to investigate feedback mechanisms of movement control. In a chapter on voluntary movement, Eccles (Ref. 1, p. 275) states that there are many hierarchical levels in the mechanisms of control of voluntary movements, and he reviews all of those known so far. Considering the most important and very complex levels of control, he refers briefly to 'speech and song and gesture, so that the whole personality can stand revealed', but this level of control is not specified in anatomical or physiological terms.

At the beginning of this contribution I presented a hierarchical schema for the control of the voice. In order to complete this schema in terms of feedback loops one must look for anatomical and/or physiological evidence that the various levels of motor integration of phonatory patterns are linked in one way or another to the auditory system in the first place and also to other systems known to be involved in movement control and thereby voice control, such as the cerebellum and the extrapyramidal system. Reviewing the topographical relationships between the aforementioned lowest integration level for call production in the periaqueductal region (see Fig. 4, III) and the auditory system in this area, one could speculate on feedback loops through which corollary discharges or efferent copies could be fed.[55,56,57] However, nothing is known about such mechanisms. The next level in this schematic representation (Fig. 4, II), the cingular area and (in humans) its extension, the supplementary motor area, is also a structure in which to look for feedback loops. If one elicits vocalizations from the precallosal cingular area in the squirrel monkey and injects tritiated leucine exactly into loci which yield vocalizations, the autoradiographic tracings lead not only to subcortical structures, as mentioned earlier, but also to a number of cortical areas other than the primary motor cortex which are known to be involved in the control of voluntary movements, such as areas 6, 8, 9, 10 (Fig. 5). Among these projections, whose neurophysiological functions are not yet known, a pathway of particular interest was discovered which runs from the precallosal cingulate cortex to the auditory association cortex.[58] Attempts to discover the function of this pathway have not yielded conclusive results, but the finding raised an important question which has since been pursued experimentally with some success (P. Müller-Preuss, in preparation).

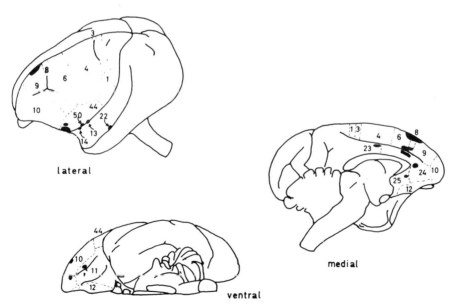

FIG. 5. Ipsilateral cortical projections with delineation of Brodmann areas according to Rosabal.[65] The curved arrows point to terminal fields buried within the lateral and superior temporal sulci.[58]

The question is simply whether the auditory system processes self-produced vocalizations differently from those produced by others. To gain experimental access to this question, the action potentials of single neurons of the squirrel monkey's auditory cortex were recorded extracellularly during self-produced vocalizations and during playbacks of the same vocalizations from a tape. Since it is difficult to evoke vocalizations reliably and repeatedly from the animal in a controlled behavioural situation, the vocalization was elicited by electrical stimulation of the central grey matter. Electrode sites were chosen which produced a vocalization 100–800 milliseconds after termination of the electrical stimulus. The monkeys received three types of auditory input, namely input during the evoked self-produced vocalization, input of the tape-recorded playback of the identical vocalization, and input of tape-recorded playbacks of other species-specific calls not identical with the electrically evoked self-produced vocalization.

Two types of responses were seen in the 210 cells tested. In the first type the cells did not change their spontaneous activity during the time from the end of electrical stimulation to the onset of the call and were strongly excited throughout the duration of the call, with no appreciable difference in the response pattern to the playback calls and other vocalizations. In the second type of response, encountered in more than 50% of the cells, there was again no change in spontaneous activity from the end of electrical stimulation to the onset of calling, but the response during self-produced vocal activity was either much weaker than during loudspeaker-transmitted vocalizations or was totally absent. By studying both auditory stimuli (the self-produced and the recorded vocalizations) during the time between the end of electrical stimulation and the onset of the evoked call (on average 400 milliseconds), Müller-Preuss[59] was able to determine that it is the self-produced call which inhibits the auditory cells and not the electrical stimulation of the central grey matter.

The conclusions drawn from these results are twofold. First, since the spontaneous activity of the auditory cells did not change during the interval between termination of the electrical stimulus and onset of vocalization, the auditory cortex does not appear to receive information from the motor structures during that time. Secondly, the auditory cortex seems to receive different information depending on whether the calls are self-produced or foreign-produced. It is suggested that the inhibition during self-produced calling is caused by corollary discharges of the vocalization structures to midbrain structures of the auditory pathway at the instant of the call production. This mechanism provides the animal with information on its own vocal activity and, at the same time, allows for the processing of incoming signals from the environment while the animal is vocally active.[59] As has been stated before, squirrel monkey infants produce their species-specific vocal patterns immediately after birth and use a great many vocal signals for social communication within the first days of life. From this it can be concluded that the brain structures involved in phonatory patterning are mature at birth. One must assume that this also holds true for the feedback mechanism which has just been described, i.e. neonates can distinguish between their own calls and calls from others. This is corroborated by the vocal behaviour of the infant which occurs in the appropriate context of social interaction with the infant's conspecifics and can be observed in combination with other complex motor signals.[46]

In line with the hierarchical model of phonation and its control, I conjecture that the brain mechanisms of vocalization which operate in the monkey are homologous to those in the human neonate, which means that human infants also make the distinction between their own vocalizations and vocal input from others. Furthermore, as recent studies have shown,[40,60,61] the very young human infant can also discriminate between species-specific sounds, i.e. phonemic sounds in speech, and non-phonemic auditory input. It is suggested that the neural mechanisms underlying phonation and voice perception serve as an early means of self-awareness.

With reference to Karl Popper, I began with the question of whether language was the first product of the human mind. The purpose of this contribution was to demonstrate that in humans vocal behaviour and the brain mechanisms involved must be considered to be prerequisites for speech.[62] Long before speech becomes possible human infants develop self-awareness and demonstrate consciousness of self by their preverbal competence in social interactions. It is suggested that the earliest and predominant means which lead to this end are the vocal–auditory feedback mechanisms. These mechanisms operate from birth but develop and mature in stages until the command of verbal utterances is achieved. The earliest of these mechanisms, especially the ability to distinguish between one's own and other voices, is shared with the other primates. But voluntary control over vocal production, fractionating fixed action patterns and moulding them into the learnt units of speech, is a new acquisition, first occurring in the human species. In view of the long natural history of vocal behaviour in vertebrates one must assume that innumerable stages in the evolution of the social communication system have a bearing on mechanisms which are involved in the emergence of human language. Thus one must assume that the transition from automatic to voluntary vocal production has taken place in slow stages. Self-awareness seems to be a constituent of such development. If one grants the human baby self-awareness, one must concede that such stages of the mind were developed before the emergence of humankind.

References

1. POPPER, K. R. & ECCLES, J. C. (1977) *The Self and its Brain*, Springer International, Berlin
2. MACLEAN, P. D. & PLOOG, D. W. (1962) Cerebral representation of penile erection. *J. Neurophysiol. 25*, 29–55
3. ROBINSON, B. W. (1967) Vocalization evoked from forebrain in *Macaca mulatta*. *Physiol. Behav. 2*, 345–354
4. JÜRGENS, U., MAURUS, M., PLOOG, D. & WINTER, P. (1967) Vocalization in the squirrel monkey (*Saimiri sciureus*) elicited by brain stimulation. *Exp. Brain Res. 4*, 114–117
5. JÜRGENS, U. & PLOOG, D. (1970) Cerebral representation of vocalization in the squirrel monkey. *Exp. Brain Res. 10*, 532–554
6. WINTER, P., PLOOG, D. & LATTA, J. (1966) Vocal repertoire of the squirrel monkey (*Saimiri sciureus*), its analysis and significance. *Exp. Brain Res. 1*, 359–384
7. JÜRGENS, U. (1976) Reinforcing concomitants of electrically elicited vocalizations. *Exp. Brain Res. 26*, 203–214
8. MAGOUN, H. W., ATLAS, D., INGERSOLL, E. H. & RANSON, S. W. (1937) Associated facial, vocal and respiratory components of emotional expression: an experimental study. *J. Neurol. Psychopathol. 17*, 241–255
9. SKULTETY, F. M. (1962) Experimental mutism in dogs. *Arch. Neurol. 6*, 235
10. SCHMIDT, R. S. (1966) Central mechanisms of frog calling. *Behaviour 26*, 251–285
11. KENNEDY, M. C. (1975) Vocalization elicited in a lizard by electrical stimulation of the midbrain. *Brain Res. 91*, 321–325
12. KELLY, A. H., BEATON, L. E. & MAGOUN, H. W. (1946) A midbrain mechanism for facio-vocal activity. *J. Neurophysiol. 9*, 181–189
13. BOTEZ, M. I. & BARBEAU, S. (1971) Role of subcortical structures and particularly of the thalamus in mechanisms of speech and language. *Int. J. Neurol. 8*, 300–320
14. SUTTON, D., LARSON, C. & LINDEMAN, R. C. (1974) Neocortical and limbic lesion effects on primate phonation. *Brain Res. 71*, 61–75
15. BUGE, A., ESCOUROLLE, R., RANCUREL, G. & POISSON, M. (1975) Mutisme akinétique et ramollissement bicingulaire. 3 observations anatomo-cliniques. *Rev. Neurol. (Paris) 131*, 121–137
16. RUBENS, A. B. (1975) Aphasia with infarction in the territory of the anterior cerebral artery. *Cortex 11*, 239–250
17. JÜRGENS, U. & MÜLLER-PREUSS, P. (1977) Convergent projections of different limbic vocalization areas in the squirrel monkey. *Exp. Brain Res. 29*, 75–83
18. JÜRGENS, U. (1974) The elicitability of vocalization from the cortical larynx area. *Brain Res. 81*, 564–566
19. JÜRGENS, U. (1979) Neural control of vocalization in non-human primates, in *Neurobiology of Social Communication in Primates: An Evolutionary Perspective* (Steklis, H. D. & Raleigh, M. J., eds.), Academic Press, New York
20. KUYPERS, H. G. J. M. (1958a) Some projections from the pericentral cortex to the pons and lower brain stem in monkey and chimpanzee. *J. Comp. Neurol. 110*, 221–255
21. KUYPERS, H. G. J. M. (1958b) Corticobulbar connexions to the pons and lower brain stem in man. *Brain 81*, 364–388
22. JÜRGENS, U. & PRATT, R. (1979) The cingular vocalization pathway in the squirrel monkey. *Exp. Brain Res. 34*, 499–510
23. ROBINSON, B. W. (1976) Limbic influences on human speech. *Ann. N. Y. Acad. Sci. 280*, 761–771
24. PLOOG, D. (1970) Social communication among animals, in *The Neurosciences, Second Study Program* (Schmitt, F. O., ed.), pp. 349–361, Rockefeller Press, New York
25. PLOOG, D. (1974) *Die Sprache der Affen und ihre Bedeutung für die Verständigungsweisen des Menschen*, Kindler-Verlag, München

26. WOLFF, P. H. (1969) The natural history of crying and other vocalizations in early infancy, in *Determinants of Infant Behavior IV* (Foss, B. M., ed.), pp. 81–109, Methuen, London

27. WOLFF, P. H. (1963) Observations on the early development of smiling, in *Determinants of Infant Behavior II* (Foss, B. M., ed.), pp. 113–133, Methuen, London

28. LENNEBERG, E. H. (1967) *Biological Foundations of Language*, John Wiley, New York

29. KOEHLER, O. (1954) Vom Erbgut der Sprache. *Homo 5*, 97–104

30. LENNEBERG, E. H., REBELSKY, F. A. & NICHOLS, I. A. (1965) The vocalization of infants born to deaf and hearing parents. *Hum. Dev. 8*, 23–37

31. BROWN, R. (1965) *Words and Things*, Collier-MacMillan, New York

32. LORENZ, K. (1937) Über die Bildung des Instinktbegriffes. *Naturwissenschaften 25*, 289–300; 307–318; 324–331

33. TODD, G. A. & PALMER, B. (1968) Social reinforcement of infant babbling, *Child Dev. 39*, 591–596

34. JAKOBSON, R. (1971) *Studies on Child Language and Aphasia*, p. 9, Mouton, The Hague

35. NAKAZIMA, S. (1975) Phonemicization and symbolization in language development, in *Foundations of Language Development. A Multidisciplinary Approach*, vol. 1 (Lenneberg, E. H., & Lenneberg, E., eds.), pp. 181–187, Academic Press, New York

36. JAKOBSON, R. (1968) *Child Language, Aphasia, and Phonological Universals*, p. 68, Mouton, The Hague (English translation of *Kindersprache, Aphasie und allgemeine Lautgesetze*, Uppsala Universitets Aarsskrift 1942)

37. WINTER, P., HANDLEY, P., PLOOG, D. & SCHOTT, D. (1973) Ontogeny of squirrel monkey calls under normal conditions and under acoustic isolation. *Behaviour 47*, 230–239

38. HUPFER, K., JÜRGENS, U. & PLOOG, D. (1977) The effect of superior temporal lesions on the recognition of species-specific calls in the squirrel monkey. *Exp. Brain Res. 30*, 75–87

39. BEATTY, J. & DEVITT, C. A. (1975) Call discrimination in chimpanzees. *Current Anthropol. 16*, 668–669

40. SINNOTT, J. M., BEECHER, M. D., MOODY, D. B. & STEBBINS, W. C. (1976) Speech sound discrimination by monkeys and humans. *J. Acoust. Soc. Am. 60*, 687–695

41. BLOOM, K. (1975) Social elicitation of infant vocal behavior. *J. Exp. Child Psychol. 20*, 51–58

42. LENNEBERG, E. H. (1975) The concept of language differentiation, in *Foundations of Language Development. A Multidisciplinary Approach*, vol. 1 (Lenneberg, E. H. & Lenneberg, E., eds.), pp. 17–33, Academic Press, New York

43. LECOURS, A. R. (1975) Myelogenetic correlates of the development of speech and language, in *Foundations of Language Development. A Multidisciplinary Approach*, vol. 1 (Lenneberg, E. H. & Lenneberg, E., eds.), pp. 121–135, Academic Press, New York

44. YAKOVLEV, P. J. & LECOURS, A. R. (1967) The myelogenetic cycles of regional maturation of the brain, in *Regional Development of the Brain in Early Life* (Minkowski, A., ed.), pp. 3–70, Blackwell, Oxford

45. TALMAGE-RIGGS, G., WINTER, P., PLOOG, D. & MAYER, W. (1972) Effects of deafening on the vocal behavior of the squirrel monkey (*Saimiri sciureus*). *Folia Primatol. 17*, 404–420

46. PLOOG, D. (1969) Early communication processes in squirrel monkeys, in *Brain and Early Behaviour. Development in the Fetus and Infant* (Robinson, R. J., ed.), pp. 269–298, Academic Press, London

47. HOPF, S. (1970) Report on a hand-reared squirrel monkey (*Saimiri sciureus*). *Z. Tierpsychol. 27*, 610–621

48. MASON, W. A. (1979) Maternal attributes and primate cognitive development, in *Human Ethology. Claims and Limits of a New Discipline* (Cranach, M. von et al., eds.), pp. 437–455, Cambridge University Press, Cambridge

49. PAPOUŠEK, H. (1961) Conditioned head rotating reflexes in infants in the first months of life. *Acta Paediatr. 50*, 565–576

50. PAPOUŠEK, H. & BERNSTEIN, P. (1969) The functions of conditioning stimulation in human neonates and infants, in *Stimulation in Early Infancy* (Ambrose, A., ed.), Academic Press, London

51. WATSON, J. S. (1972) Smiling, cooing and "The game". *Merrill-Palmer Q. 18,* 323–339

52. HELD, R. & HEIN, A. (1963) Movement-produced stimulation in the development of visually guided behavior. *J. Comp. Physiol. Psychol. 56,* 872–876

53. BROWN, R. A. (1973) *A First Language: The Early Stages,* Harvard University Press, Cambridge, Mass.

54. BRUNER, J. S. (1974/75) From communication to language – a psychological perspective. *Cognition 3,* 255–287

55. VON HOLST, E. & MITTELSTAEDT, H. (1950) Das Reafferenzprinzip, *Naturwissenschaften 37,* 464–476

56. TEUBER, H.-L. (1964) The riddle of frontal lobe function in man, in *The Frontal Granular Cortex and Behavior* (Warren, J. M. & Akert, K., eds.), pp. 410–444, McGraw-Hill, New York

57. MACKAY, D. M. & MITTELSTAEDT, H. (1974) Visual stability and motor control (re-afference revisited), in *Cybernetics and Bionics* (*Proc. 5th Congr. Deutsche Gesellschaft für Kybernetik*), Oldenbourg, Munich

58. MÜLLER-PREUSS, P. & JÜRGENS, U. (1976) Projections from the cingular vocalization area in the squirrel monkey. *Brain Res. 103,* 29–43

59. MÜLLER-PREUSS, P. (1978) Single unit responses of the auditory cortex in the squirrel monkey to self-produced and loudspeaker transmitted vocalizations. *Neurosci. Lett. Suppl. 1,* S. 7

60. EIMAS, P. D., SIQUELAND, E. R., JUSCZYK, P. & VIGORITO, J. (1971) Speech perception in infants. *Science (Wash. D.C.) 171,* 303–306

61. EIMAS, P. D., COOPER, W. E. & CORBIT, J. D. (1973) Some properties of linguistic detectors. *Percept. Psychophys. 13,* 247–252

62. PLOOG, D. (1975) Vocal behavior and its "localization" as a prerequisite for speech, in *Cerebral Localization* (Zülch, K. J. *et al.*, eds.), pp. 229–237, Springer, Berlin

63. JÜRGENS, U. & PLOOG, D. (1976) Zur Evolution der Stimme. *Arch. Psychiatr. Nervenkr. 222,* 117–137

64. JÜRGENS, U. (1970) Durch Hirnreiz induzierte Vokalisationen (vocalization elicited by · electrical brain stimulation.) *Verh. Dtsch. Zool. Ges. 54,* 253–256

65. ROSABAL, F. (1967) Cytoarchitecture of the frontal lobe of the squirrel monkey. *J. Comp. Neurol. 130,* 87–108

Language: perspectives from another modality

URSULA BELLUGI and EDWARD S. KLIMA*

*The Salk Institute for Biological Studies, La Jolla, California and *University of California, San Diego*

Abstract Human languages have been forged in auditory–vocal channels throughout evolution. This paper examines the formal properties of a communication system that has developed in the absence of speech: the sign language of the deaf. The objective is to investigate to what extent the overall form and organization of language is determined by the articulatory and perceptual modality in which it has developed (its transmission system) and to what extent its form and organization represent more fundamental aspects of the human mind (intellect). Experimental and linguistic evidence is brought to bear on the analysis of the sign: studies of coding and processing of signs in memory; of slips of the hand; of historical change in signs over time; the heightened use of language in poetry and wit. American Sign Language differs dramatically from English and other spoken languages in the mechanisms by which its lexical units are modified. For the form of its morphological processes, the mode in which the language develops appears to make a crucial difference. Finally, the issue of cerebral specialization with respect to a visual–manual language is addressed.

Human languages have been forged in auditory–vocal channels throughout evolution. In our research, we examine the formal properties of a communication system that has developed in the absence of speech. Our general objective is to investigate to what extent the overall form and organization of language is determined by the articulatory and perceptual modality in which it has developed (its transmission system) and to what extent its form and organization represent more fundamental aspects of the human mind (intellect, cognitive processes).

Until recently, all that we have learnt about human language has been learnt from the study of spoken languages. The very concept of language entails complex organizational principles that have often been thought to be intimately connected with vocally articulated sounds. History records not a single instance of a community of hearing people who have a sign language rather than a spoken language as their primary, native language: speech is clearly the preferred system.

Our research has taken an unusual point of departure for the investigation of language and its formal properties. We study a language which has developed in modalities other than auditory–vocal: American Sign Language (ASL), the system of hand signs developed by deaf people and passed down from one generation to the next. If sign languages are autonomous languages —as the mounting evidence from our research clearly demonstrates—then they constitute an experiment of nature allowing us to address fundamental issues about the human capacity for language, the general form of language, the necessary conditions for language, and the determining forces of its structural properties.

At the beginning of our research, some eight years ago, we did not know whether ASL was an independent language, nor precisely how that concept might apply to gestural communication. The available literature generally stressed the icon and image behind the global form of signs. We read that sign language is 'a collection of vague and loosely defined pictorial gestures'; that it is a 'universal' communication; that it is pantomime; that it is 'much too much a depicting language, keeping the thinking slow'; that 'sign language deals mainly with material objects, dreads and avoids the abstract'; that it is 'derived from English, a pidgin form of English on the hands with no structure of its own'.

We were then faced with a communication system that appeared totally different from speech and spoken language, a communication system that apparently violated some of the putative universal characteristics posited for human language: that language is based on speech and the vocal apparatus; that linguistic symbols are essentially arbitrary, the form of a symbol bearing no relation to the form of its referent. What aroused our interest was the opportunity to study a language that had developed fully in an unexpected and different mode.

Since that time, our investigations have covered a wide array of concerns: the linguistic structure of the sign; iconicity in signs and signing; historical change in signs; immediate and long-term memory for signs; comparison between two independent sign languages; perception of signs; studies of slips of the hand; the role of non-manual signals in the language; studies of ASL syntactic processes; studies of the rate of production of sign language and spoken language; studies of grammatical processes such as compounding, derivational and inflectional processes; studies of invented or recently coined signs; studies of the linguistic expression of category levels in sign language; studies of wit and poetry in sign language; studies of hemispheric specialization for signs.[1-10] The evidence clearly indicates that an autonomous language has developed in the hands which in its grammatical patterning is entirely distinct from that of the surrounding language community.

THE TWO FACES OF SIGN *

There is a fundamental difference between American Sign Language (and, to our knowledge, most primary sign languages) and spoken languages. The newcomer to sign language, the researcher, the analyst, and even the native signer is struck by the iconicity that pervades the language at all levels. Characteristically lexical items themselves tend to be globally iconic, their form resembling some aspect of what they denote. At the morphological and syntactic levels there is also often congruence between form and meaning. Spoken languages are not without such direct clues to meaning: reduplication processes (e.g. those expressing plurality) and ideophones, as well as ono-matopoeic words in spoken language provide direct methods of reflecting meaning through form. But in sign language such transparency is pervasive.

Until recently, the signs of sign languages were regarded as global wholes without any formal internal structure. Earlier writers focused on the physical form of the signal only to discuss the images that are generated by that form, and this apparently prevailed over any consideration of the structure of signs. Certainly mimetic representation is the *source* of many symbols used in signing

---

*The two papers (Dr Ploog's and ours) for the session on Language both use the phrase *two faces* to refer to communication signals. It is important and relevant to distinguish the uses of the phrase in these different contexts. Dr Ploog discusses social signalling processes in non-human primates (and in humans). For him, social signals are two-faced: 'the signal carries the message for the recipient and expresses simultaneously the sender's emotional state.' That is, an animal communication signal, for example, may express a holistic coded message to another animal (food, danger) while at the same time signalling the emotional state of the sender.

In our paper, when we use the term two faces to refer to the lexical items of a human visual–gestural communication, we are focusing differently. We already assume that the message in signing (the proposition or sentence) is composed of elements (signs) in differing arrange-ments which permit an infinite variety of novel messages; they are not limited to signalling the signer's emotional state (and generally do not, for the most part conveying objective in-formation). Our first question with respect to sign language had to do with the two faces of the individual linguistic symbols: their overall iconic representational character and their simultaneous decomposition into arbitrary formal elements which function as differentiators between signs. In general, this is the issue of duality of patterning of linguistic symbols.

(TIME*, 'pointing to a wrist-watch'; BIRD, 'the opening and closing of the beak of a bird'; VOTE, 'putting a vote in a ballot box').

Yet in addition to their mimetic quality and representational character, we have found that there is another aspect to the form of signs. The first serious attempt at a structural description of the basic lexical units of a sign language was made in 1960, 1965 by William Stokoe,[11,12] who posited that signs can be described in terms of a limited set of componential elements that recur across signs. To distinguish one sign from all others in the language, critical information is required about the *configuration* of the hand in making the sign; the *place* where the sign is made; and the *movement* of the hands in making the sign. Analysis of this criterial information suggests that ASL signs are not simply iconic mimetic forms but are also composed of a very limited set of recurring formal elements which function as pure differentiators between signs.

We have argued elsewhere[7] that there is a continual interplay between the representational character of ASL signs and their encoded arbitrary componential character. Much of our early research was motivated by attempts to determine the conditions under which each of the two faces of sign dominate. There are many conditions under which both faces of sign are evident: in signing conversation, in sign poetry, in plays on signs, in invented signs. But there are some specific conditions under which the arbitrary componential face of signs distinctly and clearly dominates: immediate memory processing for signs; slips of the hand; historical change in sign forms; and the operation of grammatical processes in the language. We shall consider each of these issues briefly within this paper.

PREDOMINANCE OF SUBLEXICAL CODING UNITS

Immediate memory processing

We all have a vivid impression of the immediate present, but if we are asked to recall in detail the moment just passed, we can reproduce only a

---

*We adopt some notational conventions for this paper. Words in capital letters represent English labels (glosses) for ASL signs. A gloss is chosen on the basis of common usage among deaf informants. The gloss represents the meaning of the unmarked, unmodulated form of a sign. Spoken words are represented in italics. Written word responses (as in memory experiments) are represented in quotation marks. A bracketed word following a sign gloss indicates that the sign is made with some regular change in form associated with a systematic change in meaning, and thus indicates grammatical change on signs. Modulatory forms embedded within other modulations are indicated by nested brackets.

limited part of its contents. It is a common experience for hearing people to remember sounds, such as the last few words of a sentence, when they were not paying attention to the sounds as they occurred. Such echoes are the mode in which we experience the immediate past and retain its details after it is no longer physically available. We can partially hold onto and seemingly even reinvigorate auditory experiences just passed in the time stream. Our capacity for immediate memory plays a special role in language processing. When we hear sentences, we must process and store a stream of ongoing speech until we have taken in enough to understand structure and meaning. The form in which linguistic signals are stored in immediate memory has been of much interest to psychologists and linguists and has been the focus for a large number of experiments. The form in which words and signs alike are encoded has turned out to provide evidence for the psychological reality of some levels of language structure—in particular of sublexical structure.

There is now abundant experimental evidence (summarized by Norman[13]) that hearing people code linguistic information in short-term memory on the basis of the sound-form of words or letters. Some of this comes from typical intrusion errors, misremembering, or partial remembering of a lexical item (e.g. 'tide' for *time*; 'word' for *bird*; 'vat' for *vote*), where in each instance the item presented and the error differ in only one phonological segment.

We have completed a series of studies of short-term memory for lists of signs of ASL in native deaf signers (Refs. 1, 8, 14 and unpublished work by H. Poizner, U. Bellugi and R. Tweney). All of our experiments yield one consistent result: in short-term memory, the componential face of signs is dominant, and the iconic face is submerged. We found that intrusion errors were consistently errors based on partial remembering of component elements of signs. For example, a common error for TIME was 'potato'; for BIRD was 'newspaper'; for VOTE was 'tea'. In each of these cases, the common error formed a minimal pair with the sign presented, differing only in one formational parameter. The signs TIME and POTATO are alike except for configuration of the hand; the signs BIRD and NEWSPAPER are alike except for place of articulation; the signs VOTE and TEA are alike except for movement. There was no consistent evidence of any other basis for the intrusion errors: not sound-based, not printed-word-based, not semantically based and—important for this discussion—not iconic. Consistently, the errors were based on the special organizational principles of the signs themselves: configurations of the hand, places of articulation, movements—the arbitrary components of signs.

Note an important difference between the organization of words and signs which is highlighted by the errors: the component elements of words (the segments) are essentially *linearly* organized (*time* and *tide* differ in final segment) while the component elements of signs are essentially *simultaneously* organized (TIME and POTATO differ in the configuration of the hand throughout the sign).

Our other experimental studies in immediate memory processing confirmed this finding: lists of signs which were similar in component elements (CHAIR, NAME, EGG) were remembered significantly worse than matched control lists of signs, indicating that these sublexical components have a direct effect in short-term memory. However, lists of signs that were low in iconicity (DOLL, MOTHER, PENNY) were equally well remembered as lists of signs that are high in iconicity (WINDOW, TICKET, MELON). There is apparently no effect of iconicity in short-term memory.

The results of these experimental studies provide important support for the basic finding that in immediate memory we process linguistic signals in terms of component elements, regardless of the degree of iconicity of the global symbols, regardless of the sequential or simultaneous organization of these components, and regardless of the modality of the language. Overall, then, the componential face of signs, as of words, predominates in short-term memory processing and the iconic face becomes completely submerged.

Slips of the hands

We found further evidence for the psychological reality of sublexical structure in unintended misordering errors which occur in everyday signing—slips of the hands, analogous to slips of the tongue.[1,15] We have recorded over a hundred inadvertent misordering errors from videotapes of deaf people signing. Occasionally these were transpositions of whole signs; far more frequently they were transpositions of component elements of signs. These slips of the hands, like slips of the tongue for spoken language,[16] are valuable as spontaneously occurring data from everyday signing behaviour which provide clues to the organization of sign language and to the way the signs are coded.

One person intended to sign SICK, BORED (meaning roughly the equivalent of 'I'm sick and tired of it') and inadvertently switched the hand-shapes only. The sign SICK was made with the pointing index-finger hand intended for BORED, while BORED was made with the bent mid-finger hand of SICK. No other parameters were affected in the error. Another person intended to sign RECENTLY EAT in a sentence context, and instead switched only the place of articulation of the signs—making EAT on the cheek where RECENTLY should be and RECENTLY at the mouth where EAT should be. Another person intended to sign TASTE GOOD, and in producing the signs switchcd the movements of the two inadvertently, all other parameters remaining intact. The movement of TASTE, an iterated contact, was exchanged with the movement of GOOD, a single straight diagonal movement away from signer. Thus among the collection of slips of the hands, we found exchanges of hand-shape only, exchanges of place of articulation only, exchanges of movement only, the other parameters remaining as intended. The errors produced were typically not actual signs of ASL. For the most part these sign forms with single parameters exchanged were *possible* sign forms in ASL —formed from the small set of available hand-shapes, locations and movements that comprise other ASL sign forms. In a large number of cases, we found some readjustments of parameter values accompanying some structural substitution to bring the error forms into conformity with constraints on the combination of parameter values in ASL. Slips of the hands provide striking evidence for the psychological reality and independence of individual parameters of ASL; they are behavioural evidence from everyday communication that for deaf signers a sign is organized sublexically and thus that the language of signs exhibits duality of patterning.

Historical change in signs

Studies of historical change in signs provide some clues to the coexistence of the iconic face of signs and the encoded arbitrary face of signs.[17,18] Many ASL signs in their contemporary form have lost much of their original transparency. When signs have changed, they exhibit several tendencies. One tendency is to focus information in the hands and their movements rather than in movements of the face or body; another is to displace the location of signs in regular ways within the signing space; another tendency is towards symmetry between the articulators; another is towards assimilation of the formational components of multipart signs resulting in the characteristics of unitary lexical items; and another is towards the generalization of parameter values. The direction of change in particular signs over the past century has consistently been from the more iconic and representational to the more arbitrary and constrained, conforming to a tighter linguistic system.

A classic example of historical changc is the current ASL sign HOME, which is an opaque non-transparent sign in our studies of the iconicity of signs.[7] When hearing non-signers wcrc asked to guess the meaning of the sign, they responded with guesses such as 'familiar', 'touch base', 'close to a person', 'comprehend', 'telephone', 'orange', 'communicate'. None of our subjects guessed the correct meaning of the sign, even when it was presented as an item on a multiple choice test. And none of our subjects guessed that the sign HOME is directly related to eating and sleeping. But in fact, the current opaque sign HOME is historically a merged compound, deriving from the two highly transparent signs EAT and SLEEP. In EAT an 'O' hand moves as if bringing food to the mouth; SLEEP is made with the cheek laid on the open palm. As a result of historical change the second sign has assumed the hand configuration of the first, and the place of articulation of the first contact has moved towards that of the second, so that the citation form today is a unitary sign with an 'O' hand touching two distinct places on the cheek. A consequence of these changes is a complete loss of the iconicity of the original two signs: the sign HOME is one of the more opaque signs of ASL. Such historical change in signs suggests what appear to be systematic pressures in ASL towards constraining its lexical elements, resulting in more opaque forms.

Wit and poetry

Nowhere are the two faces of the language more evident than in wit and poetry. We have completed a series of studies designed to discover how such forms of expression, which are so directly sound-based in spoken languages, manifest themselves in a language without sound.

In wit and poetry, elements of form and meaning—a linguistic system— are used to create complex many-layered expressions with multiple meanings and even to create whole new systems of form and meaning. Similarities and differences in form, function and meaning are exploited; the elements of the linguistic system are manipulated and sometimes distorted. How language is used in wit and poetry can inform us about the awareness, on the part of the language users, of regularities in the language.

We have found that one method of playing on signs is to substitute one regular ASL parameter value for another, thus using elements of the linguistic code to create new sign forms. This occurs when a signer intentionally distorts a sign by substituting a value that adds a new dimension of meaning. For example, consider the plays on the sign UNDERSTAND: by substituting the little finger for the index finger, one deaf person effectively conveyed 'understand a little'. By making the movement backwards, another deaf signer conveyed the meaning 'un-understand', or 'understand not at all'. But sign plays are not limited to substitution of parameter values. In signing, the existence of two autonomous articulators creates the physical possibility of producing two independent signs simultaneously, one in each hand. Such simultaneity is consistent with the tendency towards simultaneous expression in many regular processes in the language: the tendency to compress information into sign units and the use of simultaneous (rather than sequential) modifications of signs to modulate meaning. Double articulations of signs occur frequently in the self-conscious signing of preplanned material: in theatrical productions, in narratives, in poetic signing—and in plays on signs. One deaf signer effectively condensed into a single sign creation the ambivalence of his emotions by signing EXCITED with one hand while simultaneously signing DEPRESSED with the other.[19]

In poetic signing, deaf signers sometimes choose signs with the same hand-shape within a line or verse; such shared hand configurations in consecutive signs are analogous to such phenomena as consonance (alliteration) or assonance in the poetic tradition of spoken language. Again, in poetic signing, we also find special patterned attributes of the presentation of signs, by maintaining a balance between the two hands and creating a flow of movement between signs.[20]

Operations on signs and the submergence of iconicity

We have discovered that ASL signs undergo regular operations to change their form and meaning in a large number of ways. (We will come back to this point later.) One of the most striking effects of regular morphological operations on signs is the distortion of their form so that iconic aspects of the signs are overridden and submerged. Grammatical processes operate on ASL signs without reference to any iconic properties of the signs themselves; rather, they operate 'blindly' on the formational components. This is the case even when the operations may themselves exhibit some degree of iconicity. For instance, as a way of intensifying the meaning of a sign, a sign may be made with very rapid tense movement. The sign FAST made in this way means 'very fast', SICK means 'very sick', BLUE means 'very blue', and so on. The sign SLOW is made in citation form with one hand moving along the back of the other hand. But under the regular operation on signs resulting in the intensified meaning 'very slow', the movement of the sign is not elongated or made more slowly; rather the meaning 'very slow' is regularly conveyed by making the sign with an extremely short rapid movement. The form of 'very slow', is clearly incongruent with the meaning of the basic sign.

Other operations on signs similarly change their form in ways that obscure iconic properties. The sign BABY is a highly iconic sign, derived directly from the pantomimic act of holding and rocking a baby. By a regular process the sign can be changed in form to mean 'act like a baby', or 'babyish'. The gentle rocking motion disappears, the movement becomes an intense downward jerk repeated in a way that would be highly inappropriate for the meaning of the original sign. The change in form completely submerges the iconicity of the root form of the sign.

Thus under many conditions the iconic aspect of signs is obscured. The iconic face does not show at all in the processing of signs in immediate memory (nor, we would conjecture, in ongoing sentence processing). Historical change diminishes the iconic properties of ASL signs; some signs become more opaque over time, some completely arbitrary. Grammatical operations that signs undergo can further submerge iconicity. Thus many signs, while having their roots deeply embedded in mimetic representation, have lost their original transparency as they have been constrained more tightly by the linguistic system.

But iconicity in ASL is not a buried etymological legacy. Newly coined signs are frequently based on mimetic representation of shape, action or movement. Moreover, iconic properties of established lexical signs are always potentially available and are exploited by signers to add dimension and colour to their expressions. The two faces of this language of shapes moving in space are ever present and ever provocative. It is now clear that ASL is a highly abstract, rule-governed, combinatorial linguistic system while at the same time preserving its iconic roots and mimetic potential.

GRAMMATICAL PROCESSES IN AMERICAN SIGN LANGUAGE

In the study of a communication system that seems as markedly iconic as ASL does, we felt that a reasonable first area of attack was the internal structure of the citation-form signs—basic naked forms. We have since found that ASL has its own rules of syntax which govern sentential construction. Furthermore, we find that in sentence contexts, the basic sign units undergo meaningful modifications of form by changes in movement and spatial displacements. These modifications prove to be a key to one of the salient structural characteristics of the language: its richness in morphological processes, which result in single complex sign units—complex in form as well as in meaning.[1,3]

We have found that ASL has developed elaborate morphological devices in a form which is unique to a visual–gestural language. Morphological processes in English and other spoken languages—the means by which complex words are built from minimal meaningful units—typically involve the linear addition of phonological segments to words.* American Sign Language

---

*In spoken languages the most widespread morphological device for modification of meaning is probably affixation. Internal modifications also occur (as in *wife, wives*); other devices include reduplication as well as changes in stress or tone.

manifests no tendency whatever to build up its lexical units in this way. Rather, signs undergo a wide variety of grammatical processes—regular changes in form associated with regular changes in meaning—each of which operates by imposing different dynamic changes in movement and spatial contouring. (See Fig. 1 for examples of the sign PREACH under a variety of inflections.)

The elaborate formal inflectional devices, their widespread use to vary the form of signs and the variety of fine semantic distinctions they systematically convey suggest that ASL, like Russian, Latin and Navajo—but unlike English and Chinese—is one of the inflective languages of the world. The specification of these grammatical processes is a major thrust of our current research.

Semantic distinctions

Investigations of the semantic distinctions marked by specific morphological operations reveal the extent and variety of such processes in the language. We have found that ASL signs may undergo modulation for referential indexing; for reciprocity; for grammatical number (marking dual, trial, multiple); for distributional aspect (differentiating actions to 'each', 'any', 'certain ones'); for temporal aspect (marking distinctions such as 'for a long time', 'regularly', 'frequently', 'incessantly', 'characteristically', 'uninterruptedly'); for temporal focus (differentiating 'starting to', 'increasingly', 'gradually', 'resulting in'); for manner ('with ease', 'readily'); for degree ('a little', 'very', 'excessively'). There are also a large number of derivational processes, such as those which derive nouns from verbs, predicates from nouns, and those which signal figurative or extended meanings.

Dimensions of movement

Study of the global form of ASL morphological processes reveals that they are in form totally unlike such processes in spoken language. It appears that the key to the grammar of ASL is in simultaneous multidimensional changes in movement imposed on signs. We have found that each morphological process embeds the sign stem in a superimposed movement pattern, leaving other structural parameters (hand-shape, target locus) intact. Fig. 2 shows six different signs under a single inflectional process: a process which embeds the sign stem in superimposed triplicated smooth circles of movement. The semantic effect of this modulation is to change a transitory or temporary state into an inherent characteristic. Thus under the modulation, the sign WRONG means 'error-prone', the sign QUIET means 'taciturn', or 'quiet by nature', the sign SILLY means 'characteristically foolish'. In English such shifts can be accounted for phrasally or lexically: a person can be temporarily

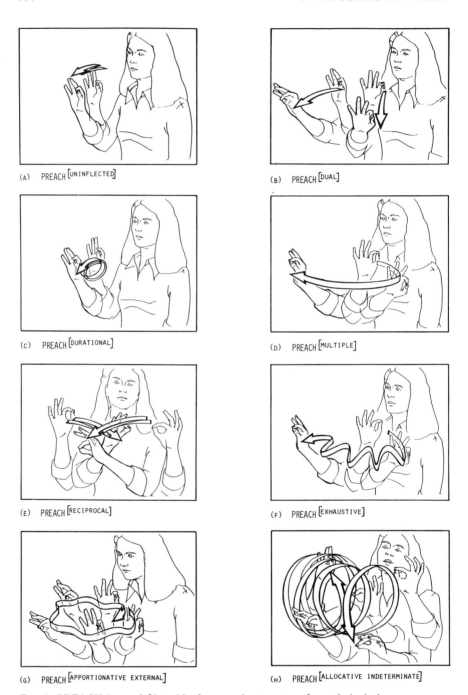

(A)   PREACH [UNINFLECTED]

(B)   PREACH [DUAL]

(C)   PREACH [DURATIONAL]

(D)   PREACH [MULTIPLE]

(E)   PREACH [RECIPROCAL]

(F)   PREACH [EXHAUSTIVE]

(G)   PREACH [APPORTIONATIVE EXTERNAL]

(H)   PREACH [ALLOCATIVE INDETERMINATE]

FIG. 1. PREACH (upper left) and its forms under an array of morphological processes.

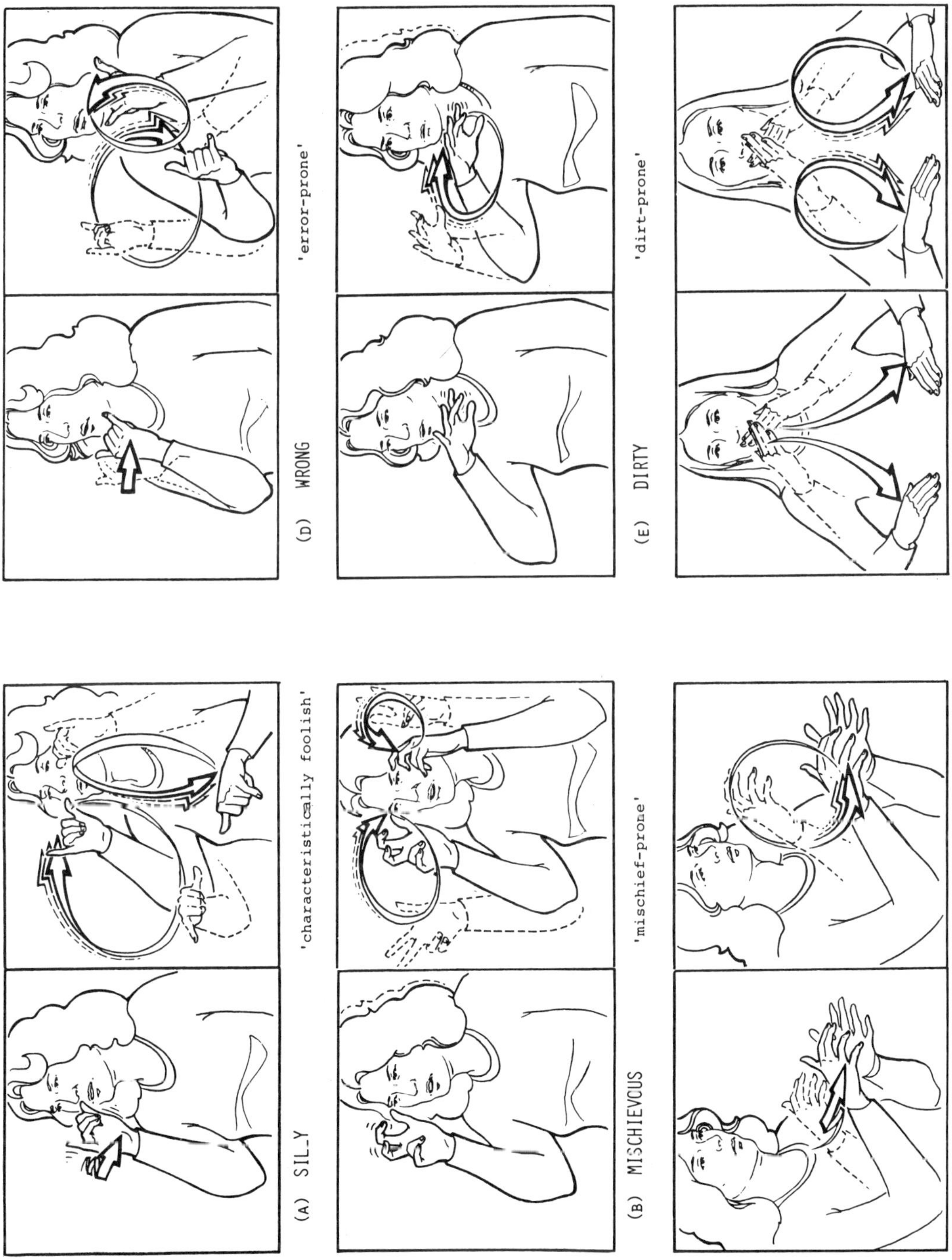

FIG. 2. An array of ASL signs and their form under modulation for characteristic aspect.

cross but characteristically *ill-natured*; temporarily *afraid* but characteristically *apprehensive*; temporarily *sad* but characteristically *melancholic*. In ASL, by contrast, the distinction is marked by a regular modulatory inflection. Note that the hand-shape and target locus are unaffected; furthermore, whatever the inherent movement of the basic uninflected sign (wrist twist, movement to contact, iterated contact, etc.), the modulation imposes a smooth triplicated continuous movement on the sign stem. Another inflectional process embeds signs in iterations along an arc of a specific plane, still another embeds signs in a single elongated lax continuous movement, and so forth.

Our linguistic analysis suggests that in their final surface form, the morphological processes we examined (over forty different ones) differ from one another on only a limited number of abstract spatial and temporal dimensions. Spatial dimensions such as geometric arrays (circles, lines, arcs); planar locus (vertical, horizontal); and direction of movement (upwards, downwards, sideways) involve primarily the manipulation of forms in space and figure significantly in the structure of inflections for indexing, reciprocity, grammatical number, distributional aspect. Qualities of movement (manner of onset and offset, rate, tension, acceleration) figure significantly in the structure of inflections for temporal aspect, focus and degree. Two dimensions (reduplication and doubling of the hands) interact with the others in the formation of inflections in several grammatical categories. We have identified within each dimension minimal pairs of inflectional forms. For example, the multiple inflection ('verb to them') and the exhaustive inflection ('verb to each') differ only in that one is made with a single movement, the other with a reduplicated movement; the exhaustive and the apportionative ('verb among the members of a group') differ only in geometric array (iterations along an arc as contrasted with iterations along a circle); and so forth.

Analysis of the linguistic dimensions of ASL morphological processes suggests that these processes exhibit internal systematicity in their dimensions of patterning. The multitude of forms exhibited by these modulations appear to differ from one another along only a limited number of dimensions. These differences in dimensions may correlate with a network of semantic distinctions, suggesting that within the language these modulations show underlying systematic relationships characteristic of grammatical processes in general.

HIERARCHIES OF FORM AND MEANING

We have also found that inflectional processes in ASL can apply in combinations to root signs, creating different hierarchies of form and meaning. In these combinations, the output of one inflectional process can serve as the

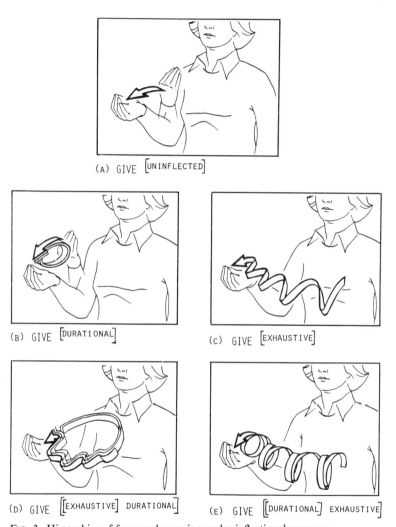

(A) GIVE [UNINFLECTED]

(B) GIVE [DURATIONAL]

(C) GIVE [EXHAUSTIVE]

(D) GIVE [[EXHAUSTIVE] DURATIONAL]

(E) GIVE [[DURATIONAL] EXHAUSTIVE]

FIG. 3. Hierarchies of form and meaning under inflectional processes.

input for another, and there are alternative orderings with different hierarchies of semantic structure as well. Fig. 3 shows the uninflected sign GIVE (a); the sign under the durational inflection ('continuously') (b); and alternatively under the exhaustive inflection ('to each') (c). The same sign can also undergo the exhaustive inflection embedded in the durational ('give to each, that action occurring continuously') (d), or the durational embedded in the exhaustive ('give continuously to each in turn') (e). Furthermore, such processes are recursive: the output of (e), for instance, can undergo the process in (b) once again (the durational of the exhaustive of a durational of GIVE), resulting in the meaning 'give continuously to each in turn, that action recurring over time'. Such cyclic application of rules to create complex expressions is characteristic of spoken language structure; the form that this takes in a visual–manual language—one inflectional process spatially and temporally nested in another—is unique.

The proliferation of components of form brought into play in morphological processes and in the language in general is consistent with our view of the tendency of the language towards conflation; towards packaging a great deal of information into a single unit form. The simultaneous use of superimposed spatial and temporal patterning in inflectional processes reflects, at this morphological level, the same principle of simultaneous organization that ASL sign units exhibit at the basic level.*

Thus we find that ASL has developed mechanisms for the regular modification of its lexical units. The morphological processes themselves are again deeply rooted in iconicity, as are the basic lexical items. The processes operate as simultaneous (not linear sequential) changes on signs, just as the signs themselves are essentially organized as simultaneously occurring components. The processes may have arisen as globally different from one another, just as signs may have their origins in global representational qualities. But the morphological processes which signs undergo have clearly been forged into a language-like system—themselves built out of a few component elements, with internal systematicity in their patterning. Furthermore, there is evidence that—as is characteristic of spoken language structure—these grammatical processes can apply in combinations to signs creating different hierarchies of form and meaning. For the form of its morphological processes, however, the mode in which the language develops appears to make a crucial difference.

---

*We have developed tests for investigating these morphological processes among deaf signers, using ASL sentential contexts which require a particular modulated form of a sign for their completion; we find that these processes are general across deaf signers of deaf parents who learnt ASL as a native language. We are now beginning a series of studies that focus on how signers encode, process and store morphologically complex forms in ASL. In one study of short-term memory for modulated signs, we find evidence that the signs and the morphological operations they undergo are stored as separable units even though the lexical and grammatical elements are simultaneously encoded. We find, for example, that subjects often remember the basic signs in the correct serial positions but transpose their inflections. Statistical analysis reveals that these rearrangement errors cannot be accounted for simply on the basis of mis-remembering movements similar in form, but rather indicate more abstract encoding of these complex forms.

CEREBRAL SPECIALIZATION FOR SIGNS

One of the most striking findings in the study of the relation between the structure of the brain and behavioural functioning is that of cerebral dominance in humans. Processing language structure has generally been considered a left hemisphere function, whereas processing visual–spatial relations has been considered a right hemisphere function. American Sign Language incorporates both complex language structure and complex spatial relations, thus exhibiting properties for which each of the hemispheres of normally-hearing people show predominant functioning. We have therefore been interested in investigating hemispheric specialization, in deaf people, for signs and for visual–spatial non-language tasks.[21]

In one study we investigated differential recognition of sign language stimuli presented to the left and right visual fields. Deaf adults showed superior accuracy in the recognition of line drawings of sign language presented initially to the left hemisphere. On a test of the localization of dots in space, these deaf subjects again showed superior left hemisphere accuracy, whereas hearing adults showed just the opposite: performance was better when the stimuli were initially presented to the right hemisphere. The data suggest that right-handed deaf people whose major form of communication is American Sign Language have the normal pattern of left hemisphere specialization for language, even though their language is acquired in a different mode. It appears, further, that in contrast to results with hearing subjects, the left hemisphere of signing deaf people is also specialized for a non-language task which has a strong visual–spatial component. These early results are suggestive: we speculate that since spatial localization is an important aspect of the grammar of sign language, it may be adaptive to bring together these two functions within the same hemisphere. The results presented here must be taken as preliminary because of their unexpected nature and because of the small number of subjects involved. Nonetheless, the evidence to date suggests that the two cerebral hemispheres are not irreversibly preprogrammed or hardwired to specialize for particular functions. The data from deaf subjects in this and other experiments[22] suggest that both biological and experiential factors, such as language acquisition and mode of language acquisition, interact in determining the functional organization of the brain. This research suggests that the linguistic function is primarily served by the left hemisphere, even when the language presented is visual–spatial in nature.

We stated in the introduction that throughout man's evolution, language has been forged in the vocal–auditory system. If, in addition, speech has been specially selected for, if sound constitutes such a natural signal for language, then it is all the more striking how the human mind, when deprived of the faculty that makes sound accessible, seizes on, perfects and systematizes an alternative form to enable the deeper linguistic faculties to give explicit expression to ideas.

ACKNOWLEDGEMENTS

This work was supported in part by National Institutes of Health Grant NS-09811 and by National Science Foundation Grant BNS-78-07225 to The Salk Institute for Biological Studies. Illustrations are made by Frank A. Paul.

References

1. KLIMA, E. S. & BELLUGI, U. (1979) *The Signs of Language*, Harvard University Press, Cambridge, Mass.
2. NEWPORT, E. & BELLUGI, U. (1978) Linguistic expression of category levels in a visual-gestural language, in *Cognition and Categorization* (Rosch, E. & Lloyd, B. B., eds.), pp. 49–71, Erlbaum, Hillsdale, New Jersey
3. BELLUGI, U. & NEWKIRK, D. (1979) Formal devices for creating new signs in American Sign Language, in *Proc. Natl. Symp. Sign Lang. Res. Teaching* (Stokoe, W. C., ed.) in press
4. LIDDELL, S. K. (1978) Nonmanual signals and relative clauses in American Sign Language, in *Understanding Language Through Sign Language Research* (Siple, P., ed.), pp. 59–90, Academic Press, New York
5. BELLUGI, U. & FISCHER, S. (1972) A comparison of sign language and spoken language. *Cognition 1*, 173–200
6. BELLUGI, U. & KLIMA, E. S. (1975) Aspects of sign language and its structure, in *The Role of Speech in Language* (Kavanagh, J. F. & Cutting, J. E., eds.), pp. 171–203, MIT Press, Cambridge, Mass.
7. BELLUGI, U. & KLIMA, E. S. (1976) Two faces of sign: iconic and abstract. *Ann. N.Y. Acad. Sci. 280*, 514–538
8. BELLUGI, U., KLIMA, E. S. & SIPLE, P. (1975) Remembering in signs. *Cognition 3*, 93–125
9. POIZNER, H. & LANE, H. (1979) Cerebral asymmetry in the perception of American Sign Language. *Brain Lang.*, 7, 210–226
10. KLIMA, E. S. (1975) Sound and its absence in the linguistic symbol, in *The Role of Speech in Language* (Kavanagh, J. & Cutting, J., eds.), pp. 249–270, MIT Press, Cambridge, Mass.
11. STOKOE, W. C. Jr. (1960) *Sign Language Structure*, University of Buffalo Press, Buffalo, New York
12. STOKOE, W. C. Jr., CASTERLINE, D. & CRONEBERG, C. (1965) *A Dictionary of American Sign Language*, Gallaudet College Press, Washington, D.C.
13. NORMAN, D. A. (1976) *Memory and Attention*, Wiley, New York
14. BELLUGI, U. & SIPLE, P. (1974) Remembering with and without words, in *Problems in Psycholinguistics* (Bresson, F., ed.), pp. 215–236, Centre National de la Recherche Scientifique, Paris
15. NEWKIRK, D., KLIMA, E. S., PEDERSEN, C. C. & BELLUGI, U. (1979) Linguistic evidence from slips of the hand, in *Slips of the Tongue, Ear, Pen, and Hands* (Fromkin, V., ed.), Academic Press, New York, in press

16. FROMKIN, V. A. (1973) Slips of the tongue. *Sci. Am. 229* (6), 110–117
17. FRISHBERG, N. (1975) Arbitrariness and iconicity: historical change in American Sign Language. *Language 51*, 696–719
18. FRISHBERG, N. (1976) Some aspects of historical change in American Sign Language. Dissertation, University of California, San Diego
19. KLIMA, E. S. & BELLUGI, U. (1975) Wit and poetry in American Sign Language. *Sign Lang. Stud. 8*, 204–223
20. KLIMA, E. S. & BELLUGI, U. (1978) Poetry without sound, *Hum. Nat. 1 (10)*, 74–83
21. NEVILLE, H. & BELLUGI, U. (1978) Patterns of cerebral specialization in congenitally deaf adults, in *Understanding Language Through Sign Language Research* (Siple, P., ed.), pp. 239–257, Academic Press, New York
22. NEVILLE, H. (1977) Electrographic and behavioral cerebral specialization in normal and congenitally deaf children: a preliminary report, in *Language Development and Neurological Theory* (Segalowitz, S., ed.), pp. 121–131, Academic Press, New York

Commentary on papers by Detlev Ploog and Ursula Bellugi

JONATHAN BENNETT

Department of Philosophy, University of British Columbia, Vancouver*

Out of the rich array of hard facts and glittering conjectures which Detlev Ploog has laid before us, I can pick up only a few. I shall offer some questions, suggestions, amplifications—perhaps even criticisms—which may help to set the direction for the discussion.

SELF-AWARENESS

For reasons which will emerge, I take first what Ploog takes last—namely self-awareness.

I am not clear what anyone means by 'self-aware' or 'self-conscious', and I suspect that there is no one hard-edged concept of self-awareness waiting to be clarified. There are many ways in which a sentient being can be cognitively related to itself; and which of these should be regarded as of prime importance —for instance in creating an interesting division within the animal kingdom— must depend upon a lot of empirical knowledge about what sorts of self-knowledge there are. Eventually the selecting and defining of a preferred concept of self-awareness will involve philosophical reflection, but for that we shall need more than we have at present in the way of facts to think *about*.

Ploog certainly gives us something to think about. When the squirrel monkey produces a call, the parts of the brain which register the call are informed of it through a short-cut which lies entirely within the brain, avoiding the detour through sound-waves, ears and acoustic nerves. These beautiful results must surely go into any informed consideration of self-awareness and its place in nature.

*Present address: Department of Philosophy, Syracuse University, Syracuse, NY 13210, USA

I have a couple of questions about those results, though.

(1) Granted that the monkey's calls are registered in its brain through a different mechanism from the calls of others, I wonder whether the monkey can *discriminate* between its own calls and those of others—taking discrimination as something cognitive which would show up in behaviour. Ploog doesn't say whether this difference of brain mechanisms is accompanied in the monkey by a cognitive difference: he cites some of his own work on one aspect of the monkey's knowledge about its vocalizations, but not an aspect which bears on my present question.

Ploog remarks that if human babies are like monkeys in the relevant respect, this 'means that human infants can also make the distinction between their own vocalizations and vocal input from others'. This seems to treat a cognitive question as automatically answered by a claim about mechanisms in the brain; but surely we need behavioural evidence too. Ploog mentions evidence (presumably behavioural) of the baby's ability to discriminate between phonemic and non-phonemic sounds, but that doesn't bear on its ability to discriminate its own voice from those of others.

When Ploog says that 'Long before speech becomes possible human infants develop self-awareness and demonstrate consciousness of self by their preverbal competence in social interactions', he is going too fast for me: I am not clear what concept of self-awareness he is using, or upon what behavioural basis. But it is evidently not a concept which owes much—directly at least—to that work on how the brain of the squirrel monkey registers its own sounds.

(2) I wonder whether there are more lowly animals in which the information about a noise the animal makes is reported to its brain along a pathway which lies wholly within the brain, by-passing the mechanisms whereby it registers noises from outside. If it turned out that birds do this too, that might lessen our inclination to think that this feature—even if reflected in a cognitive discrimination—was a very important part of that cloudy concept of self-awareness which we are hoping to capture and render precise. *Has* any work been done on this lower down the scale?

That is all I want to say about self-awareness. I now go back to the beginning of Ploog's paper.

ONTOGENY RECAPITULATES PHYLOGENY

Ploog compares the development of the human child's vocal repertoire with that of the monkey, in the light of what is known and conjectured about the cerebral control of each. The basic picture is this:

(i) One area of the brain which in many animals controls the vocal cords, etc., and organizes vocal activity, is purely a matter of 'hard wiring', owing nothing to the lessons of the individual animal's experience.

(ii) Another area, in primates only, adds a further measure of control: the same kinds of vocal performance are involved, but now they are 'instrumental', i.e. motivated by *learnt* associations between vocalization and reward.

(iii) A third area is, in humans alone, also somehow involved in vocal behaviour, in control of the facial area; and it is assumed to be involved in the processes of learning human language.

The first level

Ploog points out differences as well as similarities between the human and non-human first stages. I want to comment on the dissimilarities.

(1) The 'babbling' of the human baby is unlike the vocalizations of non-human primates both in constituting an enlargement of vocal repertoire and in having no potential signalling function. The explanation of babbling which Ploog suggests, namely that it is a kind of practice for the Herculean vocal labours which lie ahead, is presumably right. Although the babbling occurs along with vocal behaviour which *is* comparable with that of non-human primates, it is itself a sheer extra—not part of the recapitulation-of-phylogeny picture, but rather an adaptation for that special kind of vocal future which lies ahead of the young human but not of the monkey.

Babbling aside, the baby's vocalizations could be called 'signals', in the sense that much information can be inferred from them. But they differ in two big ways from the signals of non-human animals.

(2) In many non human species, some signals contain information about topics other than the present state of the signaller, in particular, about the future behaviour of the signaller or about the environment. And the behaviour which it is a signal's function to elicit is sometimes useful not to the signaller directly but rather to the audience; e.g. signals which warn of danger. In contrast, the signals of the small human baby are informative only about its present condition, and are useful—if at all—only to the baby itself. It is easy to see why: the human baby's lack of motor capacity prevents it from having behavioural intentions which others need to know about, and from having much environmental information which it would be useful for others to know.

(3) Also, most of the informative content of the human baby's signals is lost on its adult guardians. The perceptible differences between cries signalling pain, hunger, loneliness, frustration, interruption of feeding, etc., apparently aren't picked up by the parent. I don't mean just that parents aren't consciously

aware of the differences, but that there is behavioural evidence showing that 'The social influence of the different cries on the parent is not nearly as specific in the human species as it is in the lower species'.[1] This is unsurprising. With a non-human species, much adult behaviour which is essential to the survival of an infant won't occur unless triggered by signals from the infant; so a parent which isn't wired to respond to a hunger signal by feeding the infant will have a dead infant. Human behaviour is of course much less rigidly controlled than this, i.e. much more accessible to the results of individual learning; to which we can add that humans can learn faster and more copiously than can non-humans, and —uniquely amongst animals on this planet—can transmit general information to one another. So a human mother can have and act upon her society's knowledge that, for instance, babies die if they are not fed often enough, which removes the need for her to be sensitive to shades of difference amongst the baby's signals.

So human babies differ from monkeys in one respect which concerns their different vocal futures, a second one arising from their different motor capacities, and a third which reflects the different intellectual levels of their adult conspecifics.

The second level

In what Ploog says about the 'instrumental' use of vocal signals—the use which is 'learnt' or produced by conditioning—there is something I don't quite understand. He reports that structures in the limbic cortex control these instrumental or learnt vocalizations, and says that this part of the brain 'serves this function in primates only'. Is it that non-primates cannot be changed in their vocal behaviour by conditioning, or rather that when they are thus changed it is a different part of the brain that is in control?

I don't want to make anything of this: I simply want to know. Either way, an important aspect of the brain control of vocal behaviour is present in all primates and in no other animals. I find this remarkable. Given how greatly primates differ in vocal behaviour, because human beings have semantically structured languages and non-human primates don't, in the wild anyway, I can't easily get this great similarity into perspective. It might be replied that it is just a matter of a similarity conjoined with a difference: the similarity is an adaptation which we share with the monkeys and the apes, though it is no longer of much use to us, and our real linguistic capacities are simply a further feature which the other primates lack. But that picture is wrong, because Ploog tells us that 'patients with lesions in these areas have only slight difficulties in repeating sentences, but may often lose spontaneous speech completely'. So it seems that that cingulate area of the brain is involved in our strictly linguistic activities too; and I am having trouble viewing it both in this light and as something we share with the non-human primates.

Something remarkable begins to emerge. If we accept Ploog's basic comparison of the non-human primates with certain aspects of humans, the above-mentioned loss by humans of the capacity for spontaneous speech must be put on a par with—regarded as somehow comparable with—the loss by monkeys of their learnt vocal responses when they suffer destruction of the cingulate area. This need not imply that human speech *is nothing but* a repertoire of vocal signals acquired through conditioning; but it does imply that spontaneous speech *involves* learnt vocal signalling, not merely as a required stepping-stone towards full linguistic competence—something one uses for a while and then leaves behind—but rather as a crutch, which one must take everywhere if one is not to fall down. If it were merely a stepping-stone, damage to the cingulate area of the brain would not cause the loss of linguistic competence once it had been acquired.

Has the concept of a learnt vocal response any real work to do in the description of full-fledged human linguistic behaviour? Many would say No. The prevailing philosophical climate is hostile to the view that normal human language-use has any significant overlap with what goes on in conditioned responses to stimuli. If that hostility is justified, then this part of Ploog's comparison needs to be modified, e.g. so that it says that the cingulate area of the brain controls learnt vocal responses in non-humans and has in humans a function which, though doubtless an evolutionary descendant of that one, is in itself quite different from it.

I have no view about which side is right. I do think that Ploog's findings, and the persuasive general comparison which he bases on them, provide some reason to predict that the concept of operant conditioning will turn out to have a working role in the best full description of human language-use.

In any case, this matter is interesting and I am grateful to Ploog for re-raising it from this fresh angle.

The third level

This much is clear: an area in the cortex controls movements of the larynx, tongue and face; these organs are used in vocalization by humans but not by non-humans; and so this cortical area helps to govern human vocalization but not that of other primates. But I went wrong in my understanding of Ploog when I came to his added remark: 'It is assumed that these structures play a role in the process of vocal learning and mediate learned articulatory movements'. It was not clear to me in Ploog's paper how strong an assumption that was meant to be, and I was led to inflate it by my desire to connect it with a problem which interests me. I shall explain.

We know that full-fledged human languages involve complex and sophisticated structures, governed by elaborate rules which are now being discovered by the transformational grammarians; and it seems that virtually all of that structure-handling capacity is special to humans. One wonders what region of our brain controls our handlings of linguistic structure, and it occurred to me that Ploog might have been proposing that the region in question is the cortical larynx and face area which belongs on his third level.

He has explained to me that that is mistaken, and that he proposed to associate that area of the brain with the control of certain sound-producing activities but not with anything like the management of syntactic structure. So I have no comments on his third level.

But I shall, independently of Ploog's paper, briefly canvass the idea that the management of linguistic structure is indeed linked in the brain with the same aspect of the control of vocalization, so that at the level of brain control there is an intimate connection between what is *linguistic* and what is *vocal*.

CHOMSKY'S HYPOTHESIS

Of course there can be—and indeed are—languages whose modality is not vocal and auditory. But they are special cases. If Chomsky is right in his hypothesis that we have innate mental capacities whose function is solely or primarily the handling of linguistic structure, it would not be surprising if they rested upon specializations of the vocalizing parts of the brain.

On the other hand, if Chomsky is wrong, and the grammatical structures of natural languages merely reflect the application of general intelligence to problems of communication, then it would be unbelievable that our grasp of them should be localized in the region controlling the larynx and the face.

So the view which I am considering—the one which I at first thought might be Ploog's—implies that Chomsky is right. It also implies an answer to a question which is urgently raised by Chomsky's hypothesis but which he seems never to have discussed. If the brain behaves differently when handling language from how it behaves in processing practical problems generally, how does it know when it is handling language? The specifically linguistic mechanisms in the brain cannot be brought into play by a brain event corresponding to the thought *I am dealing with language:* the common concept of language is too vague and ill-defined to correlate with any characteristic kind of event in the brain which could do the triggering job. It is a bit more plausible to suppose that there is a specific kind of brain event correlated with the person's *wanting to communicate;* but it is hard to have much enthusiasm for that either.

The answer implied by the view now under consideration is that the language-structuring mechanisms in the brain are triggered by the fact that voluntary vocal behaviour is being engaged in. That answer strikes me as more inherently plausible than any alternative I can think of.

It needs to be strengthened in two ways, however, because our linguistic competence is exercised passively as well as actively, and in written language as well as in spoken. But there could well be supplementary mechanisms linking the primary vocalization trigger with secondary auditory and script/visual triggers, in the brain of someone who has learnt to correlate speaking with hearing, and to correlate speaking/hearing with writing/reading.

Incidentally, I cannot clearly link the question I have been raising with the data on hemispheric dominance. That is because Chomsky's hypothesis is as much concerned with passive as with active linguistic competence, whereas hemispheric dominance seems—judging from such reports as I have read—to be strictly a matter of active competence: the non-dominant hemisphere apparently 'understands' language as well as the dominant one does. One can envisage a primary triggering mechanism which is restricted to one hemisphere though socially linked with a secondary trigger in the other; but that presupposes that what is being triggered is itself present in both hemispheres. If Chomskyan 'universal grammar' rests on brain mechanisms belonging only to the dominant hemisphere, and if that dominance really does pertain only to active and not to passive competence, then Chomsky's whole account of linguistic capacity would have to be restructured so as to give central prominence to the distinction between active and passive competence. I have no idea of how that restructuring might go.

AMERICAN SIGN LANGUAGE (ASL)

I return now to the idea that Chomsky's hypothesis is true, and that the primary trigger is vocal. One way of testing this double conjecture would be to examine a language such as ASL, which is not vocal–auditory and has developed through use by people who have never had a vocal–auditory language. If the deep structures of vocal languages reflect mechanisms in the brain which are triggered by vocalization, or by activities which have been socially correlated with vocalization, then it is to be expected that the ASL will be structurally different from every vocal language, i.e. will not share those deep grammatical features which are supposed to reflect the specifically language-oriented systems in our brains.

That would not be so if the grammar of the ASL had been imposed upon it from the outside; we can discard that possibility if we take very literally the report of Ursula Bellugi and Edward Klima[2] that 'It became clear to us with our first encounter with the system of communication which is transmitted from one generation of deaf people to the next, that their language was not based on English in any essential way'.

The known differences between ASL and English are all at the level of noun- and verb-phrases: they concern the nature of the basic lexical units, and the ways those units are encoded, stored in the memory, built into compounds, inflected, and so on. Some of this can fairly be called grammatical. Dr Bellugi and her colleagues have done work of great power and beauty on the grammar of inflexions in ASL: they have found that the basic meanings of signs can be systematically varied—giving 'chair' from 'sit', 'babyish' from 'baby', 'habitually quiet' from 'quiet', and so on—by systematic variations of hand movements. The relevant parameters of change in the hand movements have been identified, classified and interrelated, and many results about them have been established. For instance, the iconicity of ASL signs is less important than one might think, since it is frequently submerged by the grammatical changes now under discussion.

But to my disappointment I can't bring these grammatical discoveries to bear in any significant way on the question I have been raising. The question is: do natural vocal languages reflect in their deep structures features of our minds—and thus mechanisms in our brains—which are special to language, and are these brain mechanisms primarily triggered by vocalization? Those who find Chomsky's hypothesis plausible do so mainly, I believe, on the strength of facts about the grammar of whole sentences and their inter-relationships, rather than anything which is confined to linguistic units less than the sentence. If that is right, and if I am right in believing that the transformational grammar of ASL sentences has not yet been worked on, it is premature to look to ASL for evidence bearing on my question.

Dr Bellugi's paper concludes by tentatively propounding a remarkable suggestion about hemispheric dominance in users of ASL, namely that although they resemble most of the rest of us in having a linguistically dominant left hemisphere, they are unlike us in that their visual–spatial functions are also controlled by that same hemisphere. It will be fascinating to watch further developments on that as on all other aspects of this wonderful research programme; but I have explained why the findings on hemispheric dominance seem not to bear directly on my question about the brain substratum of the special language-structuring capacities—the innate 'universal grammar'—which Chomsky thinks must be postulated to explain human linguistic competence.

Of course my question is not Dr Bellugi's: I am simply connecting her work as best I can with an issue about brain and mind which interests me and which I at first thought might link her work with Dr Ploog's.

References

1. WOLFF, P. H. (1969) The natural history of crying and other vocalizations in early infancy, in *Determinants of Infant Behaviour IV* (Foss, M. B., ed.), pp. 81–109, Methuen, London (at p. 83)
2. KLIMA, E. S., & BELLUGI, U. (1979) Properties of symbols in a silent language, in *Du Contrôle Moteur à l'Organisation Gestuelle* (Hécaen, H. & Jeannerod, M., eds.), Masson, Paris

Discussion: Language

Putnam: One of Chomsky's arguments for what he called *the language organ* was the 'what else could it be' argument. The argument was that if we had to rely on general intelligence to learn our native language, only geniuses could solve the problem. The language organ hypothesis implies that humans couldn't learn a Martian language which lacked human linguistic universals. Chomsky's argument about linguistic universals was that they were *arbitrary*, not dependent on the functional aspect of language. In his Russell Lectures, he said explicitly that it is the existence of universal features of language which are *not* functionally explainable that demonstrates the 'innateness' of language. In his view, if we found extraterrestrials they might well speak a language which could only be translated by machines or by geniuses working for years and which human beings could not learn. Ursula Bellugi's work puts this collection of ideas into very hot water. First of all American Sign Language (ASL) lacks universal features of phonology, described by Chomsky and Halle. Those features were supposed to be pretty far down the level of speech. If, as you suggested, there are two kinds of language—one which we learn using general intelligence—Chomsky is in trouble.

Bennett: It would depend on what the properties are of the language that is learnt by general intelligence. Chomsky couldn't deny that a language could be learnt by general intelligence if we made it simple enough.

Seurle: What implication do you think this research holds for the innateness hypothesis, Dr Bellugi?

Bellugi: There has been a preconception in linguistics that sound is central, if not essential, to language, and our evidence certainly calls this into question. We are now beginning to specify the complex rules which relate surface lexical forms and inflectional forms (Ref. 1, ch. 12). It appears likely that the same kinds of rule systems (phonological and morphophonemic) will underlie both spoken and sign languages, despite the fact that one is based on aural–oral signals and the other on visual–gestural signals. We are also specifying the aspects of form that appear to be specific to the modality in which the language develops; thus we are investigating how and within what limits the transmission end shapes the rest of the linguistic system. It may well be that for both sign language and spoken language certain kinds of perceptual strategies and memory processes may determine aspects of language structure that were at one time called innate.

Medawar: The existence of ASL as quite a subtle language seems to undermine Chomsky's views. One of the obvious things about ASL is that it has to be learnt. It would be absurd to suggest that any of these gestures could be preprogrammed.

Searle: I am not sure that gesture is preprogrammed.

Bennett: In Chomsky's hypothesis what are preprogrammed are some of the very general principles by which one goes from data to conclusions— principles which guide how, when you have been exposed to such and such linguistic data, you go on performing in certain ways. It seems perfectly possible that Chomsky is right that these exist and that they cover ASL as well. What I was saying was that ASL could provide a test for both whether the Chomsky hypothesis is right and whether the brain mechanisms are vocally triggered. That is possibly too specialized for us to discuss here.

Young: If Dr Bellugi could show us the signs for mind and intentionality it might help us in our discussions.

Searle: Does ASL have words for 'belief', 'fear', 'hope', 'desire' and so on, and in what sense are they iconic?

Bellugi: Perhaps I need to clear up some points before responding. There are different sign languages, as there are different spoken languages. The sign language developed by deaf people in Great Britain is entirely different from ASL, for example. International meetings of deaf people from different countries require sign interpreters, not just from spoken languages to sign language, but from one sign language to another.

Contemporary signs of ASL are generally opaque. Except for a very small proportion of signs, one cannot guess the meaning of the sign from its form alone. While there are signs of American Sign Language for concepts such as 'mind', 'information', 'belief', 'fear', 'hope', 'desire', 'lateralization', 'grammar', and 'philosophy', they are, for the most part, non-transparent signs.

Young: Do those deaf people have discussions on philosophical questions?

Bellugi: Yes, deaf people have discussions on philosophical, linguistic and metalinguistic questions, experimental design, cognitive psychology. Such discussions occur regularly within our laboratory, carried on in ASL with the deaf members of our research group. Of course, new vocabulary sometimes has to be created. We have recently completed a study of the mechanisms within ASL whereby lexical gaps are filled, including formal devices such as compounding and derivational processes.[2]

Young: Do they understand the square root of −1?

Searle: That goes with writing. That whole language was never vocal.

Bunge: Professor Ploog, what is the minimum size of a neuronal system capable of responding to a specific sentence?

Ploog: I don't think one can answer that question. Many of the 100 million or so neurons in the primary auditory cortex are involved in each answer. This is only one of several cortical areas involved in decoding auditory messages, not to speak of all the subcortical structures of the auditory system.

Blakemore: The question is certainly difficult to answer. The number of neurons involved in the recognition of any event depends on the type of expression to which that recognition is being put. There is no unique end to a process of recognition somewhere in the nervous system. Recognition is defined by the action it produces. The minimum number of neurons that can potentially be involved in setting off a behavioural response may be one alone, since a single photoreceptor in the eye is capable of responding to a single quantum of light.

Bunge: The answer betrays a reductionistic confusion between levels of nervous system activity. My question did not concern the detection of stimuli —which even unicellular organisms can do—but the production of sentences.

Blakemore: I think that you should also specify by what kind of outward response you wish to judge the response of the nervous system. There is no single level at which one can say that an event has been recognized by some hypothetical internal analyser.

Bunge: Surely between one neuron and the whole nervous system there are neuronal systems of intermediate size?

Searle: Did you ask the question just to get a quantitative estimate?

Bunge: No. Some people think that single neurons can think of their grandmother, the so-called pontifical neuron. Others say that the whole brain is needed for that. I was asking whether there was some subsystem that could do the trick.

Ploog: If you take out the whole auditory cortex of a monkey bilaterally, the monkey is unable to distinguish between noises and calls. That is, if you take out that cortical area the capacity for recognizing not only the animal's own calls but all other noises is lost. The animal can then respond only to noise or not-noise. It is not deaf. If you condition it to do a certain task, it will do that task on hearing any noise.

Bunge: So there is sensation but not perception?

Ploog: You might call it sensation. At any rate, this area is necessary for decoding acoustic energy, including species-specific calls. The intact monkey can distinguish between hundreds of variations of species-specific calls and all other sounds and noises presented to him. The animal can probably also distinguish between different members of the group without needing to see the other animals.

Bunge: Dr Bellugi, you said that ASL is at the same time iconic and abstract.

Do you mean 'abstract' in the sense that grammar is not visual and not perceptible?

Bellugi: The language as it has evolved today has aspects that are both formally and conceptually abstract. For example, morphological processes operate on abstract structures such as compounds and noun-phrases in different ways. There are processes for deriving predicates from nouns, for forming nominalizations of verbs, for forming conditional sentences and relative clauses. There are also processes for the syntactic realization of abstract concepts, such as the one that transforms temporary states into inherent qualities.

Crown: I suggest that the philosophers are making the area of self-awareness too simple. In clinical work, and also in the observation of normal persons, certain areas have to be accounted for when we are thinking about self-awareness. Take the creative person, for example: when musicians, poets or playwrights are asked how they create they say they don't know. They just go along with the process and it seems to come; they must not question it too much or it stops. In hypnosis, particularly the form of self-awareness known as post-hypnotic suggestion, people may demonstrate the remarkable phenomenon of a negative hallucination—they report that someone they are apparently observing is not there. In clinical psychiatry schizophrenic patients demonstrate bizarre disorders of body image. And what is the state of self-awareness in schizophrenic patients apparently in a catatonic stupor with grossly reduced awareness who, when the stupor remits, can report accurately what has gone on around them? Finally, to return to the other pathological phenomena: one resembles hospital addiction and is sometimes called the Munchausen syndrome. The person comes into hospital repeatedly with simulated disorders which may even lead to their being operated on. These people appear to be in a state of normal awareness. The other area is the Ganser state in which persons in stressful situations, particularly in courts of law, give approximate answers, such as $2 + 2 = 5$, to simple questions.

It was said in discussion that communication between human adults and young babies may be less complicated than among animals. I question this. There is increasing convergence of view between ethologists, child developmentalists and psychoanalysts that the first year of life is crucially important. For example, whether a person develops a basic trust in other persons or not may arise in the first year, and may relate to how sensitive parents are in interpreting communications of need from the cries of their babies.

Dr Bellugi, how subtle is communication between people using American Sign Language? Would they communicate sexual desire or would some sort of inhibition exist in ASL as in normal speech?

Bellugi: Communication between deaf people using American Sign Language is capable of a wide variety of nuances, just as is any spoken language. We have not focused, in our research, on conditions of language use or inhibition, so I cannot directly answer your question.

Crown: Which side of the brain is most basic for ASL?

Bellugi: There is some preliminary evidence that for right-handed native deaf signers, signs are processed better by the left hemisphere than the right, as I mentioned in my paper. We are now embarking on a series of studies of cerebral specialization for other aspects of sign language (e.g. grammatical processes). The clinical evidence for effects of cerebral lesions among deaf patients is not definitive (see Poizner & Battison[3] for a good review of this area).

Towers: Is the right hand used more in signs than the left?

Bellugi: A one-handed sign has the same lexical meaning regardless of which hand is used. One hand is more active than the other for the majority of ASL signs, but which one depends on the handedness of the signer.

Cooper: With the new non-invasive techniques such as computer axial scanning, if you followed a large enough population for long enough you could determine whether different areas are involved when these people become unable to speak.

Bellugi: We are planning studies of signing skills of elderly deaf people before and after cardiovascular accidents.

Cooper: A very unappreciated fact characteristic of the nervous system which was noted in Dr Ploog's study is that no sound could be produced from stimulation of the cortex, yet sounds could be inhibited by stimulation of a relatively small area in the cortex which resembled Broca's area. Am I correct in thinking that when you anaesthetized the cortex, stimulation of lower centres no longer produced vocalization?

Ploog: No, I said that single units in the auditory cortex can be inhibited if the call is a self-produced one and they can be excited if the same call is played back on tape. The same cell responds in two different ways.

Cooper: Yes, I understood that. Did you make any ablative or temporarily ablative lesions in the cortex?

Ploog: Yes; as I said, if we take off the auditory cortex completely, the monkey is not able to distinguish between its own calls, the calls of other monkeys, and any other noises. It can distinguish only noise and non-noise.[4]

Plum: Are the lesions unilateral or bilateral?

Ploog: Bilateral. In addition, if one takes out the analogue to Broca, the facial motor area and the lateral frontal cortex, the monkey is able to vocalize or even be conditioned to external stimuli. If one takes out the cingulate area bilaterally the monkey loses the ability to respond to conditioned stimuli; one might say the monkey is not able to use its voice voluntarily.[5]

Creutzfeldt: Did you say that if you electrically stimulate the Broca analogue, you are not able to elicit the same type of vocalization as after cingulate stimulation?

Ploog: If one stimulates the facial area in the monkey one sees a movement of the vocal chords but there is no vocalization.[6] If one does the same thing in human beings there is both vocalization and movement of the vocal chords.[7]

Young: But that is not Broca's area.

Ploog: Stimulation of Broca's area in humans does not yield vocalization. I mean the facial–laryngeal area.

Warrington: Dr Bellugi, I was particularly interested in your description of visual errors on short-term memory tasks in subjects using ASL. Have you estimated the capacity of their visual short-term memory system? Do you think they use the same structures as we do? There is some evidence for different anatomical structures sub-serving auditory short-term memory and visual short-term memory in normal subjects. The capacities of these two systems seem to be rather different, the capacity of the visual short-term memory system being rather less than the capacity of the auditory short-term memory.

Bellugi: In a study comparing short-term memory among hearing and deaf subjects,[8] we presented the same lists of items to hearing people in spoken English and to deaf people in ASL at the rate of one item per second. We found that the memory span was one item shorter on average for deaf people than for hearing people. But the two situations were in fact not entirely comparable since the signs took up twice as much of the one-second interval as the words, and thus the deaf people presumably had less rehearsal time than the hearing people. The possible connection between memory and grammatical structure is intriguing; the answer must await further research.

Warrington: So memory in the deaf people approximated this magic figure of seven plus or minus two, did it?

Bellugi: In our study, hearing subjects had a memory span of about six items; for deaf subjects it was about five items.

Towers: One item about human vocalization which has always intrigued me has been lost sight of in the last twenty or thirty years. That is, when we vocalize we set up sound waves in the larynx which we then manipulate on the mucous membrane of the pharynx and the mouth cavity. We manipulate those sounds by use of the tongue against the palate, teeth, lips and so on. That is only possible because the human larynx is situated so far down in the neck. In all other mammals the larynx is very much higher in position. In some mammals such as sea-dwelling mammals the larynx is permanently situated in the nasal cavity, so when they set up sound waves all they can do is to set up blips or noises through the blow-hole. They cannot manipulate those sound waves to make different sounds as we do. Grazing mammals almost always breathe through the nose; when they graze the food goes back and round the epiglottis, through the lateral food channels, as we call them. In other words, food particles for them meet the front of the larynx at the back of the mouth. For all non-human mammals, including higher primates, it is only possible to vocalize through the mouth by opening the mouth wide, very often by throwing the head back, as the dog does when it bays or barks at the moon.

In the human fetus the larynx is situated in the same position as in all other mammals. The epiglottis rests above the soft palate in the human fetus and in the neonate. The human neonate is an obligatory nose-breather; if it is born with a blockage of the nostrils it dies unless a tube is put down its larynx. It cannot breathe through its mouth other than by having the jaw and other structures pulled down. Only after six to eight months, when the larynx begins to drop down, is it possible for the baby to begin to vocalize in the normal human way. Even if it had the wit to vocalize, it would be anatomically impossible. That has been a very important feature in the development of human language in evolutionary terms. Whether the dropping of the larynx stimulated the brain in evolution I don't know, but the larynx had to drop before human speech became possible.

Ploog: This has been a major issue ever since Philip Lieberman[9] advanced his hypothesis comparing Neanderthal Man, the human neonate and apes in this regard. In mongol children (Down syndrome), for instance, the larynx doesn't descend and the upper airways do not function properly.

The issue of what is first, the egg or the hen, has been with us since Darwin. According to ethological theory, the adaptive function of the signal requires not only the development of the appropriate signalling apparatus of the sender but also the development by the receiver of proper means of decoding that signal. Brain organization and motor behaviour correspond to each other. I don't think one can decide which comes first.

Crow: How much is known about the precise anatomical structures involved in the vocalization pathways you described, Dr Ploog? In this caudal brain-stem there is the nucleus ambiguus in the diagram you showed. At the next stage up there are cells in the central grey matter and there are cells lateral to the central grey matter. Do we know what these structures are?

Ploog: The parabrachial nuclei are involved and below those there is a fractionating of natural calls. That is, the integration level for natural calls must be not lower than the parabrachial nuclei.

Crow: At a higher level the loops you drew didn't include the basal ganglia, did they? I am wondering whether these pathways are analogous to those involved in the control of voluntary movement. For example speech is affected in Parkinson's disease and this suggests that the basal ganglia are included in the control mechanism for speech in the same way as they are involved in the control of voluntary movements.

Ploog: The cingular vocal pathway accompanies the corticospinal tract down to the caudal diencephalon; the pathway then ascends dorsally into the periaqueductal grey matter and follows this structure to its end, where it sweeps laterally to the parabrachial area.[10]

Crow: So you would say it was part of the pyramidal tract, in some sense?

Ploog: Yes, partly, until it leaves the cerebral peduncle.

Plum: Dr Bellugi, how many people do you have available to study?

Bellugi: I have worked with more than 400 deaf people.

Plum: If there is ever any reason to justify a cerebral arteriogram for one of these people, the so-called Wada test which anaesthetizes the speech mechanism with a unilateral injection of sodium amobarbital might give useful information.

Recent techniques suggest that different thoughts may be the product of different areas in the brain. Current studies of cerebral blood flow[11] seem to show that if someone thinks internally, for example if they silently count numbers in the mind, the regional metabolism of the brain is distributed differently than if the person thinks about moving the hand or actually moves the hand. There is even some evidence that more emotional thinking—imagery or drifting reverie, as it were—commands different levels of metabolic responsibility in different structures from mathematical activity. David Ingvar,[12] using the same technique, even finds that patients with schizophrenia have a regional cerebral blood flow (and, by inference, metabolism) different from that in normal people. The implications are that normal and abnormal thought processes reflect grossly different brain mechanisms. If so, the finding forces an entirely new approach to the biology of our conscious behaviour.

Cooper: I have had the misfortune, in operating on many cases of neurological disorders and placing discrete lesions, particularly in the thalamus, to encounter a few cases where aphonia was a consequence of the bilateral operation. It has never occurred with unilateral operation but there is a 13% chance of temporary but recognizable dysphonia or dysarthria when bilateral lesions are placed in the thalamus. Out of thousands of operations we have seen six cases of aphonia in which the pyramidal tract was most certainly not invaded—the lesions were well within the thalamus. I know of no one who can explain that unfortunate phenomenon. Also, a lesion in the dominant ventrolateral nucleus of the thalamus not infrequently produces a temporary aphasia which, if it is not recognizable clinically, is picked up by the pathologist. Except in the aged, this disappears in a few weeks. Our clinical psychologist has found a very notable fall-off in abstract thinking in the older patients after a small lesion in the right thalamus, again in the ventrolateral nucleus which is theoretically a motor relay nucleus but is in fact a sensory structure. Those unfortunately negative observations somehow have to be put into the scheme of vocalization and probably of speech too.

Ploog: I agree fully. All I am saying is that parts of the limbic system of the caudal diencephalon, midbrain and pons are involved in vocalization. Motor aphasia was for a long time thought to be a merely cortical or sub-cortical phenomenon but it is now more readily explained by including structures which are part of the vocal system.

Marsden: In human beings bilateral damage to the corticobulbar portions of the pyramidal pathways not only causes difficulties in speech but also produces emotional incontinence. People laugh when they are not happy and cry when they are not sad. Does something similar happen in animals?

Ploog: There is no way to judge that but of course the rudimentary vocalizations of people with motor aphasia almost always consist of emotional curses and other kinds of vestigial speech they wouldn't make otherwise. That is certainly tied to damage in limbic areas.[13]

References

1. KLIMA, E. S. & BELLUGI, U. (1979) *The Signs of Language*, Harvard University Press, Cambridge, Mass.
2. BELLUGI, U. & NEWKIRK, D. (1979) Formal devices for creating new signs in American Sign Language, in *Proc. Natl. Symp. Sign Lang. Res. Teaching* (Stokoe, W. C., ed.), in press
3. POIZNER, H. & BATTISON, R. (1979) Cerebral asymmetry for sign language: clinical and experimental evidence. *Langages*, in press
4. HUPFER, K., JÜRGENS, U. & PLOOG, D. (1977) The effect of superior temporal lesions on the recognition of species-specific calls in the squirrel monkey. *Exp. Brain Res. 30*, 75–87
5. SUTTON, D., LARSON, C. & LINDEMAN, R. C. (1974) Neocortical and limbic lesion effects on primate phonation. *Brain Res. 71*, 61–75
6. JÜRGENS, U. (1976) Projections from the cortical larynx area in the squirrel monkey. *Exp. Brain Res. 25*, 401–411
7. PENFIELD, W. & ROBERTS, L. (1959) *Speech and Brain Mechanisms*, Princeton University Press, Princeton, N.J.
8. BELLUGI, U., KLIMA, E. S. & SIPLE, P. (1975) Remembering in signs. *Cognition 3*, 93–125
9. LIEBERMAN, P. (1973) On the evolution of language: a unified view. *Cognition 2*, 59–94

10. JÜRGENS, U. & PRATT, R. (1979) The cingular vocalization pathway in the squirrel mon-monkey. *Exp. Brain Res., 34,* 499–510

11. LASSEN, N. A., INGVAR, D. H. & SKINHOJ, E., (1978) Brain function and blood flow. *Sci. Am. 239* (4), 62–71

12. INGVAR, D. H. & FRAUZEN, G. (1974) Distribution of cerebral activity in chronic schizo-phrenia. *Lancet 2,* 1484–1485

13. ROBINSON, B. W. (1976) Limbic influences on human speech. *Ann. N. Y. Acad. Sci. 280,* 761–771

Representation of reality in the perceptual world

COLIN BLAKEMORE*

Physiological Laboratory, University of Cambridge†

Abstract What contribution can neurobiologists make to the philosophical issues involved in the Theory of Knowledge? The sensory physiologist or psychologist must start with the assumption (albeit philosophically naive) that the biological function of sense organs is to act as transducers of genuine events in the outside world, and thus to contribute to an internal description of external reality. Although visual perception seems to its introspecting owner to be a unitary process, involving an integrated and complete description of all the properties of the visual scene, there is now good evidence that sensory processing of messages from the eyes involves a great deal of filtering of information and anatomically segregated analysis of such features as shape, colour, movement and distance.

Sensory neurobiology can say little about the way in which conscious perceptions are synthesized from the heap of features into which the sensory signals are shattered, about how the inherent ambiguity of messages from sensory neurons is overcome, or about how the ultimate percepts are externalized. Finally, the evidence that the nature of the sensory world varies from species to species forces us to re-examine the theory of solipsism in biological terms.

> *'What is Matter? – Never mind.*
> *What is Mind – No matter'.*
> *Punch, 1855*

The so-called Theory of Knowledge is a central problem in philosophy, ancient and modern. It is a curious fact that neurobiologists of the sensory systems have (with some notable exceptions) had little more than a tug at this conceptual knot; yet one might imagine that they are able to answer, or at least address, some fundamental questions that the philosopher might ask. A deep yearning

---

*Royal Society Locke Research Fellow
†Present address:* University Laboratory of Physiology, Parks Road, Oxford OX1 3 PT

of philosophers, from at least the time of Heraclitus, has been to find what is permanent, what is real, what is valid. The philosopher might then demand of the sensory physiologist or psychologist:

'In what form is the real world represented in the brain?'
'To what extent can we learn from our own perceptions that the external world *is* real? How valid is perception?'
'Are there structures or activities in the brain that are equivalent to Platonic *universals?* How does the brain categorize and name?'

I cannot claim that any of these enquiries can yet be answered in full, but in this brief paper I shall try to point out some of the successes of sensory neurobiology, as well as prise open some of the gaps in our understanding.

THE NEUROBIOLOGICAL APPROACH TO EPISTEMOLOGY

We should certainly not have got far in the study of sensory pathways if we held, with Gorgias the Sophist, that 'Nothing exists and if it did no one could know it'! The brain researcher's approach is necessarily more empirical and pragmatic. Perhaps that is because biologists are fond of comparing animal functions to those of physical instruments. The physiologist treats sense organs as if they were physical transducers and compares their design and performance with idealized detectors of physical events. So rather than asking whether the world that we apprehend is real, the scientist asks how efficiently the senses analyse those attributes of the world (whether real or not) that can be estimated with physical devices.

If we sidestep the disturbing circularity caused by the fact that physical instruments can, in turn, only be interpreted through the use of those very sense organs[1] whose performance we wish to judge, this approach is reasonable enough. It has certainly provided an adequate foundation for the experimental study of sensory systems.

The sense organs form an interface between the behaviour of the organism and the environment within which it can operate. Hence the required function of those sense organs, in the biological and evolutionary context, is to provide descriptions of external events that are adequate to permit the animal to guide its behaviour, to survive and to reproduce. Equally important (since animals can act as homeostatic and servo-controlled devices), the senses inform the organism of the environmental consequences of its own actions. This begs the question of the *absolute* validity of sensory signals and defines reliability in terms of functional *utility*—a theme to which I shall return later in attempting to arrive at a biologically based definition of knowledge.

THE FUNCTIONS OF VISION

The different senses clearly play different roles in the process of guiding behaviour, and it is not surprising that both biologists and philosophers have paid disproportionate attention to the sense of vision, being, as it is, the supreme 'distance receptor'[2]. For most land-dwelling animals it is visual information that gives the most complete advance warning of approaching danger, that guides hunting, and that provides a spatial representation of the environment in which the animal operates.

Our conscious visual experience is usually a unitary one and gives no hint of some kind of fragmentary, piecemeal, even incomplete analysis. An object within our field of view has place as well as form and colour, has distance as well as motion. However, one currently fashionable view of neurobiologists is that the various attributes of the visual world are analysed separately within the brain. The evidence comes partly from perceptual studies of various visual illusions and after-effects (such as those shown in Fig. 1), where certain

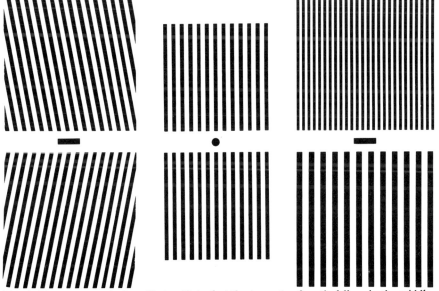

FIG. 1. Two perceptual after-effects. Note that the two sets of vertical lines in the middle, with the dot between them, are identical in orientation and line width. Now, with the book at arm's length, stare for about 30–60 seconds at the short horizontal bar between the two patterns on the left, moving the gaze back and forth along the bar, thus exposing the region of retina above and below the fovea to lines of opposite tilt. At the end of the period of adaptation, quickly glance back at the central dot, and while holding fixation there, compare the lines above and below. They should appear slightly inclined in opposite directions.

After a pause of at least a minute, repeat the procedure with the gratings of different bar width on the right. These should induce an apparent change in bar width for the two central patterns (see ref. 3).

attributes of a visual stimulus, such as its size, orientation, position or movement can be altered independently of other qualities by prior adaptation or by simultaneous stimulation with surrounding patterns.[3]

There is further support for the notion of segregated analysis of the visual scene from the differential effects of damage to the two major visual centres: the visual cortex in the cerebral hemispheres, and the superior colliculus in the midbrain. It is usually held that cortical damage, in a variety of mammals from rats to humans, abolishes the capacity to discriminate visual stimuli on the basis of shape. In other words, lesions of the visual cortex interfere with identification. On the other hand, in the golden hamster (the species on which Schneider[4,5] has built the theory of 'two visual systems'), lesions in the superior colliculus prevent the animal from localizing objects in space and from orienting the body, head and eyes towards novel peripheral visual stimuli. This has led Schneider to propose that two different aspects of visual perception (crudely speaking, the 'what' and the 'where' of a visual stimulus) are dependent on the integrity of different parts of the brain.

Phylogenetic comparisons of visual pathways lend support to the theory of two visual systems. In fish, amphibians and reptiles the midbrain visual area, the optic tectum, is massive and the forebrain visual structures non-existent or poorly developed. Through the mammalian line the proportionate sizes of forebrain and midbrain areas shift, until, in humans, the pathway to the visual cortex takes roughly two-thirds of the nerve fibres in the optic tract. This fits nicely with the fact that identification and categorization of objects have become an increasingly dominant aspect of visual function in higher mammals, whereas spatial localization and orienting are the primary visual functions in lower vertebrates.

A corollary of this approach is that the more 'cognitive' aspects of vision, and in particular conscious visual perception, depend on the cerebral cortex. Electrical stimulation of the occipital or temporal lobes in human patients gives rise to apparent visual sensations[6,7] and damage to the occipital lobe is usually reported to cause total blindness in the part of the visual field represented there.[8] In golden hamsters, damage to the superior colliculus has no obvious effect on the animal's ability to orient to moving peripheral stimuli and it therefore appears, at first glance, to be quite normal. However, closer testing shows that such an animal is quite unable to discriminate shapes.[4,5]

Recent work on residual visual function in patients with cortical lesions[9,10] has revealed that in some cases of indubitable injury to the visual cortex there is a subtle and apparently unconscious form of residual vision—'blindsight' as it has been called.[10] These patients, presumably using the pathway from the eyes to the midbrain, can, to some extent, guide their eyes to look towards lights briefly flashed within the 'blind' part of their visual field; they can point with accuracy at some lights; and can even 'guess' with reliability the orientation of a patch of stripes projected into the unseen area.[10] The most remarkable thing about these results is not so much that the 300 000 or so optic nerve fibres from each eye that go to the midbrain are able to mediate some kind of visual function, but that the patients remain apparently consciously unaware of the stimulus even when they are able to react appropriately to it.

These intriguing observations seem to me to pose problems for almost any view of consciousness: what is one to make of a man who is able reliably to describe a visual stimulus, who is aware that he is doing so, and yet denies being able to see it?

THE NATURE OF IDENTIFICATION

The recognition and identification of objects are primary tasks of the visual system, especially in higher animals. During the past fifty years great advances have been made in the understanding of how these functions are performed. Most of the experimental evidence comes from the technique of electrical recording from individual nerve cells or fibres in the eye or the brain. The picture that emerges is of massive compression of information, wholesale abstraction and selection from the flood of signals, in order to reduce the enormous informational load at the photoreceptors to a level acceptable to the limited channel capacity of the organism as a whole.

When Adrian & Matthews[11] first put an electrode into the optic nerve of a conger eel they must have been amazed to discover that most of the axons seemed not to respond simply to the presence of light but to give a brisk, brief burst of impulses whenever a light was turned on or off in front of the eyes. The general principle, amply confirmed by subsequent research, is that the nerve cells of the visual pathway tend to respond best to *change* in the stimulus rather than to steady states. (Heraclitus would presumably have been delighted to learn this!) Indeed, in the cat and probably in other species, there is one class of ganglion cell in the retina, the so-called Y cell, that responds almost exclusively at the onset or end of illumination.[12]

If this kind of rapid temporal adaptation ensures that signals that are unchanging in time are eliminated, another property of the retina tends to filter out signals that are steady in space. Barlow[13] and Kuffler[14] discovered that ganglion cells in frogs and cats can be excited by either illumination or darkening of a local point on the retina (in other words by the appearance of a light or dark stimulus at a particular point in the visual field). But simultaneous stimulation of the surrounding part of the so-called *receptive field* reduces or abolishes the response, due to the presence of an 'inhibitory surround'. The optimal stimulus for such cells is thus a localized contrast in the visual field, such as occurs at the boundary of an object. Barlow[15] has pointed out that this process of lateral inhibition reduces spatial redundancy, eliminating signals about uniformly illuminated areas of the retina, and allowing through messages mainly about the information-rich borders of patterns, in the same way that temporal adaptation reduces redundant signals about stimuli that do not change in time.[16]

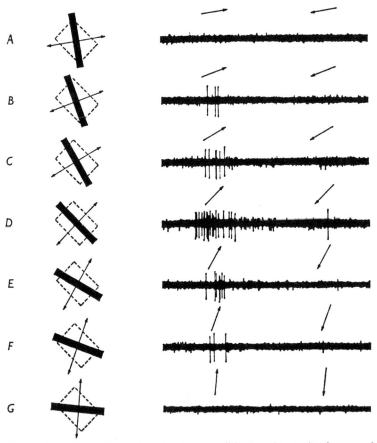

FIG. 2. Recordings of nerve impulses from a cell in the primary visual cortex of a monkey.[21] The traces on the right are photographs from an oscilloscope, showing, as a function of time, each individual impulse (a vertical deflection). The cartoons on the left show the stimulus presented on a screen in front of the animal's eyes—a bar of varying orientation moved in the directions shown by the arrows. The cell, in record D, responded best to a diagonal line moving upwards. (Redrawn, with permission, from records of D. H. Hubel and T. N. Wiesel.)

The physicist Ernst Mach predicted some kind of inhibitory network within the retina on the basis of his observations of various illusions of apparent brightness caused by certain distributions of light.[17] Most, if not all, of the classical visual illusions may be the consequences of operations within the visual system whose functional value is the elimination of unwanted signals and the sharpening of the abstraction process.[3]

Beyond the retina in mammals (and even in the retina itself in lower species[18,19]), the process of sorting, selecting and characterizing continues, as demonstrated most fully by the well-known work of Hubel and Wiesel[20,21] on the primary visual cortex of the cat and the monkey. Here individual neurons are often highly selective for the orientation of lines and edges presented in their receptive fields (Fig. 2): the neurons are almost totally unresponsive to gross overall changes in illumination of the visual field and even to boundaries of the inappropriate orientation. It is generally assumed that neurons like this are involved in the analysis of shape and thus in the identification of objects from their boundaries.[22]

Other aspects of the visual world, such as colour, movement and distance, are also selectively detected by neurons with differential sensitivity to wavelength, direction and velocity of motion, and retinal disparity. Indeed the current work of Zeki[23] in the monkey suggests that different component features of the visual image are analysed piecemeal in separate small regions of the cerebral cortex in front of the primary visual cortex.

One present view of visual analysis is, then, that it proceeds as the selective extraction of component features, or points of high informational content, from the complete retinal image: it is a decomposition of the visual scene, not into any kind of simple geometric description, but into the coordinates of a feature-space whose many axes are inscribed in different and independent regions of the brain.

LOGICAL PROBLEMS

Externalization and localization

Our present understanding of sensory analysis in the brain tells us nothing about the vital process of externalization—the referral of sensed events to the outside world. We are rarely aware that the source of our visual sensations is our eyes. Our conscious awareness is of the objects themselves that produce or reflect the light that enters the eyes, not of incomplete, second-hand, internal reports of those objects. Nor have we an adequate explanation of how the localizations of objects in space are interpreted from the pattern of activity within the distorted spatial representations in the visual areas of the brain.

These cannot be discounted as simple 'given' functions that require no explanation. Both complete externalization and appropriate spatial localization may depend at least in part on a gradual learning process mainly occurring during early visual development. A common problem in blind people to whom vision has been restored is that visual stimuli are perceived as touching the eyes, like objects on the skin.[24] In the same way, although the visual phosphenes produced by electrical stimulation of the eye or the visual cortex, by pressure on the eyeball or a blow to the head, appear to most people to be externalized visual sensations, with their own existence in the outside world, stimulation of the cortex in a patient blind for many years produced sensations that seemed to come from the eyes themselves.[25]

Brain lesions in the right parietal lobe can upset grossly but quite selectively the sense of spatial localization,[26] and occasionally patients even see some part of the visual field apparently inverted without any obvious effect on the quality of the objects lying within that portion of the field.

Even Descartes, who first suggested that there might be a spatial representation of the retina in the brain (Fig. 3), was (unlike certain of the *Gestalt* psychologists) not so naive as to think that the isomorphism of the central representation was of itself helpful in the perception of space or form:

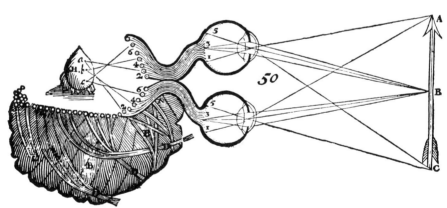

FIG. 3. Descartes' diagram, from *Traité de l'Homme*, of his model of connections between the eyes and the walls of the ventricles, with influence passing, in a pattern similar to the retinal image, to the pineal body.

'Although this little picture still retains some resemblance to the objects from which it originates, as it passes to the back of our head, we should not fall into the error of thinking that it is by the means of this resemblance that we see the objects; for there is not another set of eyes inside the head with which we could see the images' (from *Dioptrique*, 1637, quoted in translation by Morgan[27]).

Descartes thought that the intrinsic connectivity that 'Nature has determined' ensures that activity in such and such a part of the visual representation in the brain will automatically evoke such and such a perception of position in the field. But there are operational problems with this view. If we study one visual area after another, in their serial order from the retina through the brain, we find that the sizes of the receptive fields of neurons increase and the precision of the topographic map of the visual field decreases. How can activity in such a network of cells specify the position of a target with the precision that we know we have in localizing objects?

My reason for believing that the interpretation of spatial relationships may depend on a learning process comes from the many experiments in young animals and even in adult humans showing great capacity for adaptation of visuomotor behaviour to prismatic displacement, rotation and even inversion of the visual field.[28]

Kittens can learn to cope remarkably well if one eye is surgically rotated early in life, even though there is no obvious compensatory reorganization of the representation of the retina in the visual cortex.[29] When a cat that has had one eye rotated by 90° early in life has that eye covered, and learns an orientation discrimination (by being trained to jump onto a platform covered with vertical stripes and avoid one with horizontal stripes), not only can it immediately perform the same task if the normal eye is covered and the rotated one opened, but it continues to respond to the same orientation *in space*, despite the fact that the vertical lines on the platform now lie on the innately *horizontal* meridians of its twisted retina[30] (Fig. 4).

The meaning of nerve impulses: the ambiguity of signals

Nerve cells communicate principally by firing impulses in bursts, at frequencies up to about 1000/second. In general, at least for peripheral sensory nerves, the firing rate is found to correlate with the physical strength of some external stimulus,[31] or to vary systematically with variation of the stimulus along some particular dimension. But the fact that such correlations can be detected by an experimenter eavesdropping on the activity does not, of course, mean that all these correlations can be interpreted by the brain.

Indeed some workers have emphasized the way that sensory neurons select one particular absolute feature and maintain an invariant response as other characteristics of the visual stimulus are changed.[18] The contrast-detecting retinal ganglion cells of the cat[14] are a fine example, for the inhibitory surrounds

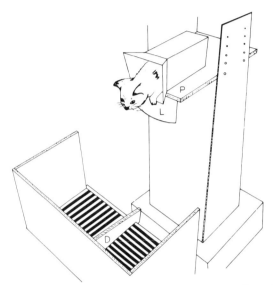

FIG. 4. Jumping-stand apparatus used by Mitchell *et al.*[30] to test interocular transfer in eye-rotated cats. The animals were trained to jump from the platform, P, onto one of the two patterns of stripes placed on the trapdoors below, which were separated by a divider, D. The cat was petted as a reward for jumping to the correct stimulus, which was randomly varied from side to side.

of their receptive fields make them relatively insensitive to change in overall illumination and their firing activity is thus related to local contrast or intensity difference. Another classical example is the group of so-called direction-selective ganglion cells of the rabbit's retina,[32] which respond selectively to objects moving in one direction across the receptive field. This property is maintained if the size, shape or velocity of the moving object is varied, and even if its contrast is reversed.

Barlow[33] has taken the extreme view that variation in the firing rate of a sensory cell might convey no information about variation in the strength or quality of the stimulus but might merely determine the certainty with which a particular encoded feature could be said to be present. This view, though attractive to the theory of selective feature detection, is weakened by the fact that individual sensory cells often have their responses 'gated' by a large number of different variables in the stimulus and show correlations in firing rate with more than one attribute of the stimulus. Thus any level of firing in any particular neuron is inherently ambiguous, in that it could be set up by an infinity of different stimulus conditions.[16] Feature detection must be a function of populations of nerve cells. But how is activity in a population analysed without the extra 'set of eyes inside the head' that Descartes warned us about?

This problem becomes even more daunting when we move from the analysis of features (decomposition) to the interpretation and identification of whole objects. The existence of orientation-selective cells in the visual cortex may explain why I am able to detect the similarity between a satirical cartoon of President Carter and a photograph of him, and in turn recognize the relationship of identity between the photograph and the group of bright and dark dots on my television screen that the commentator's voice assures me is Mr Carter. It does little to explain how the Mr-Carter-ness of any of these stimuli persists as I turn my head or as I vary my distance from the image. Despite the speculation about pontifical grandmother-detecting neurons, or cardinal cells,[33] I think that we are still far from understanding how objects are perceived as separate from their background, how they are recognized and how their identification remains constant despite enormous variation from moment to moment in the features that define those objects.

The distinction that Wittgenstein[34] draws between 'seeing' and 'seeing as' is an important one but it does not help us to understand the physiological nature of interpretation. It is difficult enough to see how a variety of different assemblies of features can at different times be analysed to produce the *same* interpretation (e.g. a grandmother); it is doubly difficult to understand how a single pattern of lines can evoke at different times differing interpretations. What we *see* is our derived interpretation of the object in that it is that interpretation which determines our reaction to the supposed object. If our interpretation is wrong its wrongness can only be estimated by the discovered inappropriateness of the behavioural actions evoked.

Innate and environmentally induced variations in sensitivity

If the inherent ambiguity of nerve signals, because of their multiple sensitivity to different aspects of the stimulus, provides problems for models of perception, the growing evidence that systems of central sensory neurons can be modified by unusual forms of early experience poses even more difficulty. To take a particular example, it is now firmly established that if a kitten is reared in an environment that restricts its visual experience to lines of one orientation, the orientation-selective neurons in its cortex become highly biased in their sensitivity towards that particular orientation[35,36,37] and such an animal is behaviourally relatively more sensitive to the orientation experienced than to any other.[38] There is an analogous condition in human patients who have been relatively deprived of contours of one orientation because of a large astigmatic refractive error in their eyes.[39] The relevance of these results to the nativist–empiricist debate seems obvious, but interestingly the interpretation is not yet entirely clear. Although it is possible that these effects imply an actual *determination* of neuronal properties purely by the pattern of stimulation that the cells receive, some recent evidence[37] suggests that the results are at least partly caused by selective visual experience producing differential retention of those cells *innately* predisposed to respond to that particular pattern and degenerative failure of those cells pre-specified to prefer the wrong orientation.

Whatever the mechanism of such developmental changes, their undoubted effect on the organism makes doubtful any view of perceptual analysis as a rigid system of interpretation. The output of populations of sensory cells is unstable during development and is inevitably ambiguous even in the mature animal.

Finally, and of particular importance in discussion about the validity of perception, it must be said that comparative sensory neurobiology does not lend weight to Protagoras's view that 'Man is the measure of all things'. A number of other species, much lowlier than the human species, seem to be the measure of a variety of things that are unperceived and unperceivable by humans. For instance, several species of insects can sense the plane of polarization of light, bats can detect ultrasound much higher in frequency than we can hear, some birds can feel the direction of a magnetic field, and many animals respond to wavelengths of light too low or too high to fall within the so-called visible spectrum of man. The pit organs under the eyes of certain snakes are sensitive to infrared light and there is even a spatial representation of the infrared world in their tectum, in the layers below the conventional visual map.[40]

BIOLOGICAL SOLIPSISM

Berkeley himself admitted that it was logically possible that there could be unperceived things (such as spiritual objects and events). Perceived events are presumed by their perceiver to have occurred, but not all occurrences, even within the field of observation of the viewer, are necessarily perceived. If a man blind from birth cannot conceive of the notion of seeing, how can we comprehend the sensation of a bat or a rattlesnake, responding to stimuli that are undetectable to us? Common sense, not introspection, is the only way that I see of overcoming the conceptual dilemma that unperceived things pose for the concept of perceptual reality.

The perceived environment is what it *needs* to be for the animal in question. Behaviourally, things indeed do not exist if they are not perceived, because if they go undetected they cannot play a part in guiding the animal's behaviour. Since the spectrum of sensory capacity varies from animal to animal, and even from individual to individual within one species, this implies that one animal's reality need not exist for another. Knowledge is interpretation adequate to guide behaviour. Validity is utility.

References

1. MACH, E. (1914) *The Analysis of Sensation and the Relation of the Physical to the Psychical* (Williams, C. M., transl., Waterlow, S., rev.), Open Court Publishing Company, Chicago
2. SHERRINGTON, C. S. (1906) *The Integrative Action of the Nervous System*, Yale University Press, New Haven
3. BLAKEMORE, C. (1973) The baffled brain, in *Illusion in Nature and Art* (Gregory, R. L. & Gombrich, E. H., eds.), pp. 9–47, Duckworth, London
4. SCHNEIDER, G. E. (1967) Contrasting visuomotor functions of tectum and cortex in the golden hamster. *Psychol. Forsch. 31*, 52–62
5. SCHNEIDER, G. E. (1969) Two visual systems. *Science (Wash. D.C.) 163*, 895–902
6. PENFIELD, W. & RASMUSSEN, T. (1955) *The Cerebral Cortex of Man: A Clinical Study of Localization of Function*, Macmillan, New York
7. BRINDLEY, G. S. & LEWIN, W. S. (1968) The visual sensations produced by electrical stimulation of the medial occipital cortex. *J. Physiol. (Lond.) 194*, 54–55P
8. HOLMES, G. (1918) Disturbances of vision by cerebral lesions. *Br. J. Ophthalmol. 2*, 353–384
9. PÖPPEL, E., HELD, R. & FROST, D. (1973) Residual visual function after brain wounds involving the central visual pathways in man. *Nature (Lond.) 243*, 295–299
10. WEISKRANTZ, L., WARRINGTON, E. K., SANDERS, M. D. & MARSHALL, J. (1974) Visual capacity in the hemianopic field following a restricted occipital ablation. *Brain 97*, 709–728
11. ADRIAN, E. D. & MATTHEWS, R. (1927) The action of light on the eye. I. The discharge of impulses in the optic nerve and its relation to the electrical changes in the retina. *J. Physiol. (Lond.) 63*, 378–414
12. ENROTH-CUGELL, C. & ROBSON, J. G. (1966) The contrast sensitivity of retinal ganglion cells of the cat. *J. Physiol. (Lond.) 187*, 517–552
13. BARLOW, H. B. (1953) Summation and inhibition in the frog's retina. *J. Physiol. (Lond.) 119*, 69–88
14. KUFFLER, S. W. (1953) Discharge patterns and functional organization of mammalian retina. *J. Neurophysiol. 16*, 37–68
15. BARLOW, H. B. (1961) Possible principles underlying the transformations of sensory messages, in *Sensory Communication* (Rosenblith, W. A., ed.), pp. 217–234, M.I.T Press, Cambridge, Massachusetts
16. BLAKEMORE, C. (1975) Central visual processing, in *Handbook of Psychobiology* (Gazzaniga, M. S. & Blakemore, C., eds.), pp. 241–268, Academic Press, New York
17. RATLIFF, F. (1965) *Mach Bands: Quantitative Studies of Neural Networks in the Retina*, Holden-Day, San Francisco

18. LETTVIN, J. Y., MATURANA, H. R., McCULLOCH, W. S. & PITTS, W. H. (1959) What the frog's eye tells the frog's brain. *Proc. Inst. Radio Eng. 47*, 1940–1951

19. MATURANA, H. R. & FRENK, S. (1963) Directional movement and horizontal edge detectors in the pigeon retina. *Science (Wash. D.C.) 142*, 977–979

20. HUBEL, D. H. & WIESEL, T. N. (1962) Receptive fields, binocular interaction and functional architecture in the cat's visual cortex. *J. Physiol. (Lond.) 160*, 106–154

21. HUBEL, D. H. & WIESEL, T. N. (1977) Functional architecture of macaque monkey visual cortex. *Proc. R. Soc. Lond. B Biol. Sci. 198*, 1–59

22. CREUTZFELDT, O. D. & NOTHDURFT, H. C. (1978) Representation of complex visual stimuli in the brain. *Naturwissenschaften 65*, 307–318

23. ZEKI, S. M. (1974) The mosaic organization of the visual cortex in the monkey, in *Essays on the Nervous System* (Bellairs, R. & Gray, E. G., eds.), pp. 327–343, Clarendon Press, Oxford

24. VON SENDEN, M. (1960) *Space and Sight*, Methuen, London

25. RUSHTON, D. N. & BRINDLEY, G. S. (1978) Properties of cortical electrical phosphenes, in *Frontiers of Visual Science* (Cool, S. J. & Smith, E. L., eds.), pp. 574–593, Springer, New York

26. CRITCHLEY, M. (1953) *The Parietal Lobes*, Edward Arnold, London

27. MORGAN, M. J. (1977) *Molyneux's Question*, Cambridge University Press, London

28. HOWARD, I. P. & TEMPLETON, W. B. (1966) *Human Spatial Orientation*, John Wiley, London

29. BLAKEMORE, C., VAN SLUYTERS, R. C., PECK, C. K. & HEIN, A. (1975) Development of cat visual cortex following rotation of one eye. *Nature (Lond.) 257*, 584–586

30. MITCHELL, D. E., GIFFIN, F., MUIR, D., BLAKEMORE, C. & VAN SLUYTERS, R. C. (1976) Behavioural compensation of cats to early rotation of one eye. *Exp. Brain Res. 25*, 109–113

31. ADRIAN, E. D. (1947) *The Physical Background of Perception*, Oxford University Press, Oxford

32. BARLOW, H. B., HILL, R. M. & LEVICK, W. R. (1964) Retinal ganglion cells responding selectively to direction and speed of image motion in the rabbit. *J. Physiol. (Lond.) 173*, 377–407

33. BARLOW, H. B. (1972) Single units and sensation: a neuron doctrine for perceptual psychology. *Perception 1*, 371–394

34. WITTGENSTEIN, L. (1967) *Philosophical Investigations* (Anscombe, G. E. M., transl.), Blackwell, Oxford

35. HIRSCH, H. V. B. & SPINELLI, D. N. (1970) Visual experience modifies distribution of horizontally and vertically oriented receptive fields in cats. *Science (Wash. D.C.) 168*, 869–871

36. BLAKEMORE, C. & COOPER, G. F. (1970) Development of the brain depends on the visual environment. *Nature (Lond.) 228*, 477–478

37. STRYKER, M. P., SHERK, H., LEVENTHAL, A. G. & HIRSCH, H. V. B. (1978) Physiological consequences for the cat's visual cortex of effectively restricting early visual experience with oriented contours. *J. Neurophysiol. 41*, 896–909

38. MUIR, D. W. & MITCHELL, D. E. (1975) Behavioral deficits in cats following early selected visual exposure to contours of a single orientation. *Brain Res. 85*, 459–477

39. MITCHELL, D. E., FREEMAN, R. D., MILLODOT, M. & HAEGERSTROM, G. (1973) Meridional amblyopia: evidence for modification of the human visual system by early visual experience. *Vision Res. 13*, 535–558

40. HARTLINE, P. H., KASS, L. & LOOP, M. S. (1978) Merging of modalities in the optic tectum: infrared and visual integration in rattlesnakes. *Science (Wash. D.C.) 199*, 1225–1229

Neuropsychological evidence for multiple memory systems

ELIZABETH K. WARRINGTON

National Hospital, Queen Square, London

Abstract Neuropsychological data provide strong support for the existence of multiple memory systems. The distinction between short-term memory and long-term memory has been discussed in the experimental literature for some years. More recently it has been argued that the concept of long-term memory is misleading in that it fails to differentiate between semantic memory and episodic/event memory. The independent and selective impairment of multiple memory systems, each with its own functional and structural properties, has been recorded in patients with cerebral lesions and the evidence for impairment of such systems is reviewed. It is argued that the cerebral organization of short-term memory, long-term (non-individual) semantic memory and long-term (individual) event memory is highly differentiated.

Neuropsychological data provide strong support for those experimental psychologists who postulate not merely two memory systems but multiple memory systems. Differences in kind as well as extent are crucial for any multi-system memory theory; to reject the unitary theory of memory it is necessary to specify the properties of each separate memory system which is identified. The independent and selective impairment of different memory systems, each with its own functional and structural properties, has now been recorded in patients with focal cerebral lesions. The aim of this presentation is to give a brief account of the concepts short-term memory, semantic memory and event memory and to review the neuropsychological evidence that these systems can be selectively impaired. Each system will be considered from the point of view of its capacity, temporal properties and the code of the central representation, with some indication of the anatomical substrate.

SHORT-TERM MEMORY

Short-term memory is held to be a system of limited capacity. The immediate memory span, one measure of the capacity of the system, is in the order of seven (plus or minus two) items or 'chunks' of information. Thus there is a strict limitation to a normal subject's performance on tasks requiring ordered verbatim recall. It is a labile or transient memory system, there being little or no permanent record or memory trace. Thus, if there is no delay between presentation and recall, strings of numbers can be recalled repeatedly without there being any decrement in performance or interference from previous items.[1] The central representation of short-term memory has been shown to be based primarily on an acoustic (or alternatively an articulatory) code. Thus performance in tasks testing immediate memory span is worse if the individual stimulus items are acoustically similar (e.g. mad, map, man) than if they are semantically similar (e.g. huge, big, great). This type of evidence is interpreted as indicating that linguistic and semantic factors are not directly implicated in the operation of this short-term memory system (for detailed review see Baddeley[2]).

Although a reduced immediate memory span for verbal material is commonplace in the context of aphasic difficulties, a relatively selective impairment of immediate memory span occurs in patients with posterior left hemisphere lesions. This phenomenon was first reported by Luria and colleagues,[3] who described two patients in whom the main symptom was an inability to repeat strings of digits. Dr T. Shallice and I have investigated in some detail a patient (KF) with a profound inability to repeat verbal material. He had a digit and letter span of between one and two items (see Table 1). At the same time he could comprehend spoken speech without difficulty; his own speech, although halting and hesitant, was adequate for conversational exchanges; and perhaps most impressive was his excellent performance in a variety of verbal learning tasks. We argued that a selective

TABLE 1

Repetition of numbers and letters presented auditorially and visually to patient KF (derived from Warrington & Shallice[4])

| | String length | | | | | |
| | Auditory presentation | | | Visual presentation | | |
	1 Item	2 Items	3 Items	1 Items	2 Items	3 Items
Numbers						
Items correct	20/20	28/40	37/60	20/20	39/40	48/60
Strings correct	20	12	6	20	19	10
Letters						
Items correct	19/20	21/40	26/60	20/20	37/40	48/60
Strings correct	19	7	2	20	17	11

impairment of auditory–verbal short-term memory could account for his selective impairment on verbal span tasks.[4,5]

Our interpretation was strengthened by this patient's very impaired performance on a short-term forgetting task. Peterson and Peterson[6] have demonstrated that for normal subjects a marked decrement in recall of sub-span items (e.g. the letters X R S) presented auditorially occurs up to 30 seconds if rehearsal is prevented by an intervening task. This decrement is held to reflect the short-term memory component of the task. Patient KF forgot *single* letter stimuli abnormally rapidly when intervening intervals as short as 5, 10 and 15 seconds were used (see Fig. 1). When a single stimulus item was presented visually, neither normal subjects nor KF showed any decrement in performance. Thus for KF it would appear that information in some auditory–verbal short-term store is more transitory than normal.[7]

KF's deficits appeared to be modality-specific in that his auditory–verbal memory span was worse than his visual–verbal memory span (see Table 1); the converse holds for normal subjects. Furthermore, it was shown that there

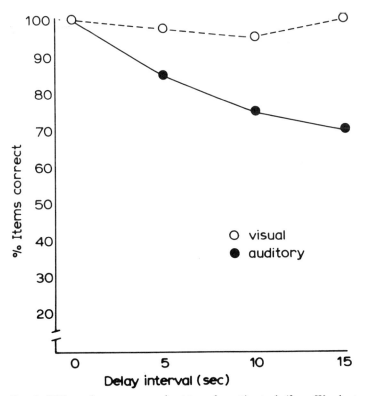

FIG. 1. KF's performance on a short-term forgetting task (from Warrington & Shallice[7]).

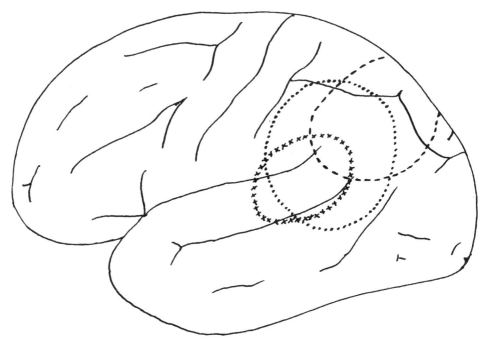

FIG. 2. Schematic diagram of location of lesion in patients with a selective impairment of auditory-verbal short-term memory (patients KF, JB and PH).

was a significantly higher incidence of acoustic confusion errors on auditory span tasks than on visual span tasks (for a full discussion of the significance of this finding see Warrington and Shallice[7]).

These early experiments with KF have now been confirmed in other patients,[8,9] and it appears that critical anatomical structures in the left inferior parietal lobe are responsible for this syndrome (see Fig. 2).

In summary, those properties which are considered to characterize the short-term memory system are all implicated in these patients. Thus there is a marked reduction in the normal capacity of the auditory memory span, the decrement in performance after short intervals is abnormally great, and there is an increased incidence of acoustic errors. The existence of this group of patients provides both functional and structural grounds for differentiating short-term memory as a distinct system. The relationship between this short-term memory system and other memory systems is of some interest and will be discussed briefly in the last section.

SEMANTIC MEMORY

The distinction between short-term memory and long-term memory has been discussed in the experimental literature for some years now.[2,10,11] More recently, however, it has been suggested that the concept of long-term memory is misleading in that it fails to differentiate between semantic knowledge—that is memory for words, facts and concepts—which is a pool of knowledge shared by individuals, and event memory, that is memory for events or experiences resulting in a pool of memories unique to the individual. Earlier a point was reached when simple reaction times for letters or words were reported under the guise of long-term memory. At this stage Tulving[12] made a very timely intervention by arguing on theoretical grounds that a distinction should be drawn between episodic memory (referred to here as event memory) and semantic memory. I hope to demonstrate that this distinction between event memory and semantic memory is valid in the context of neurological deficits.

Semantic memory is a system of very large but probably limited capacity. To give but two examples, normal subjects have a large but limited vocabulary, and learning a second language presents difficulties for most adults. The time course of semantic memory appears to be very stable. Indeed it can be argued that it is a memory system which provides a 'durable' trace relatively unchanged by use or disuse; our vocabulary, knowledge of word meanings, is for practical purposes a permanent and readily accessible acquisition.[13] The central representation of semantic memory has been considered to be categorically and hierarchically organized. Verbal category effects are robust and the effects of subordinate and superordinate categories can be differentiated (for detailed discussion of these issues see Tulving and Donaldson[14]).

Selective impairment of semantic memory can occur in patients with cerebral lesions. I would argue that the somewhat obscure and rare agnosic syndromes can be identified with the impairment of some facet of semantic memory. These agnosic syndromes almost certainly subdivide into a vast number of modality-specific and category-specific deficits in semantic memory, which it is beyond the scope of this paper to discuss. In order to achieve comparability with the other memory systems being considered, I will restrict my comments to deficits of knowledge of word meanings.

Comprehension of word meanings can be impaired in patients in whom other aspects of language function are relatively well preserved. Especially striking is their ability to express themselves fluently and lucidly within the limitations imposed by their restricted vocabulary.

I have investigated word comprehension deficits in three patients who were selected for detailed study on the basis of semantic deficits in the visual modality (though of great interest, their visual agnosic deficits are not strictly relevant to the present discussion). It was observed that these three patients, unable to comprehend the meaning or significance of objects or pictorial

TABLE 2

Picture and word recognition tests in three patients (derived from Warrington [15])

	AB	EM	CR
Picture recognition	19/40	37/40	13/40
Word recognition	27/40	26/40	21/40

representations of objects, had comparable difficulty in understanding the spoken word. All three had received a university education and two of them (AB and EM) were still able to score at a relatively high level on intelligence tests. They were able (at least at a superficial level) to read, write and talk within the limits of their impoverished vocabulary (for further details see Warrington [15]).

To document this phenomenon, objects of medium frequency (e.g. camel, kite, harp) were presented pictorially and auditorially and the patients were asked to identify the picture or define the spoken word. The numbers of items correct for each condition of presentation are given in Table 2. It can be confidently assumed that all items had been well within each patient's vocabulary. Although the problem of the modality-specificity of these agnosic deficits will not be discussed further, it is worth noting that there was not a one-to-one correspondence in the comprehension of 'concepts' in the visual and auditory modes. Thus a drawing of a basket might be identified, whereas the spoken word 'basket' could not be understood, and conversely, in the same patient a drawing of a gate might not be identified though the spoken word 'gate' could be.

The most striking example of category-specificity noted in these patients was in the concrete/abstract dimension. Seventy-five words from the Brown and Ure list (for which concreteness ratings are available) had been defined by all three patients. A very lenient scoring criterion was adopted and the numbers of words (low and high frequency, and low and high concreteness) correctly defined are given in Table 3. The effect of frequency for word

TABLE 3

Concrete and abstract word definition test in three patients [15]

Patient	High frequency		Low frequency	
	High concrete words	Low concrete words	High concrete words	Low concrete words
AB	14/15	10/10	6/25	17/20
EM	14/15	10/10	14/25	9/20
CR	15/15	9/10	15/25	12/20

comprehension is very clear in all three patients. For CR there was no effect of word concreteness, but for EM comprehension of abstract words was significantly worse than for concrete words. AB is of special interest in this regard as his comprehension of concrete words was much more impaired than that of abstract words. Some examples of AB's attempts to define concrete and abstract words were as follows:

Concrete words	Patient's response
Blacksmith	'I've forgotten'
Hound	'An animal' (no further details on questioning)
Macaroni	'No idea'
Carrot	'Don't know'

Abstract words	Patient's response
Soul	'Your basic interior element'
Knowledge	'Make oneself mentally familiar with a subject'
Opinion	'Having own view'
Perjury	'People behave in damaging manner—telling untruths'.

The selective preservation of abstract words observed in AB renders untenable any explanation of word comprehension deficits in terms of generalized intellectual failure, either at the level of 'abstracting' a concept or at the level of linguistic explanation. It is reasonable to assume that such factors would be maximized in abstract word definition; yet for AB there was a remarkable preservation of abstract words compared with concrete words. It is therefore suggested that not only are there functional and linguistic differences between concrete and abstract words, but also that these differences have a structural basis in the brain.

The impairment of individual word meanings displayed by these patients was not an absolute all-or-none phenomenon. In many instances they appeared to have preserved partial or incomplete comprehension of words. It was observed that subordinate (fine-grain semantic details) information was more vulnerable than superordinate information (broad category knowledge). It appeared that the patients had no access to a sufficiently specific or precise semantic representation for adequate comprehension. For example a 'bucket' was defined as a container but on further questioning no details of its function, size or weight were known.

An attempt was made to quantify these observations of the ordered or hierarchical organization of semantic memory. The results of probing the same superordinate and subordinate categories for 20 animal names are given

TABLE 4

Auditory recognition by semantic probe in three patients [15]

	Animals and objects		Animals	
	Animals?	Bird?	English?	Size?
AB	29/40	15/20	14/20	13/20
EM	34/40	13/20	12/20	11/20
CR	26/40	9/20	9/20	5/20
Controls (mean score) $n=5$	39.8/40	19.4/20	18.8/20	15.2/20

in Table 4. The overall level of performance for all three patients was very poor; nevertheless there was a trend for superordinate judgements to be more accurate. In a further experiment with EM more compelling evidence for the relative vulnerability of subordinate information was obtained. It was shown that even for words she apparently 'knew', there was loss of specific semantic information, and conversely for words she had apparently 'forgotten', there appeared to be some preservation of superordinate category information (for further details see Warrington[15]).

These patients all had diffuse brain disease and therefore cannot provide us with information on the anatomical correlates of the syndrome. However, evidence from other patients presenting with similar syndromes but investigated in a different context suggest that the left temporo-occipital region of the brain is critical. This anatomical correlation has also emerged from a group study of patients with unilateral lesions: on word comprehension tests the left temporal lobe cases were impaired relative to the left non-temporal cases.[16]

EVENT MEMORY

Long-term retention of events, as distinct from facts, is of memories unique to the individual, and it can only be investigated rigorously by providing an experimental event as the starting point. The capacity of event memory, like that of semantic memory, is probably very large; indeed it has no known limits. It is not impossible that event memory, with its power to reorganize and amalgamate, may have for practical purposes an infinite capacity. The time course of event memory is neither as transient as in short-term memory, nor as stable as for semantic memory. Rather event memory appears to reflect a dynamic trace which can provide a continually changing and reconstructive long-term record of events experienced by the individual. It is a system which involves the use, reuse and reorganization of the elements or components of semantic memory. A conversation could be considered a verbal event. It is clear that the same vocabulary is used repeatedly in different contexts and with the passage of time memory for such verbal events may be condensed, amalgamated or perhaps forgotten. (For a full discussion of this issue see Bartlett[17] and Neisser[18]).

The selective impairment of event memory can occur in patients with cerebral lesions. The amnesic syndrome, known to neurologists since Korsakoff's original description in 1889 (cited by Talland[19]), is characterized by a severe impairment of memory for ongoing events in patients whose performance on cognitive tasks is otherwise normal. The severe amnesic is the patient who, although able to score normally on intelligence tests, is not only unable to recall ongoing events but is also unable to refer forwards or backwards in time to personal events and experiences. The difficulties of these patients appear to be global in that memory for both verbal and non-verbal events is impaired; typically they forget new names, new faces and new places.

Anterograde amnesia, the central component of the amnesic syndrome, can be documented and quantified using the classical techniques of verbal learning experiments. Free recall of word lists, paired associate learning, yes/no recognition and forced-choice recognition are all equally and markedly impaired in patients with the amnesic syndrome.[19,20] However, it has now been demonstrated that the apparently severe anterograde deficits in amnesic patients are not so absolute as either their behaviour in daily life or their performance on conventional verbal learning experiments would suggest. Strikingly different results are obtained when retention is tested by cued recall. retention scores of amnesics can then under certain testing conditions be normal. This phenomenon has now been observed with different types of cue. Word fragments, initial letters of a word and category information are all effective in demonstrating relatively good retention by the amnesic.[21,22] Different methods of retrieval can be compared directly and it has been found that there is a significant differential effect of methods of testing retention, cueing recall of the first three letters being advantageous for the amnesic but not the normal subject (see Fig. 3).

Retrograde amnesia, the forgetting of events before the onset of illness, is a constant feature of the amnesic syndrome, though estimates of its duration are very varied. Obvious difficulties are encountered in attempts to quantify this condition and until recently much of the evidence has derived from anecdotes and unsystematic observations. There was clearly a need for some more objective method of assessing the duration and time course of retrograde

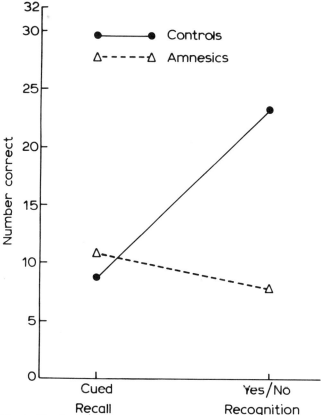

FIG. 3. Number of correct responses when retention was tested by cueing with the initial three letters of words and by yes/no recognition. (From Sanders & Warrington.[24])

amnesia. Recognition of photographs of faces of contemporary personalities, well known either in the present or in the past, provided our most satisfactory test. On the recall version of this test our small group of amnesic patients ($n = 6$) had a very profound deficit, being virtually unable to score on any of the time periods sampled. Similarly, on the multi-choice version of the test the amnesic scores were no better than chance for either contemporary faces or for faces from the past.[23] However, as with the anterograde deficits, a dramatic improvement in performance was obtained by adopting a cued-recall method of retrieval. For each face in the test a prompt of the first two or three letters (e.g. ST for Stalin, WIL for Wilson) was given. The amnesic patients tested with this method ($n = 3$) obtained very similar scores to those of normal subjects tested by recall, at all the time periods sampled[24] (see Fig. 4).

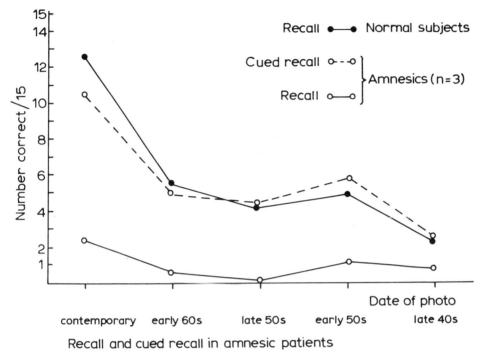

Recall ●——● Normal subjects

Cued recall ○--○ ⎫
                   ⎬ Amnesics (n=3)
Recall ○——○ ⎭

Recall and cued recall in amnesic patients

FIG. 4. Recall and cued recall in amnesic patients. (From Warrington & Weiskrantz.[30])

Lastly, turning to the problem of the central representation of event memory, there are strong indications from the experimental literature that both recall and recognition memory are mediated by associative retrieval mechanisms. Thus for normal subjects visual associations (imagery) and verbal associations are powerful determinants of efficient retention (for review see Baddeley[2]). Though the operation of such retrieval mechanisms in normal subjects is not yet understood, some form of associative retrieval deficit would seem to be the most plausible explanation of the amnesic syndrome, and it can to some extent account for what an amnesic can and cannot remember. It has been shown that amnesic patients gained no advantage from visual imagery on a verbal learning task, though for normal subjects this was a very effective mnemonic strategy. The patients were, however, able to take advantage of both acoustic similarity and taxonomic grouping (categorical information), as were normal subjects.[25] Similarly, in paired-associate learning tasks, amnesic patients were able to take advantage of strictly semantic links but not associative links (e.g. fruit—apple, but not grass—green).[26,27] Can the cued-recall phenomenon also be encompassed by this distinction between associative and categorical dimensions of verbal events? It could perhaps be argued that effective cues for amnesic retention are those in which the cue and the response can be 'matched' in the domain of semantic memory. Cued recall, whether by initial letters (acoustic), fragmented words (visual) or taxonomic category (semantic), might be thought of as a response reflecting the differential strength of items stored in the verbal knowledge systems. Perhaps the associative retrieval mechanisms, so important for many verbal learning and retention skills, are by-passed by the cued-recall paradigm, and therefore for normal subjects and amnesics alike cued recall may be mediated by facilitatory effects in the semantic memory system.

The anatomical basis of the amnesic syndrome is complex and it seems likely that at least two, possibly interconnected, regions of the brain are involved. The septo-hippocampal-fornix-mammillary body system as well as the midline nuclei of the thalamus have been implicated.[28] It seems fairly certain, however, that bilateral lesions must be present for the classical severe amnesic syndrome to emerge.

THE INTERRELATIONSHIP OF VERBAL MEMORY SYSTEMS

I have attempted to review the evidence for selective impairment of short-term memory, semantic memory and event memory. Not only are these deficits selective; they are also dissociable. If these three memory systems alone are considered, there is fairly good evidence for not just a double dissociation but for a triple dissociation.

First, the short-term memory system: it has been shown that knowledge of word meanings (and other aspects of verbal knowledge) and performance on verbal learning tasks can be quite normal in patients with short-term memory deficits. In contrast it has been firmly established that patients with the amnesic syndrome can perform normally on short-term memory tasks.[20] Furthermore, it is generally agreed that verbal vocabulary is intact in the amnesic patient although other aspects of semantic memory have not yet been systematically investigated. One amnesic patient, however, with an extensive retrograde amnesia, has been described as having 'extremely intact' scholastic knowledge of history, geography and literature.[29]

The patients described here as having semantic memory deficits all performed at an average or above average level on verbal span tasks. The assessment of event memory in these patients was more problematical. It would seem to be formidable for them to attempt a conventional verbal learning task when many or most of the items are meaningless, and indeed, on verbal memory tests, it was found that their performance was very poor. Yet these patients were by no means amnesic—they were well orientated and they were able to recall past and present events and anticipate future events, constrained only by the limitations of their impoverished vocabulary. It is of some interest to note that though their recognition memory for common words and new faces was very poor, on a recognition memory task for paintings their performance was comparable to that of normal subjects. (It may be significant that these reproductions were in colour and colour was the only visual category for which these patients [AB and EM] were not agnosic.) It would appear, then, that the processes sustaining event memory are intact in these patients even though the impairment of semantic memory systems may constrain its level of operation where the items to be remembered are meaningless to the subject.

CONCLUSION

These examples of different memory systems are illustrative of a strategy useful in neuropsychological research along a much broader front. The strategy is not only to examine and characterize each deficit, but also to look for dissociations of functions as a method of determining what capacities can be independent of each other. On the one hand one infers the properties of the various dissociable systems and, on the other hand, one relates these systems to our anatomical and physiological knowledge of the brain. Thus disorders may not only selectively affect particular regions or neural systems of the brain; they can also selectively disrupt mental phenomena. When this selectivity of functional impairment can be 'mapped' onto the categories postulated by experimental psychologists working with normal subjects, as in the examples of the memory systems discussed here, the constructs of both disciplines gain in validity and at the same time can be linked to the organization of the brain itself.

ACKNOWLEDGEMENTS

I am grateful to Dr R. T. C. Pratt and Professor L. Weiskrantz for their advice in the preparation of this manuscript.
I wish to thank Dr A. M. Whiteley who prepared the brain diagram (Fig. 2).

References

1. MELTON, A. W. (1963) Implications of short-term memory for a general theory of memory. *J. Verb. Learn. Verb. Behav.* 2, 1–21
2. BADDELEY, A. D. (1976) *The Psychology of Memory*, Harper Row, London
3. LURIA, A. R., SOKOLOV, E. N. & KLIMKOWSKI, M. (1967) Towards a neurodynamic analysis of memory disturbances with lesions of the left temporal lobe. *Neuropsychologia* 5, 1–10

4. WARRINGTON, E. K. & SHALLICE, T. (1969) The selective impairment of auditory verbal short-term memory. *Brain 92*, 885–896

5. SHALLICE, T. & WARRINGTON, E. K. (1970) The independence of the verbal memory stores: a neuropsychological study. *Q. J. Exp. Psychol. 22*, 261–273

6. PETERSON, L. R. & PETERSON, M. J. (1959) Short-term retention of individual items. *J. Exp. Psychol. 58, 193–198*

7. WARRINGTON, E. K. & SHALLICE, T. (1972) Neuropsychological evidence of visual storage in short-term memory tasks. *Q. J. Exp. Psychol. 24*, 30–40

8. WARRINGTON, E. K., LOGUE, V. & PRATT, R. T. C. (1971) Anatomical localization of selective impairment of auditory-verbal short-term memory. *Neuropsychologia 9*, 377–387

9. SAFFRAN, E. & MARIN, O. S. M. (1975) Immediate memory for word lists and sentences in a patient with deficient auditory short-term memory. *Brain Lang. 2*, 420–433

10. WAUGH, N. C. & NORMAN, D. A. (1965) Primary memory. *Psychol. Rev. 72*, 92–93

11. ATKINSON, R. C. & SHIFFRIN, R. M. (1968) Human memory: a proposed system and its control process, in *The Psychology of Learning and Motivation*, vol. 2 (Spence, K. & Spence, J., eds.), Academic Press, New York

12. TULVING, R. (1972) Episodic and semantic memory, in *O·ganization of Memory* (Tulving, E. & Donaldson, W., eds.), Academic Press, New York

13. NELSON, H. E. & MCKENNA, P. (1975) The use of current reading ability in the assessment of dementia. *Br. J. Clin. Psychol. 14*, 259–267

14. TULVING, E. & DONALDSON, E. (eds.) (1972) *Organization of Memory*, Academic Press, New York

15. WARRINGTON, E. K. (1975) The selective impairment of semantic memory. *Q. J. Exp. Psychol. 27*, 635–657

16. COUGHLAN, A. & WARRINGTON, E. K. (1978) Word-comprehension and word-retrieval in patients with localized cerebral lesions. *Brain 101*, 163–185

17. BARTLETT, F. C. (1932) *Remembering*, Cambridge University Press, Cambridge

18. NEISSER, U. (1967) *Cognitive Psychology*, Appleton-Century Croft, New York

19. TALLAND, G. A. (1965) *Deranged Memory*, Academic Press, New York

20. BADDELEY, A. D. & WARRINGTON, E. K. (1970) Amnesia and the distinction between long- and short-term memory. *J. Verb. Learn. Verb. Behav. 9*, 176–189

21. WARRINGTON, E. K. & WEISKRANTZ, L. (1968) New method of testing long-term retention with special reference to amnesic patients. *Nature (Lond.) 277*, 972–974

22. WARRINGTON, E. K. & WEISKRANTZ, L. (1970) Organizational aspects of memory in amnesic patients. *Neuropsychologia 9*, 67–71

23. SANDERS, H. & WARRINGTON, E. K. (1971) Memory for remote events in amnesic patients. *Brain 94*, 661–668

24. SANDERS, H. & WARRINGTON, E. K. (1975) Retrograde amnesia in organic amnesic patients. *Cortex 11*, 397–400

25. BADDELEY, A. D. & WARRINGTON, E. K. (1973) Memory coding and amnesia. *Neuropsychologia 11*, 159–165

26. WARRINGTON, E. K. & WEISKRANTZ, L. (1970) Amnesia: consolidation or retrieval? *Nature (Lond.) 228*, 628–630

27. WINOCUR, G. & WEISKRANTZ, L. (1976) An investigation of paired-associate learning in amnesic patients. *Neuropsychologia 14*, 97–40

28. BRIERLEY, B. (1977) Neuropathology of amnesic states, in *Amnesia* (Whitty, C. W. M. & Zangwill, O. L., eds.), Butterworths, London

29. SIGNORET, J. L. & LHERMITTE, F. (1976) The amnesic syndromes and the encoding process, in *Neural Mechanism of Learning and Memory* (Rosenzweig, M. R. & Bennett, E. L., eds.), MIT Press, Cambridge, Mass.

30. WARRINGTON, E. K. & WEISKRANTZ, L. (1974) The effect of prior learning on subsequent retention in amnesic patients. *Neuropsychologia 12*, 419-428

Do philosophy and the brain sciences need each other? [Commentary]

SUSAN KHIN ZAW

Bedford College, London and The Open University, Milton Keynes

Dr Blakemore raises various questions of philosophical interest and suggests that while some may safely be ignored by the practising scientist, others may actually be solved by science; that is, by empirical enquiry. This raises immediately the question of the relation between philosophy and science. If one views philosophy as essentially a conceptual inquiry—which I do—what relevance can any empirical discovery have to a philosophical problem? It is true that there are philosophical problems which are not amenable to solution merely by empirical discoveries which do not disturb the prevailing scientific theories (and some would claim that just this imperviousness to new facts is the mark of a truly *philosophical* problem). It is also true that there are scientific questions which, because they are firmly lodged within the framework of a prevailing scientific theory, have no marked philosophical resonance. It does not follow from this that philosophy and science can safely ignore each other. For particular scientific theories represent particular past philosophical decisions, and philosophical problems arise within systems of belief now largely constituted by or deriving from science. The distinction between scientific and philosophical problems tends to blur where a science is in a state of theoretical uncertainty or fluidity—as now seems to be at least partly the case with the brain sciences—when a philosophical decision may be crucial for the direction of future development, and may be taken partly on the basis of the available facts. Also, if scientific theories change, so bringing about a change in the sustaining system of beliefs, philosophical problems arising within that system may need to be reformulated, or may even cease to be statable, or just no longer seem urgent or interesting. (The question whether the mind is a different substance from the body is a case in point.) This is not the same thing, strictly speaking, as science solving a philosophical problem, in the sense that I think Dr Blakemore intends, but it remains true that advances in science may make philosophical problems fade or disappear, and we may accept such transformations as solutions of a kind. My comments are addressed to placing the questions raised by Dr Blakemore within the framework I have just sketched. I want to ask, first: are the philosophical questions which trouble him likely to be settled by scientific discoveries in the way he envisages? And second: do the theoretical difficulties he finds in the scientific study of perception have a philosophical source or component, and if so what is it?

The philosophical problem which chiefly seems to worry Dr Blakemore is some problem about reality. I infer that he regards this as a serious problem from the fact that he produces an analysis of 'perceptual validity' as functional utility which seems intended both to answer to philosophical qualms and to assist the scientific understanding of perception, and which has the consequence that 'one animal's reality need not exist for another' (p. 151). This analysis strikes me as more in the nature of a contribution to philosophy than one to science, because I can't think of a scientific question to which 'what is real for an animal is that which is functionally useful to it' is an answer—though I can think of investigations which might find heuristic value in some such assumption as 'What is perceived by an animal is that which is functionally useful to it'. Moreover, the point of introducing the notion of perceptual validity seems to be to avoid taking the question 'How good is an animal's knowledge of its environment?' in the form 'Does the animal perceive what is really there, and perceive it accurately?' The question in this form might seem to present philosophical difficulties if the nature of objective reality is thought of as essentially inaccessible to perception—any perception, including ours. Nevertheless, I think Dr Blakemore's analysis, far from avoiding the question about reality, in fact presupposes an answer to it: which is not to deny that asking the question in terms of perceptual validity may well be a better scientific bet than asking it in terms of the animal's grasp of reality. But asking the question in terms of perceptual validity does not mean that, philosophically, the scientist can dispense with, or has dispensed with, the notion of objective reality. If Dr Blakemore holds that there are strong philosophical objections to this notion, talking about perceptual validity instead does not overcome them; nor do I think that they are likely to be overcome by further discoveries about the mechanisms of perception, for the following reasons.

It is true that the history of philosophy abounds with arguments from commonplaces of perception to sceptical conclusions about reality, and perhaps this is the area Dr Blakemore has in mind when he alludes to philosophers' yearnings to know what is real. But we need to distinguish between different sceptical conclusions which have been derived from perception. Perception has standardly been thought of by inserting an intermediary—the percept—that causally links the perceiver and the external object which is the object of perceptual knowledge; though at times something not so linked to external objects may be indistinguishable by the perceiver from a percept. This constitutes, if you like, a rudimentary theory of perception, and has seemed to some enough grounds for a rational doubt about the reality of the external world. But this problem has more to do with the nature of rational doubt than with the details of perception (albeit a rational doubt which presupposes the rudimentary theory), and as such is a candidate for philosophical rather than scientific treatment. For whatever modification future theories may make to our understanding of perception, there doesn't at the moment seem to be the slightest prospect that some future theory will deny any of the elements of the rudimentary theory. I think myself that careful examination of the sceptical arguments (something not easily accomplished by common sense alone) shows that they are not valid, so in my view this particular problem about reality is not one that Dr Blakemore or any scientist studying perception need worry about.

But perhaps this is what Dr Blakemore means to suggest in any case, when he rejects Gorgias the sophist on reality and says that the brain researcher's approach is necessarily more empirical and pragmatic (p. 140). Since Dr Blakemore's object in providing an analysis of perceptual validity seems to be to purge scientific discourse of a suspect notion of 'absolute' reality, perhaps what impress him are, rather, the philosophical arguments designed to show the impossibility of knowing, not that the external world exists, but what it is like independent of our perception of it, what is its nature. There are various ways one might take this. It could be Kant's problem; but then one wonders why Dr Blakemore does not avail himself of Kant's answer—though we cannot know the objects of experience as things in themselves, we are yet in a position to think them as things in themselves. (If we were not, *any* science would be impossible.) Of course we might be rationally entitled to think things in themselves and yet not achieve more in so doing than to establish the common world of objects distinct from percepts. To do this is a prerequisite of establishing a science of objects, but it is not yet a science of objects: for that we must think them in the right way. And philosophy can provide no *a priori* guarantee that there will be a right way, that the attempt to found a science will succeed—even if it manages to show that the attempt itself is not irrational. Perhaps it is rather this problem which Dr Blakemore is addressing: perhaps his concern is not so much with whether we may think things in themselves but rather with how we should do so, with which predicates we should attribute to things in attempting a scientific account of them. This, perhaps, is the point of his question about whether there exist in the brain structures or activities equivalent to Platonic universals. If we understood the brain well enough to see how its structure limited or determined thought, we might thereby have discovered the limits or determinants of or conditions on the structure of science. But such questions—questions about the 'right' way to think things in themselves—can only be answered by the future development of science, not by philosophy. For our confidence in the legitimacy of such questions, our belief in the possibility of understanding the world better as distinct from merely constructing endless alternative descriptions of it, rests both on the actual success of physics, and on the way it has succeeded—both of which, so far as philosophy is concerned, might have been otherwise. *Pace* Kuhn,[1] the succession of theories in physics has not been a succession of revolutions, but a subsumption of special cases under wider theories, accompanied by increases in the range of prediction and control. Because of this, we are inclined to say that physics tells us what is real: in as 'absolute' a sense of reality as we are ever likely to get. Now this is a notion of reality which Dr Blakemore himself makes use of in rejecting reference to reality in favour of functional utility: for only by tacitly appealing to the framework provided by physics is he able to refer to the features of the world sensed by other animals though not by us, and state his arguments for perceptual validity as functional utility. If his own species-relative account of what is real depends on the account of objective reality given in physics, his account cannot compete with the physical one—as, philosophically, it seems intended to do. If he explains the physical account in terms of his own, as what is functionally useful to *us*, then, contrary to what he says, the human species is indeed the measure of all things; for the realities ascribed to other species are in fact all fragments of our (scientific) reality. Dr Blakemore's relativism thus turns out to be more apparent than real—if I dare use such a phrase.

There still remains, however, the question of whether the study of the brain could yield up the limits of thought. I doubt the intelligibility of this, remembering Wittgenstein's remark that to think a limit you have to be able to think on both sides of it, which in this case would be *ex hypothesi* impossible. But could understanding the structures of the brain yield up any further understanding of the structures of thought? The difficulty with this seems to be that surely what would count as understanding the brain would be understanding how it did what it does, e.g. think: which would mean that the brain was only to be understood in terms of thought, and not the other way about. We cannot say how the brain does what it does without first having some sort of a description of what it does. It seems likely that the success of that enterprise will depend partly on finding the right terms for that description. This, I think, is the real challenge to the brain sciences, and perhaps it is to this area that Dr Blakemore's analysis really belongs. For the difficulty is not a lack of possible descriptions but an embarrassing profusion of them. How is one to pick out from these, that description of what the brain does which could be explained in terms of the structure of the brain? This seems to me a crucial scientific question with an evident philosophical component. Dr Blakemore's answer to it seems to be: think biologically, rather than neurologically or psychologically. If this is what he is saying, I can see why he might be right, and even how philosophy might help: for might not there be a connection here with the various philosophical arguments against the reduction or identification of mental states or events to or with brain states or events?

I turn now, with some diffidence, to the theoretical difficulties raised by Dr Blakemore. There are so many of these that it seemed best to consider only one or two in detail. Dr Blakemore sees difficulty with explanations of externalization and localization of objects in space in terms of activity in particular areas of the brain, preferring an account which provides some role for learning. However these two accounts aren't necessarily competitors, since he points out elsewhere that perceptual history may affect the development of functional units in the brain. What then is the source of his objections? With reference to localization, I think I can see two possible grounds of objection. First, he mentions as a difficulty the fact that the perceptual fields of individual neurons get larger the more distant their serial position from the retina; and he asks, 'How can activity in such a network of cells specify the position of a target with the precision that we know we have in localizing objects?' Now, if I have understood the literature correctly, the specific localizing information is available at the retinal or near-retinal level in the small size of the retinal and lateral geniculate receptive fields; I take it that the objection is that this specificity is lost with the larger field sizes at higher levels, as cells produce a response to a stimulus of the right shape and orientation wherever that stimulus is in a relatively large area of the retina.[2] But it seems to me that this explanation can only be a difficulty for a rigidly sequential model which accommodates the neurological counterparts of all the functions to be explained in a single causal chain, a single series of events which terminates in fully achieved perception. If the pathways envisaged by Hubel and Wiesel[2] from the retina to the cortex are conceived as the locus or embodiment of part of this one series, then it will look as if greater refinement in feature extraction proceeds with loss of localization information: so that by the time the final stage of perception is reached, the wherewithal to perceive position has been lost. The explanation of perception of localization then becomes a problem.

The problem, however, is surely either with this one-track serial model, in which perception is an ultimate goal, or with the identification of the path from the retina to the form-discriminating cells with the locus of a temporal part of the series of events terminating in perception. If one assumes, for instance, that perception is not the final stage of the process but the process itself, or that there are many parallel paths from the receptors to the pen-ultimate stage, the difficulty vanishes. If we adopt the first alternative, perception of position in the visual field would be localized at the retinal or near-retinal levels where position is an important parameter, just as form perception is localized in those neurons for which shape is an important parameter. In the second alternative, the penultimate stage would presumably be conceived as an integrative process occurring at some part of the brain where inputs from all the different strands of the visual network converged, and which also received inputs from higher-level cognitive functions. It is true that there are further difficulties with these solutions. One trouble with the first is that the phenomenon of blindness resulting from damage to the cortex might seem an objection to any visual function being located elsewhere, and there are notorious philosophical difficulties with the final stage of the second solution. But whether either solution is worth discussing rather depends on whether the problem they are devised to solve is indeed Dr Blakemore's problem.

But perhaps it is not: perhaps the ground of his objection is not so much the fate of topographical information in this particular network but the impossibility of explaining localization of objects in space by any network of this kind. The question then arises, of what kind? I hesitate to say more without knowing the answer: but clearly some general difficulty is seen here (perhaps related to his earlier plea for biological thinking about the brain?) which seems to crop up again in Dr Blakemore's remarks on the meaning of nerve impulses. Individual nerve impulses are inherently ambiguous: therefore feature detection must be a function of populations of nerve cells (presumably because the collective impulses of populations are *not* inherently ambiguous). But activity within a population would require further analysis, i.e. an 'extra set of eyes inside the head'. I must confess I cannot see why further analysis is called for here if the output of the population is no longer ambiguous. Why shouldn't detection of a particular feature (represented in the cortex) just *be* the unambiguous firing of that collection of cells? Both philosophers and psychologists sometimes feel that they cannot just say that, and if Dr Blakemore could expand on the reasons for his unwillingness to say it, we might find it led somewhere. To return to localization: is there a difference between form perception and the localization of objects in space that calls for different kinds of explanation for the two cases? Here Dr Warrington's findings may perhaps be brought to bear.[3] These support the division of visual recognition into a stage of achievement of an adequate percept and a subsequent stage of the endowment of percepts with meaning by linkages with memory images. Perhaps localization can be divided along similar lines, so that locating an object in the visual field is related to locating an object in external space as achieving an adequate percept of an object is related to recognizing an object for what it is. Transition from the one to the other might then be understood in the same way: by linkage of the location in visual space to visuomotor memories. I certainly agree with Dr Blakemore that what we know of form perception in no way explains object recognition, and that we don't understand localization of objects in external space any better than object recognition. I don't think, either, that we have anything like a complete explanation even of form perception, though whether we agree about what is still missing I am not sure: it seems to me that we are beginning to understand how both form perception and localization in the visual field take place, and to have some idea of the kind of explanation that will eventually emerge.

References

1. KUHN, S. T. (1962) *The Structure of Scientific Revolutions*, University of Chicago Press, Chicago
2. HUBEL, D. H. & WIESEL, T. N. (1962) Receptive fields, binocular interaction and functional architecture in the cat's visual cortex. *J. Physiol. (Lond.) 160*, 106–154
3. WARRINGTON, E. K. (1975) The selective impairment of semantic memory. *J. Exp. Psychol. 27*, 635–657

Discussion: Perception and memory

Blakemore: The sensory mechanisms for analysis of the world are highly specialized from species to species as well as being modifiable, to some extent, during the early experiences of any one animal. There are some very impressive examples of sensory systems that exist in other species but that human beings simply don't have; and we have no concept of what the perceptual appreciations involved would be like.

The point I wanted to make, which is perhaps philosophically naive, is that reality can be defined as that which it is biologically necessary for a particular animal to detect. We believe that our perceptual world is complete, in the sense that it provides us with all the information that we could know about the physical world. But it does not. We have no way of understanding the sensations associated with a flash of infrared light or a flood of magnetism. I suppose one could argue that the physical devices we have manufactured to detect radiations or energies for which we ourselves have no sense organs qualify in a way as cultural sense organs or perceptual devices. Through artificial transducers we may gain a little perceptual insight into the alien world that lies beyond the capacities of our own cluster of sense organs.

One can, then, define validity and reality in terms of the behavioural needs of each particular animal. The world is as complete as it needs to be for the animal in question.

Susan Khin Zaw is right to worry about how animals are able to localize objects in space accurately despite the fact that the receptive fields of visual neurons become sequentially larger through the visual pathway. The only objective way of knowing whether an animal can perform a particular action is to demonstrate that the animal can do something with the information it has. A monkey, for instance, can be trained to judge whether two lines, one above the other, are offset or not (the so-called vernier acuity task). The monkey can do that when the lines have an angular offset of only a few seconds of arc, which is much smaller than the angular size of a single receptor in the animal's eye. How can we account for that extraordinary performance in terms of the way in which neurons are hooked up all the way from the retina to the muscles that the animal uses to press the appropriate button or to make some other overt indication of its perceptual judgement? That question has by no means been answered by neurophysiological studies. How can such localization be achieved when receptive fields get bigger and bigger through the sensory pathway? There appears to be no point at which signals with the necessary spatial precision could be tapped off and sent to the motor system for the external expression of knowledge.

Perception is so much tied up with response that it could be defined as the ability to organize a particular response—perception is functionally a plan (or set of plans) of action for dealing with the world. If the perception of animals is to be discussed, it must be discussed in these terms, rather than our speculating about the ability of animals to introspect.

Searle: At some points you were talking in what I would call a homunculus vocabulary, that is you talked about the perceptual apparatus of the animal providing an internal description, and you seemed to attach significance to the isomorphism between the pattern of neurons in the rat's brain and the structure of the rat's sensitive vibrissae.

Blakemore: Everybody, including Descartes, would surely reject the idea that simple isomorphism *per se* is an *explanation* of perception. Nevertheless, it is interesting to see that there is an anatomical representation of the vibrissae, and I think it is reasonable to ask why it occurs.

Trevarthen: I am an isomorphist. I think there is a little man in the head. In fact I think there is a whole crowd of people. They all understand each other perfectly well, they are innate, they make decisions in a properly formed hierarchy, they disagree occasionally but they know how to resolve their disagreements, and they also have specialized occupations which are at least as sophisticated as anything that has been created by technology. I could show you a picture of a little 'man' in the brain of a fish, but all I want to say now is that the task of getting about in space is solved morphologically by all active animals, and even by active plants.

Some plants can perceive things in different locations relative to their plans for action. There is a plant called *Monstera gigantea* that steers its growth around the forest floor as a juvenile to find a tree of the right size and it definitely perceives a spatial field of light intensity to do this. It seeks a dense shadow, actively turning to reach towards it. It has the opposite type of phototropism—negative—to most plants until it finds a tree, then it switches its phototropism to positive and climbs the tree using a kind of tactile perception to regulate its grip.

Everybody admits there is a problem with connecting these little bits of information encoded in edge detectors. I used to call it the dustpan theory of perception: the more of these little fragments you get, the less you know how to fit them into a picture. If the grid of coordinates was removed from the picture (not reproduced here) of the bird that Colin Blakemore's cat had 'seen', those little spots would all be lost. To solve this problem we must seek widely in the brain. The midbrain of all vertebrates has a coordinated map of behaviour-space that represents the body's field of action.

You referred to my interest in relating perception to action. Then you spoke about vernier acuity and the space for localizing things around the body. The scales of movement related to these functions are very different. We cannot act with vernier acuity in manipulation, but we can use that degree of spatial resolution predictively for discriminating textures, discontinuities of structure features and so on. With respect to localizing things in the behaviour field of the whole body, this is clearly related to the bisymmetry, polarization and well-ordered arrangements of nerve connections in the projection fields throughout the nervous system.

The fact that the somatotopic principle, used as a common code for information transmission throughout the nervous system, may differ in magnification is clearly important in relation to acuity. The striate cortex in which the foveal part is greatly magnified has evolved as a kind of lens: it is a second retina with special resolving properties that somebody, some homunculus, has to use with intelligent eye movements. You cannot get vision of space or objects from such a device unless you know what question to ask it, and that question will be posed relative to a spatial field for action and to objects represented in an orderly nerve net somewhere else in the brain.

Armstrong: The traditional worry of philosophers is that if we say there is a homunculus in the head we simply reproduce exactly the same problem that the homunuclus was supposed to solve. If the homunculus has to be as sophisticated as the original task was difficult, then you will need another homunculus to perform the task of the first homunculus, and so on *ad infinitum.* But Dan Dennett (W. Lycan, personal communication) now suggests that this regress is not vicious provided that the homunculi are progressively more stupid, undertaking more and more specialized and limited tasks until in the end, perhaps, the little man does nothing more than alter a switch on a 'gate'. It is a real insight to have pointed this out, and it has more or less converted me to homunculi.

Young: What do you mean by 'more stupid'?

Searle: That they are simpler mechanisms.

Brazier: Do you mean that they lose information?

Armstrong: I mean being able to perform less and less sophisticated tasks, in a much narrower range, being able to do one specific task only, a bit like a worker on an assembly line.

Young: But selecting which task to do is not stupid.

Searle: I think 'stupid' there was intended as a metaphor.

Armstrong: To avoid the regress, in the end the task will have to be simpler.

Bunge: Dr Blakemore, I am uneasy about your use of the word 'depends' when you say that conscious visual reception depends on the cortex. If you use that vague word, which is not vague in a mathematical context, you may be taken for either a monist or a dualist. You should be more specific. If you were to say, for instance, that visual perception *is* a certain activity of certain neural systems in the cortex, that would be a different thing.

Secondly, if you are serious in characterizing reality for an animal as the sum total of all the events perceptible to the animal, you run into conflict with the physicist's perception of reality. For a physicist a thing may exist whether or not it can be perceived. The physicist's concept of reality is more inclusive than the notion of appearance. If you don't accept physics I don't think you can build good neuroscience or good psychobiology. It is one thing to perceive reality and quite another to say that that is all there is.

Thirdly, you spoke of 'operational definitions' but I am sure you don't mean that. Definitions are identities and defining is a conceptual operation, not a laboratory operation. You probably mean an indicator or an objectifier but not a definition.

Putnam: I disagree with Susan Khin Zaw's attack on Colin Blakemore. She said that we shouldn't worry about absolute reality because all the shells are blank, but when you are firing at a chimera all it is worth is blank shells. It seemed to me that Susan was representing the traditional view in philosophy that we don't need to know any empirical science, although maybe we need to know that there are illusions, that perception isn't 100% perfect, and that tables and chairs exist. The work of psychologists on the theory of perception, both of Blakemore's kind and of the experimental behavioural kind, is tremendously relevant to disputes about realism.

On the antirealist side, the work of Hubel and Wiesel, Blakemore and others shows that the brain itself constructs a version of the world which has rules of representation which are as complex as those of a scientific representation or a legal representation or a representation by an abstract artist. In comparing the scientific representation of the world with perception we are comparing one representation with another—we are not comparing science with a mythical 'absolute reality'.

The discussion of realism today centres on whether the realist notions of *truth* and *reference* are notions that can do explanatory work. The dispute in philosophy and cognitive psychology is over whether notions like truth and reference belong only to a very abstract kind of logic, or whether those notions help to explain the success of human beings in dealing with the world. On the prorealist side, people like to argue that the correct model is a computing system that constructs a complex internal representation of the external world. Work in cognitive psychology is cited in support.

Wall: I sympathize deeply with Susan Khin Zaw's puzzlement. Much of modern brain science is moving rapidly away from the very problem that you and many scientists think they are addressing. We have just heard two splendid expositions of the new phrenology. Nineteenth-century phrenology argued that bumps on the skull represented bumps in the brain and that each bump represented a function. Now we are down to a microphrenology in which each whisker has its bump. Let us think about the illustration [not printed here] shown by Blakemore of results by Creutzfeldt of a cell responding to a picture of a bird. In the experiment, the picture was moved past the animal and every time the cell fired a recording was made. The experimenter knows which way the animal and the eye were pointing but the cell does not. Next we were shown three pictures of the responses of three cells. Colin Blakemore says one just adds the pictures together. This is very easy for us to do mechanically but we haven't the foggiest idea of how the brain does it. Clearly the brain must be capable of integration but the result of much modern brain research proves disintegration by showing special functions to be isolated.

Young: But we do know something from successive scanning. Nobody has mentioned that there is an active process, except that Colin Blakemore began by saying that vision is a constructive process. Wiesel's point is only subsidiary, in a sense. The real point that we have learnt is that perception is a constructive active process.

Bunge: But the problem is how to bind the various maps into a single atlas.

Searle: Or even into a single picture. This goes back to the dustpan problem as well.

Blakemore: Many of the things that I talked about, such as isomorphism between the sensory stimulus and its central representation and the way in which the neurons of the visual cortex seem to disassemble the features of the visual scene, were put up as straw men, for the sake of discussion. An important question is: what does the brain do with the visual information after it has taken the image apart? If it only reassembles the features in some way to recreate the image, then why did it take it apart in the first place?

Searle: All that does is reformulate the question that is on my mind. It is a plausible hypothesis that if you have enough cells you could reconstruct the original picture, but of course the fact that you could reconstruct the picture on the basis of the neuron firings doesn't yet show that that's how we do it.

Ploog: What do you mean by 'how we do it'?

Searle: We have the feeling that something has been explained because we have slowly simulated the original picture. That doesn't explain how we or the animals see the bird. The animal doesn't superimpose a whole lot of photographs of neuron firings—that is what the experimenter does. How do you see the problem of what we might call the integration of the neuron firings? Professor Young had a suggestion which I think was being rejected.

Creutzfeldt: I shall discuss the problem of integration of the distributed representations of the dissected points and contours to a unity of perception in my presentation. But I may refer, here, to the conclusions we drew from our 'scanning' experiments.[1] We argued that features that are being extracted from the physical environment and represented by the activities of single neurons may not necessarily be directly relevant features in perception. For orientation-sensitive neurons in the visual system it was demonstrated that the function of such a neuronal operation may be relevant for visuomotor fixation, binocular fusion and convergence rather than for perception *per se*. In fact our present knowledge about representation of sensory stimuli by neuronal activities allows us only to formulate stimulus-response sequences, i.e. sensory-motor circuits and behavioural responses to sensory signals, rather than perception. In this respect, neurophysiology provides us only with data on the limitations of the system for information transfer (data on minimum energy that can still be perceived, i.e. threshold; maximal resolution of the various sensory systems, i.e. modulation transfer; etc.). But it has as yet failed to explain how the unity of the world that is pulled to pieces is brought together into a unity of perception.

Towers: We have heard here about the interesting phenomena of blind sight and amnesic memory, where patients have the ability to do things but deny that ability. In other words they know something but they don't know that they know it. This was thought to be the distinction between perception and conscious perception, but that is too simple. I think we must have three tiers of perception rather than two tiers. I would speak of awareness in an animal that responds to something (and therefore shows itself as being aware of it), versus conscious awareness and this in turn versus self-conscious or reflective awareness at the highest level. For instance when you shine a light into an animal's eye the pupil responds by constriction. Human beings are totally unconscious of that response. That reflex is mediated or integrated at the midbrain-stem level through the superior colliculi. Then I would suggest that conscious awareness of things that we know but don't yet know that we know could well be mediated and integrated at the forebrain level, but in the diencephalon, not in the telencephalon. In other words conscious awareness of vision is being integrated in the thalamic level, in the lateral geniculate body perhaps. In order to get self-conscious awareness or reflective awareness it seems to me that a further spin-off is needed to the telencephalon of the forebrain and to the use of the cortex. This would represent both an evolutionary sequence and an ontogenetic sequence.

Khin Zaw: Some of you now seem to be claiming that all that stuff about form perception doesn't explain perception but explains being able to get around in the world, whereas what Colin Blakemore and others are saying is that it explains form perception but doesn't explain being able to get around in the world.

Blakemore: There isn't yet an adequate explanation of how sensory information allows an animal to move around in the world. Providing such an explanation could be the appropriate ambition of neurophysiologists working on sensory systems.

Animals have to have a symbolic model of the world, which allows them to identify each object regardless of the array of sensory features that defines that object from any particular viewing point. This is true whether the animal is merely going to sit back and contemplate that object, as we might, or is going to respond to it, for instance by picking it up and eating it.

Khin Zaw: What does the homunculus do that a neuron doesn't do? If a homunculus gets that stupid, why couldn't it be a neuron?

Armstrong: I expect that they are neurons, at the very bottom level.

Crown: In a discussion like this we need bridges. One bridge between brain and mind is emotion. A great enigma in psychiatry is hysteria, for example hysterical blindness. This is a reversible phenomenon, so it is in a sense a functional deficit. I wonder where one would place the 'lesion' for that, between the peripheral receptor and the visual cortex?

Elizabeth Warrington differentiated episodic or personalized memory from semantic memory. These observations are relevant to an area of psychiatry usually called 'events research'. In this, criteria are established for classifying life events according to their significance; such events are differentiated from events that are not significant. It has been shown that more events as so defined precede breakdowns such as recurrent schizophrenic episodes or depressive illness. There is also current interest in whether more life events of significance precede physical breakdowns such as appendicitis.

Warrington: I don't think that in our patients anyone has succeeded in quantifying memory for personal events as distinct from public events. Presumably what you are suggesting is that systems subserving memory for public events and personal events can be differentiated.

Ploog: I am puzzled by the arguments about picturing reality. Ever since Jakob von Uexküll[2] it has been clear that each animal has its own world and that the world one has depends on the make-up of the nervous system. It is likely that the human nervous system is not the last word in evolution, so we have limitations to the cognition of our world, just as the shrew and other animals have. Our world is certainly more complex and much more elaborate in terms of functional utility than the worlds of other species. If neurophysiologists and neurobiologists can show which mechanisms are used for mapping this world, and if the philosophers say they don't care whether the nervous system is arranged in such and such a way, then I think it is the task of the philosophers to tell us why this very unlikely brain organization is as it is. They must explain why the processing of the outer world is done in that way. The discussion on reality or non-reality is a discussion between those people who describe a machine or try to find out how and why the machine works the way it does and those who say they don't care how the machine is constructed but want to know what the machine is. The question is inadequate to natural science.

Putnam: I didn't say that knowing how the machine is constructed, or how the representation of the world is constructed, was irrelevant. I criticized Susan Khin Zaw for saying that. Philosophers do need to have this information.

Secondly, I want to take a minute to describe experimental work being done in cognitive psychology and artificial intelligence on the so-called image problem. It is clear that the mere construction of an image can't be the solution of the integration problem. The brain or nervous system already has an image on the retina and constructing another image inside the head wouldn't integrate things. Zenon Pylyshyn[3] argues that integration at the functional level has to involve judgements. Somehow the picture has to be turned into various propositions, various categories have to be imposed. Nobody in this field thinks that just recognizing verticals and horizontals solves the problem. There is more to be done.

Some studies in artificial intelligence turn on the very difficult problem of how you know which piece of the picture from the left eye corresponds to which piece of the picture from the right eye, even when the room has as uniform and confusing a pattern as you can make. Although the construction of a picture cannot be the *solution* of the integration problem, it doesn't follow that the brain can't use images, even representations which are spatial. The evidence for this from Shephard's original experiment[4] is that the time people take to rotate an image through a given distance is proportional to the objective optical angle.

Wikler: When we speak of reality as being that which is biologically necessary for the animal to perceive, we must be using 'reality' metaphorically, because I think we would all take it as axiomatic that we are living in the same reality. The theoretical content of the metaphor, I take it, is the idea that it is adaptive for the animal to perceive exactly what it does perceive.

On that view, the rest of the world, which the animal is not equipped to perceive, in a way doesn't enter into the animal's reality because there is no need for it to do so. This seems to exclude the possibility, though maybe not for any serious theoretical reasons, that if an animal were to have had the ability to perceive other parts of reality, that ability might also answer to certain of its needs. Yet, if a human being lost in the wilderness had the ability to sense a magnetic field, he or she might have a better chance of survival. The absence of the ability of certain organisms to perceive these parts of reality might be more of an evolutionary accident than any kind of functional adaptation to the world. If that were so, then the idea of reality being that part of the world that the animal needs in order to survive loses some of its force. Since an animal may need to perceive more than it does if it is to survive and reproduce, it would then perceive only part of its 'reality'.

Creutzfeldt: In response to Professor Young's earlier remark I should like to add that although scanning is an important aspect of perception, it does not explain the problem of integration in perception. It becomes even more complicated, since we now have to integrate not only over space but also over time: we added one dimension but haven't solved the problem.

Dr Warrington gave us a fascinating illustration of localized memory functions in various cortical systems. (I prefer not to use the term memory stores because it reminds one immediately of computer memory boxes, which is not how our memory works.) Since the neocortex shows, *in principle*, an identical anatomical and functional organization in all areas (see Ref. 5)— including, presumably, adaptive functions, i.e. memory—I am tempted to generalize your findings by saying that any cortical part that is connected with a given function has 'memory' for that function. This is, at least, the conclusion I would draw from what you have presented to us.

Warrington: I took my examples entirely from verbal semantic memory but Susan Khin Zaw referred to the other side of this coin, that is to semantic knowledge for visual objects. The patients I mentioned in my concluding remarks had extremely interesting deficits in comprehending the significance of objects which had been adequately perceived; for example, they could draw them beautifully and they could 'match' different views of the same object but they didn't know what those same objects were used for. Difficulties arise in trying to deal with event memory in similar terms. I don't think we have the faintest idea of where or how event memory is stored. All that the amnesic syndrome demonstrates is an inability to retrieve, but we still don't know what is doing the retrieving and where it is being retrieved from.

Blakemore: Mario Bunge pointed out the conflict between physical evidence about the world and reality as the sum of perceived events. One can argue that the physical detection of events, using instruments as cultural extensions of our sense organs, is itself part of our perceptual analysis of the world. Perception includes our interpretation, through physical instruments, of the world. Putting on a pair of glasses does not alter the world itself but adding this physical instrument can change one's perception because it affects the way light reaches the eyes.

Daniel Wikler questioned whether reality could be equated with need because under certain circumstances any animal would be better off if it possessed additional kinds of sensory apparatus. This is certainly true, but natural selection has made sure that what animals *have* is what they *most often* need. For any particular animal, reality is that fraction of the physical world that natural selection has 'decided' it needs to deal with.

Another area that has been interestingly discussed here is the relationship between the study of sensory neurobiology and the question of consciousness. For those who hold the view that consciousness is an epiphenomenon a perceptual system need not have conscious experience attached to it in order to provide an individual with the capacity to respond to the environment. That approach is weakened by the evidence from 'blind sight'. Even without the visual cortex some people still have the ability to describe what objects are in front of them, to respond to them appropriately on command, yet they deny *perceiving* them and under normal circumstances they appear completely blind in that part of the visual field. That seems to be the only piece of evidence that would allow one to reject the epiphenomenological approach to the question of consciousness.

Warrington: I don't think the patients could describe what they saw. That is a misunderstanding.

Blakemore: They can say whether a pattern of stripes presented to them is vertical or horizontal.

Warrington: They have to be told the choice and they have to be forced to make a choice. I don't think that counts as description in any sensible use of the word.

Cognitive psychologists have a concept which is perhaps helpful, since most of this discussion has been about the visual cortex and vision. They make a subdivision between what they call pre-categorical perception and post-categorical perception. The interpretative aspects of perception, which the philosophers seem to think are missing in Colin Blakemore's and Hubel and Wiesel's account, are relevant here. We now know something about these post-categorical stages of object perception and how the brain handles them. The next important stage in object recognition (after primary visual cortex processing) is perceptual categorization.[6] That is, there seems to be some mechanism whereby stored internal representations of the outside world find a 'match' with objects, even though the stimulus deviates from its prototype. Our patient who did not comprehend objects was shown a series of objects photographed from an unusual view. He said he could not recognize them but when we showed him the same objects photographed from the usual view he got very cross and said 'you have already shown me these objects but they were photographed from a different angle. I have already told you I don't know what they are'. He was able to make this perceptual categorization quite normally. In group studies we have shown that this skill of being able to allot stimuli to the same perceptual category is subserved by the right parietal area. This is a fairly strong and robust finding. As this is in the right hemisphere I would suppose that this stage is relatively independent of language or meaning.[6]

Further, we have been able to demonstrate a double dissociation between this skill, perceptual categorization, and the skill of interpreting an object in terms of its function. Left hemisphere patients can do this perceptual categorization task perfectly normally but are impaired on a task demanding comprehension of function. The patients with the right parietal lesions who are unable to make perceptual categorizations have no difficulty in saying which objects have similar functions. These stages of perception are probably organized in series, the end product being a percept that has meaning and significance.

Khin Zaw: I think I now have an answer to what I wanted to ask Colin, namely what exactly is the problem about the current candidates for explanation? It is indeed the problem of integration, but it is more than that. It seems as if what some people regard as possible explanations of how the brain works—the splitting of large-scale functions into a series of subsidiary functions probably localized in specific areas of the brain—others regard as posing a problem, while others again don't regard it as problematic exactly but don't regard it as explaining much either. The difficulty, for those that see one, doesn't now seem to be *just* that the direction of the process, where this has been identified, is towards greater fragmentation, so that the problem would be solved if a later, integrative stage in the process could be identified. It seems to be rather that the direction of the process together with other things has suggested that it is a mistake to look for an integrative stage at all, that the kind of fragmentation of function that has been found is not the right *kind* of thing to be an explanation of something as global as perception, which includes the recognition of objects for what they are. If that is the situation I think there is a philosophical question mixed up in it, namely the one suggested in my paper: what is the correct form of the explanandum, and what kind of explanans is appropriate to what kind of explanandum? This seems to me the problem that Colin Blakemore and Colwyn Trevarthen are addressing, and it seems to me to fall exactly between science and philosophy: pure conceptual analysis won't solve it, but neither will the addition of facts without some sort of explanatory scheme to make sense of them.

Medawar: One of the difficulties about this conference is that we need to discuss a draft solution of the mind–body problem. So let me give you a draft solution. Suppose a man has an electronic bonnet on his head and somebody is reading his electroencephalogram, and that his malevolent aggressive thoughts looked very spiky, while his loving tender thoughts were more gently sinuous, would not an infinitude of such correlations provide a solution to the mind–brain problem? If it isn't a solution, what is? And if it *is* an answer, what does it answer? We must be able to envisage some solution to this problem, otherwise it is no good discussing it at all. In all scientific research one has to start with a draft solution or hypothesis.

Bennett: That question presupposes that this conference is addressed to some one problem. If that is so, nobody has informed me of this. I don't think there is just one problem.

Searle: I think there is a serious question that has been a kind of *Leitmotiv* of today's discussion. That is, we are not quite sure what counts as an explanation. But that is not a barrier to further research. On the contrary, the research has to be concerned with the question of what is supposed to count as an explanation, and that itself is a mixture of empirical and philosophical questions. I welcome that situation.

References

1. CREUTZFELDT, O. D. & NOTHDURFT H. C. (1978) Representation of complex visual stimuli in the brain. *Naturwissenschaften 65*, 307–318
2. UEXKÜLL, J. VON (1909) *Umwelt und Innenwelt der Tiere* (2nd edn., Berlin, 1921)
3. PYLYSHYN, Z. W. (1973) What the mind's eye tells the mind's brain: a critique of mental imagery. *Psychol. Bull. 80*, 1–24
4. SHEPHARD, R. N. & METZLER, J. (1971) Mental rotation of three dimensional objects. *Science (Wash. D.C.) 171*, 701–703
5. CREUTZFELDT, O. (1977) Generality of the functional structure of the neocortex. *Naturwissenschaften 64*, 507–517
6. WARRINGTON, E. M. & TAYLOR, A. M. (1978) Two categorical stages of object recognition. *Perception 7*, 695–705

The tasks of consciousness: how could the brain do them?

COLWYN TREVARTHEN

Department of Psychology, University of Edinburgh

Abstract According to Darwin's theory of evolution by natural selection, the existence of mental operations proves their usefulness. Darwin called himself a mental materialist. This is one scientific theory of consciousness.

Human consciousness has three useful aspects: awareness, intentionality and sharing with others. All have simple equivalents in animals. The latter two are neglected in neurophysiology and experimental psychology.

Developmental, neuroanatomical and neuropsychological evidence shows that the human brain has innate structures of awareness, intentionality and interpersonal sharing. Human life depends on interpersonal cooperation. We may have a conscious self, but consciousness of others is essential in us.

Studies of commissurotomy patients demonstrate the elaborate interconnected neural organization of consciousness and provide evidence of underlying and necessary levels of motivation, perception and motor integration below consciousness. Additionally, they show that awareness may be split into two different modes. These regulate one another during development and are complementary in culturally sophisticated adult life. One hemisphere, usually the left, has responsibility for expressing ideas and purposes in language. The other responds to the phenomenal context and the subjective situation. Both have human experiences and purposes. Both still collaborate in a unified intentional system after commissurotomy.

Infant studies reveal that language develops out of an interpersonal mental process. This seems to control development of thinking. Thus notions of the newborn as an isolated amoral id, and of the infant as an egocentric discoverer of the object concept, must be rejected. Cultivation of moral awareness and a sense of purpose guided by meanings and values depends on innate organization of the human brain for interpersonal consciousness.

LIMITS IN THE SCIENTIFIC STUDY OF THE MECHANISMS OF CONSCIOUSNESS

In Darwin's theory of evolution by natural selection, all actions of life have usefulness to life.[1] It is important that the theory sees consciousness as necessarily beneficial in human living, certainly not an epiphenomenon.[2] It implies that mental processes are governed by adaptive brain mechanisms that evaluate life circumstances and make demands on them, and do so effectively and with benefit.

All the evidence from brain research indicates that any act or state of consciousness will involve most of the brain in excitation patterns of fantastic complexity. Analysis by the methods of neurophysiology determines how neurons excite one another and generate patterned forces of behaviour. But neurophysiology is not intended to be a science of the mind and it may offer little to such a science. Claude Bernard[3] advocated an experimental medicine that would aim at 'regulating the hidden springs of living machines'. However, the discoverer of homeostatic regulation of the *milieu interne* was eloquent in his criticism of reductionism in his subject. He would, I think, agree that modern neurophysiology is a very specialized science among the possible sciences of the brain, which is, above all, the regulator of the *milieu spirituel* or *l'esprit humaine*.

Comparative anatomy of brain systems and neuropsychology are more germane than nerve cell physiology to questions about mechanisms of consciousness. The study of brain development has special importance. It shows that the total brain cannot be considered apart from the body which performs actions, and that the body and brain are adapted by evolution to interact or resonate conjointly in response to the resources of an intricately structured world: a world that must, in consequence of evolution, have high potential usefulness for the conscious state.

THREE INSEPARABLE ASPECTS OF CONSCIOUSNESS

Dictionary definitions of the word consciousness imply that a human bein lives with immediate experience of unity of purpose. We each perceive th⌄ world relative to what we want to do, we are conscious of having acted in a chosen way, and we know what in principle we are going to do next, or later on. Perception, utilizing diverse arrays of sensory information, is unified with the single centre of purpose we have most of the time. Experience of acting affirms the same unity. Movements that orient body parts and control uptake of perceptual information are coordinated in one agency.

Consciousness also has a sense of sharing awareness; hence the use of 'we' when speaking of consciousness. In the Shorter Oxford English Dictionary, for example, the first definition is of a Middle English usage of consciousness to mean 'mutual knowledge'. In French *conscience psychologique*, concerned with a sense of purpose and of unified awareness, is distinguished from *conscience morale* which has inherent response to the life of others. It would appear that, in modern usage, there are three main strands to definition of the human mental condition.

(1) *Conscious intentionality* is knowing what one is doing, and why. It is animated by regulatory states of excitement which estimate the risks of acting in particular ways and feelings about the vital benefits or threats that may be given by the objects and milieu of performatory action.

(2) *Conscious awareness* is being perceptive of reality here and now, knowing what is being seen, heard, touched, etc. While frequently dispassionate it takes pleasure from the recognition of familiar harmony and resists confusion. It selectively attends, and usually appears to have a single channel for information uptake, but may quickly change either the concentration or the direction of attending.

(3) *Conscious sharing* of knowledge and personal feelings is having intimacy with the consciousness of others and awareness of affectional and moral responsibility to them. Personal relations are animated by intense emotions which are expressed to others involuntarily.

A psychological study of consciousness must keep interest in all three of the above natural functions of consciousness if it is to match up to facts about human brain activity. Philosophical investigations often reject one or two of them. The empiricists, for example, have little interest in (1) or (3), yet these two aspects have great importance in every free manifestation of human life where the benefits of consciousness are most obvious.

Consciousness is unified about a self. It has a centre, a direction of movement and a memory of a past. Rational philosophers tell us that a concept of 'self' is the source of unity in purpose and of experience. Self awareness is said to be acquired from experience in society. Unity of consciousness appears, in the empiricist view, to depend on the coherence of a personal itinerary of events perceived and responded to. But there are two difficulties with the idea that memory of sequences of experiences on its own makes unity in consciousness. One difficulty is that neonates do not appear purposeless or disunified in purpose, and they have little history of experience. The other is that we often find very similar patterns of consciousness in one another while having the chance of very different trails of experience. Both of these issues will be discussed below. The evidence suggests that the brain and body together form a system with unity put into it by natural selection, and well established at birth. The self which gains experience is not entirely a consequence of experience.

The interpersonal drive of human consciousness is quite at odds with any view that the self is the primary, solitary, autonomous and private core of life.[4] We may understand one another. As Buber[5] asserts, the existence of 'I' is contingent on the existence of 'You'. Interpersonal understanding is seen in the intense cooperation of human action and in the transmission of experience and knowledge. It is aided by language and other artificial systems of communication, but it is dramatically potent in infancy and childhood before these artifacts are understood.

Now there is doubt among psychologists concerning the role of words in *bringing about* community in awareness. They see abundant evidence of 'non-verbal' signals or signs in human action that serve the transmission of meanings. Infants achieve a surprisingly effective level of interpersonal understanding before they know or use any words.[6,7,8] Animals show complex joint awareness and perception of one another's motives without words.[9] Some animals achieve intimate understanding with humans, who may benefit emotionally or practically from the association.

Philosophers of language have moved away from logical positivism to Speech Act Theory.[10] This philosophy recognizes a system of intentions in each subject, as well as a fundamental, subverbal intersubjectivity that knows the kinds of relationships ('dialogue constituent universals'[11]) which intentions may build up when persons interact. In speaking we seek to influence, obstruct, help, entertain, annoy, etc., those whom we address, and we do this with attitudes, gestures, mannerisms, tone of voice, dress and choice of occasion.

I conclude that, in addition to an innate unity of intentional command and of a phenomenal awareness, we humans have an innate intersubjectivity. I believe that an 'I' or 'me' that wills and experiences inside my body, and a 'you' and 'others' that do these mental things in other bodies, are somewhat separate in the brain. The brain is moved to persistently relate the two images of personality.

Evidence will be presented for the existence of this intersubjective mechanism in the mental processes of infants, and there are some neuropsychological and neuroanatomical data which support this hypothesis too. The brain seems to have anatomical readiness before birth to set up acts of solitary purpose and acts of understanding with others. These functions, with differentiated cerebral embodiment, are reintegrated in consciousness. Much postnatal development of the mind appears to be an outcome of the mutual interaction and harmonization of processes for the self and for others.

IMAGES FOR MOVEMENT IN CONSCIOUSNESS

Control of human action is miraculously efficient. The brain processes that govern the whole body movement must be highly predictive of the physical conditions for its realization. The same goes for the temporary displacements of each of the special perceptual mechanisms such as the eyes and hands. The greater part of this control is carried out unconsciously, by a regulator of skill with a motor memory that is conscious only of resultant acts or shifts of awareness, not of constituent forces and displacements. Finally, human interpersonal behaviour is supported by a highly specialized set of mobile organs, notably the face and hands, that have a special anatomical design for promoting signalling behaviour.

Laboratory experimental psychology of perception, concentrating on a physical analysis of sensory input, nearly always with flat visual stimuli or short sounds, has neglected all forms of motive in the subject other than those directly respondent to discrete stimuli from outside the subject, or simple change of physiological state in that person's body or brain. However, headway in a general theory of intentional movement and of active perception has been made recently by attempts to record and analyse the conditions of more natural acts that interest subjects more. The dissatisfaction of one cognitive psychologist with the linear processing model of perception and thinking, according to which chunks of informational structure or configurations of neural disturbance are filtered and recoded, then processed as in an automated manufacturing process, is expressed by Neisser.[12] He invokes strategies of action that the subject contributes centrifugally to the getting of stimuli, calling them 'schemata', a term from Frederick Bartlett who in his early days was interested in explaining how a cricketer could possibly control his actions in hitting a ball. Bartlett took the term 'schema' from Henry Head who was intrigued with phantom limbs and pathological distortions of the body image produced by brain injury. Applications of experimental psychology to practical fields require that movement be taken into account because intelligence is only rarely and artificially inactive.

The place of consciousness in 'information uptake' is indicated by recent experiments on the retrieval of sensory data when the stimulus is confused by 'noise' or masked. The subjects may gain knowledge of the meaning of the stimulus relative to their experience and motives, but have no awareness of the 'real' stimulus itself. For example, they may think of the object but not see the word that brought it to mind.[12a]

Precise measurements of event perception by Michotte[12b] indicated that standards internal to the subject form the basis for judgement of various kinds of animate and inanimate causality. This line of research has been taken up with great success by Johansson,[13] among others. Clearly we perceive the aims and motivations of human movement with ease. This ability to perceive acts rather than movement patterns or physical motion, of clear adaptive value, is probably related to the long-neglected function of the senses in keeping track of the relation of one's own body-flight to surroundings in locomotion, and in recording change of posture and of limb displacement relative to the body.[14]

Skilful acts must be regulated by images of what is to be performed. That there is such an image has been proved by the bioengineering studies of Bernstein[15] and his successors. Investigation of how the eyes move in the field of light has forced both psychologists and physiologists to recognize that the brain can and constantly does make up a representation of acts of visual prehension and eye–hand coordination, and that these acts predict the layout of information in a coherent motor space.

For all acts in awareness there must be precise and well-integrated representations in the brain of goals in a single 'space' of movement, or 'praxic space'. The coherence and reliability of this space, as well as its momentary adaptation to a new perceptual array, require sensory information, but there must also be a considerable central core in the specification for movement which is not a direct impression from afference. In other words, we have to admit that intentions are being generated in well-ordered systems of our brains all the time we are experiencing. This is not the same as a motor theory of perception, because the intentions may not include a complete description of conditions for actual movement. Nor is it a reafference theory—for the same reason. It is a theory of cerebrally integrated general motives.

Image-forming systems that form motives are of embryonic origin.[16] There is anatomical evidence that motivational systems form in the brain before birth. Experiments with fetuses confirm the initial autonomy of these systems. Change of their structure in response to experiences must be with respect to an organization which is initially independent of sensory input.

Electrical activity of the brains of adults solving perceptual puzzles indicates that widespread neuronal activity occurs before the moment of stimulation.[17] This activity is involved in setting the form of consciousness and its readiness for change.

FITNESS OF THE WORLD FOR CONSCIOUSNESS

The logic of evolutionary theory is reciprocal. Forms of life inhabit a world that is fit for their adaptations. This has important implications for a theory of awareness as well as for explaining how intentions arise. It is the central theme of ecological theories of perception.

Gibson[18] has elucidated the general nature of environmental information for perception, emphasizing the rich orderliness and reliability of the informational array. Perception need not detect all the dimensions of reality that a physical meter might detect because there is a redundancy of data for verifying invariant rules about the kind of understanding that a subject is trying to get from perception. Thus the geometry of light rays which stimulate the eye is changed in invariant ways when the subject moves, when an object approaches or rotates, when a surface displaces or when it is deformed. Recently Gibson[19] has recognized that another vital factor in the use of perceptual information is the motive of the subject. Perception is not decided by the useful resources of stimulation alone; it requires an approach by the subject's mind, a latent purpose or proposition in relation to which the stimulus affords a setting for activity. What Gibson calls *perceptual affordances* are relative to what the perceiving subject is ready to do and the specific dependence of this readiness on knowing about external circumstances.

Human consciousness is supported by a space for action (extracorporeal space in general), surfaces for holding and limiting action, objects that are separate from their locations on or among surfaces, and properties of objects that permit their use by a diversity of consummatory acts. And then there are other human beings who offer interpersonal activity towards which the human mind leans strongly.

Perception arises out of a partnership of organism and environment, the subject and the world, that has been created by evolutionary adaptation of brains and bodies.

MODES OF CONSCIOUSNESS TO BE SEEN IN BEHAVIOUR

The fundamental constraints and adaptations of consciousness may be described in terms of modes of acting or perceiving in a field of behaviour centred on the body. These modes of function, which imply anatomical systems in the brain, are explained more fully elsewhere.[6]

(1) Locomotion and posture are guided by wide perception in the space round the body. They involve the whole body in integrated patterns of muscle activity. Accurate fit to the array through which progress is being made requires proprioception to detect errors of displacement of the body relative to itself and exproprioception of any consistent external reference features. Such regulation will be aided by retention of sensory–motor images or formulae for skills that apply to many situations.

(2) Orienting accomplishes choice of direction or location in surroundings. A specialized receptor locus of the body of high sensitivity is aimed at

informative loci in the stimulus array by rotating the whole body, or by rotating a part which bears the receptor. For example, the foveae scan the light array by eye rotations. Fitting selective focal orientation into the general ambient spatial field of awareness of surroundings is aided by a motor function which scans at a regular rate in measured steps (e.g. oculomotor saccades). Each locus sampled by an act of focal attention must relate to all other similar acts and to the field in which body progression is guided.

(3) Identifying objects and events is a mode of cerebral action that measures up to how much intelligence a living being has. The more a species can do, the more important is the recognition of the right goal or target object. In each species the power to perceive identities (i.e. to cognize) matches the capacities for differential praxis (skilful use of objects).

Distinguishing things requires the detection of local features or microstructures of the world and their organization in objects that can be separated from their situations. Useful things recur in the world and defining features become perceptual signs for objects. Cerebral mechanisms for focal perception have feature-detecting elements adapted to defining edges, changes of substance, and the physical and biological potentialities of things in the clutter of surroundings. These elements have been evolved to distinguish objects. But feature detectors cannot work in loose aggregates. Features can only represent objects if the feature detectors are related to each other by some space-defining set of links in the brain. Presumably the links that represent objects are analogous to the space-defining network for control of locomotion and orienting.

Perceiving specific, local detail requires extra cognitive work and precise movements of attending, focalizing, etc. Consciousness of the significance of events by the subject relative to his or her purpose may bypass this detailed apprehension: hence there may be consciousness of a judgement without retention of the evidence.[12a] Like perception of things, perception of forms and symbols requires detection of features in their relations within a space of praxic behaviours, but forms and symbols also relate to a space of communicative behaviours—i.e. to meaning.

(4) The final mode of intelligent action with special importance in human consciousness is that which causes imaging of others in relation to the self. I propose that evolution 'discovered' intersubjectivity by extending the essential benefits of intentional subjectivity. Intentionally coherent and aware subjects who are built on the same organizing principles would tend to strongly interact or resonate. The receivable output of one, disturbances created by movements, would stimulate the self-regulatory

mechanisms of others nearby, although there would be special invariants of this alteroceptive function. Most importantly, stimuli from others do not necessarily follow from one's own impulse to be active. They may happen to one, or may even deliberately elude or nullify one's purpose. The idea of an intersubjective resonance which couples patterns of intentional action has been developed elsewhere to explain communication between an infant and its mother.[7,20]

Levels of consciousness may be related to the above modes in a systematic hierarchy. Awareness may be absent from the automatic adjustments of locomotion, orienting and object recognition and from emotional responses to others.

CORRELATIONS BETWEEN THE FORMS OF EMBRYO BRAINS AND BEHAVIOUR

Adaptive modes of behaviour are embodied in visible structures of central nervous systems which emerge in embryo stages of development. General mobility within a behavioural field is reflected in the bilateral symmetry and antero-posterior polarization of the brain and spinal cord. The central nervous system of the early embryo has in it an image of the body and its main organ systems, i.e. a somatotopy. This determines basic integrative nerve activities.[16]

The brain receives input from a set of paired or midline special sense organs—eyes, vestibular organs, cochleae, lips, tongue, nostrils. Each of these includes a receptor epithelium which is patterned to give a somatotopic image in the brain of one field of experience. The collective field of experience must relate directly to the whole field of action. Both input and output of behaviour are relative to the form of the body and to the position and mobility of the satellite systems such as limbs, head, receptor organs, etc. Unified perception arises by the collective influx of excitation in all the different receptors. They map into the brain in such a way as to correspond with each other and with the motor or efferent systems, while serving as channels for selective attending.

In the course of brain development each sensory or motor map is specified to a first approximation by the splitting up of the primary embryogenic neural representation of the total body field. Several satellite partial fields are formed, each with its organizer, comparable with the primary organizer of the body and neural plate. Each partial field has a receptor array, sampling a set of directions in the body central field (e.g. an eye), and a motor structure (e.g. the extrinsic eye muscles) that can change the position of the receptor relative to the main body axis and the direction and distance of loci outside the body. Thus are created a number of *partial-orienting systems* inside the

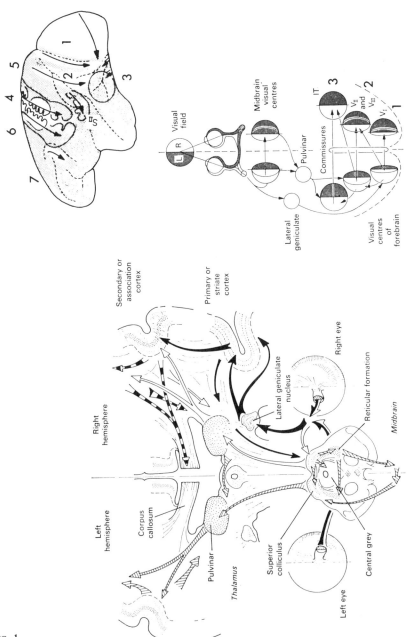

FIG. 1.

total orienting system of the whole body. Integrity of exploratory behaviour requires that each partial orientation be congruent with orientation of the body. If all the partial orienting systems are accurately specified as equivalent in their space of action to the appropriate part of the full orienting system, they will be equivalent to each other. This ensures an intermodal integrity of perception and memory, different receptor modalities being with reference to one and the same full field of experience and potential action.

Somatotopic neural arrays are macroscopic modules of the brain. Brain parts are interconnected with precise respect for a common body-field representation invisibly impressed on their constituent cells and their extensions. There is a paired chain of sensory fields, all somatotopically mapped, corresponding by orderly projection systems with the paired receptor epithelia. These in turn feed into internuncial systems that carry an orderly mapping to the connected segmental motor fields that together constitute a single efferent mechanism that projects the body into the fields of action. Stimulation and recording studies prove that these systems function to regulate orientation and selective attending.

Evolution of terrestrial and aerial life is correlated with an increase in size and complexity of the cerebral and cerebellar cortices. Both cortices represent, many times, the images of the body that are integrated in the brain-stem and spinal cord (see Fig. 1). The cerebrum is most concerned with exteroceptive information, elaborate states of motivation and retention of a memory record of significant experiences of the world. The cerebellum is organized to represent the motoric potentialities and inertial properties of the whole body. It is proprioceptive and exproprioceptive. It is involved in formation of the motor memories essential to skilled action.

Consciousness must depend on all these levels of neural process. The lower levels of the hierarchy of brain mechanisms are the essential factors for the knowing and intending of the top levels.

←

FIG. 1. Maps in the brain.[31, 44]
The rhesus monkey brain (right) shows the main cortical areas: 1: Striate cortex, unilateral retinotopic map, with foveal area magnified. 2: Prestriate belt cortex. Many maps. 3: Inferotemporal cortex. Large bilateral receptor fields all including fovea. 4: Post-central somaesthetic cortex, with enlarged hand area. 5: Dorsolateral parietal 'command' cortex, extracorporeal space coordinating eye with hand. 6: Precentral motor cortex. 7: Prefrontal cortex and frontal oculomotor field. Arrows: orientational meridian, from lateral to central. Left: Anatomical scheme for the human visual system to explain unity of ambient vision after commissurotomy, and bisection of visual awareness that depends on striatal input to the secondary or association cortex. It also explains the phenomenon of 'blind-sight' after loss of the striate cortex. Visual input to the ambient visual process, white arrows; geniculo-striate input to focal vision, black arrows.

CONSCIOUSNESS OF SPLIT-BRAIN SUBJECTS

Important information about how the human brain maintains consciousness has come in recent years from animal and human subjects after surgical disconnection of the cerebral hemispheres. The elements destroyed by surgery belong to what is presumed to be the integrative machinery of consciousness. The nerve cells and endings directly affected are in the cerebral cortex layers where responses to stimulation from different modalities overlap and where motivational sets determine how those regions will react and what they will transmit towards control of motor actions.

Most neocortical commissure neurons are in the so-called 'association cortex'. Now neurophysiologists are revising their ideas of how these tissues function, attributing to them much greater responsibility for active selection of perceptual information and initiation of movements. Cells in these cortices become active when a sentient and freely moving subject decides to aim a preformative movement to a particular place, and makes appropriate exploratory or attending movements in preparation for the move.[21] This fits with the complex psychological consequences of lesions in those regions of the human brain[22] and with electroencephalographic records of mass activity of cortical neurons.[23] Where anatomical studies show that the interhemispheric connections are richest, and in cortical tissue zones that are unique to human beings, brain lesions may cause profound disturbances in visualizations of spatial relations, loss of perceptual distinctness between objects and the surroundings, poor coordination of manipulative behaviour, loss of speech, distorted comprehension of words, inability to recognize persons by sight, or defects of planning or memory for a wide range of behaviours.[24]

After commissurotomy, cortical processes of mental integration go on separately in the two hemispheres. What in fact is the consequence of this for manifestations of consciousness? Most of our knowledge comes from intensive psychological study of a few patients at the California Institute of Technology.[25,26] Research with human subjects, who were operated on so that epilepsy could be controlled by stopping the interhemispheric build-up of seizure activity, followed a systematic investigation of the effects of commissurotomy on cats and monkeys. The main finding with the animals was that perception and consolidation of memories were split in two by the operation, but coordination of a unified purposiveness in action was only slightly affected.[27]

The human patients gave dramatic confirmation of the split-brain effect seen with animals.[28] Conscious awareness was divided completely in two. Objects to the left and right of the fixation point of the two eyes were separately perceived, and so were objects held in the left or right hand. Within each half perceptual world the modalities were equivalent—something felt in the left hand was immediately identified with the same things seen in the left visual field, and vice versa. Split awareness was also demonstrated for hearing and olfaction. Touch, temperature, pressure sense and pain on the proximal limb segments and to the face and trunk were less clearly separate for left and right of the midline, but these kinds of experience are normally less vivid in awareness and, above all, less rich in meaning.

The commissurotomy patients retained fluent motor coordination for walking, handling objects, visually exploring and attending generally. Speech was disturbed for only a short time after surgery. It became normal within a few days. Some exacting tests of bimanual coordination requiring synchronous and complementary arm and hand movement under visual guidance have revealed losses attributable to separation of the cortical motor systems, and occasional episodes of divided volition were recorded. But, on the whole, conscious intentionality seemed remarkably intact.

Commissurotomy patients show two defects in strength of consciousness. In vigilance tests they are easily overwhelmed, failing to detect stimuli when these are appearing over a wide range of space and being easily bewildered by quick and frequent changes of stimuli. They also show a memory deficit in formal tests, and considerable weakness of memory in daily life.[26] Both disorders are more pronounced than anything attributable to epileptogenic pathology or inadvertent surgical damage added to the division of the commissures. We may conclude, therefore, that maintenance of normal fluency and retention in consciousness requires close, direct interhemispheric interaction. Hemispherectomy patients and persons with congenital absence of the corpus callosum show that such interaction is probably essential to full development of complementary functions in the two hemispheres.[24]

When attempts were made with the commissurotomy patients to define the seat of feelings and emotions, the results are harder to understand. Some observations indicated that embarrassment, fear, excited happiness or sadness affected both hemispheres when precise perceptual information about the cause of change in feeling was restricted to one hemisphere, as if the emotional self was still united. Other observations indicate that feelings of pleasure or disgust on perceiving an emotive object may remain locked up in association with the lateralized percept. The great speed with which feedback cues to object identity—sounds emitted by metallic objects being turned in one hand, or movements of the lips in silent pronouncing of the name of an object seen in the right visual field—are picked up in awareness by the hemisphere that is being deprived of the critical stimulus information proves that general readiness to be aware can be shared by the two halves of the brain.

Both halves of the brain can be told how to do a task. Verbal instructions, spoken or written, can be understood to a limited extent by the hemisphere that cannot emit speech. Evidently this understanding of language depends on a high degree of awareness of the whole context of the test situation by both hemispheres. Another kind of evidence for subhemispheric involvement in conscious experience and cognition comes from tests where mental abilities of the dissociated hemispheres are put in conflict. Some of the responses indicate that functional sets in the brain-stem can prevent a hemisphere from functioning in the normal way. This has been named 'metacontrol'.[29]

All the evidence points to a whole-brain view of the neural networks of consciousness, recalling Penfield's[30] concept of centrencephalic control. Conscious intentionality must be confluent in the nerve networks in the brain-stem, cerebellum and spinal motor system. Perceptual guidance of locomotion and posture as well as orientation of gaze, hearing, or haptic prehension are

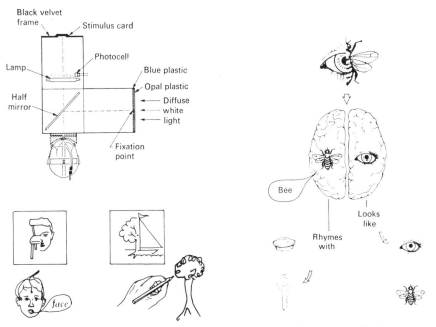

FIG. 2. Tachistoscopic presentation of small (5°) visual stimuli to test focal vision of commissurotomy patients. The phenomenon of visual completion means that two complete pictures are perceived by the disconnected hemispheres if a bilateral stimulus chimera is centred on the fixation point. Verbal report ignores the left side of stimuli, drawing reveals a preference for the left half. Appearance matching favours the right (non-speaking) hemisphere. The left, speaking, hemisphere is capable of rhyming 'in the head', but the right is not.[32, 34, 39]

essentially undivided after hemisphere disconnection. Mood and appetite can evidently be specified within undivided levels of the brain, while at other times they are coupled to a one-sided hemispheric awareness. The divided awareness shows that knowledge of the specific identity of objects and readiness to manipulate them for the special uses is built up in the cortex. These cannot be transmitted across the brain-stem. In consequence, recognition of the meaning of objects is duplicated by commissurotomy.

Experiments on awareness of spatial relations of the whole body and of peripheral events lacking definition and having only general orienting value for praxis show that there is an undivided brain-stem 'ambient' vision in commissurotomy patients[31] (Fig. 2). This mechanism may edit out local elements in the awareness of one hemisphere in relation to purpose formulated in the other hemisphere.[32] Nevertheless, none of the results of tests designed to bring out brain-stem functions proves that they make a detailed contribution to the contents of consciousness.

The most significant effects of commissurotomy on consciousness concern the human skills of language. Conscious sharing is found to be grossly one-sided in all these patients after surgery. All the experiences of the right field, which informs the left hemisphere, are spoken about normally as before the operation, but the patient can say nothing clear and well-defined about experience in the left visual field or in the left hand, both of which project to the right hemisphere. Sorting tasks and tests of object manipulation show that the mute right half-brain can grasp meanings and solve cognitive puzzles. It can match words in most semantic classes, but not on abstract criteria. The left hand connected to this hemisphere is skilful in drawing and in manipulating familiar objects and tools. Nevertheless, only the left hemisphere can speak and there is a severe loss of writing ability for the left hand. These findings are a clear confirmation of the century-old discovery from the effects of one-sided brain lesions that most human beings have language lateralized in the left hemisphere.[33,34]

Two kinds of motor patterning are associated with the hemisphere traditionally called dominant. These are the rapid and precise articulations of speech, and similarly complex activities of the hand that is preferred for fine manipulation under immediate visual and auditory guidance, as in writing, conducting an orchestra or bowing the violin. Left hemisphere control of speech seems mainly concerned with the lips and tongue, for which sensory-motor control is bihemispheric. The non-preferred hand, usually the left which is more completely under right hemisphere control, is no less sensitive or subtle than the dominant hand in its movements of manipulation. Both speech and actions of the right hand in gesture and manipulation involve the rapid sequencing of acquired stereotyped elements in infinitely varied combinations. There is evidence that the posterior temporo-parietal cortex of the left hemisphere in right-handed people, which is anatomically different from the corresponding region of the right hemisphere even before birth,[35] is a nerve centre adapted to control such complex and rapid motor sequencing.[36]

The above account fits the predominant view of the past century that the left hemisphere is the most human hemisphere, specially adapted for the skills of language and manipulative techniques that have been cultivated in the history of civilized and rational society. One may easily conclude that the contributions of the right hemisphere to consciousness are secondary and perhaps a residue of more primitive functions. Investigations during the last three decades cast doubt on this view, and the findings have most interesting implications for philosophy.

The commissurotomy patients give powerful confirmation of right hemisphere dominance for non-verbal consciousness. Tests of right hemisphere comprehension show that it has a considerable linguistic faculty and a semantic store permitting understanding not much inferior to that of the dominant hemisphere for situations where symbolic representation of decontextualized concepts is not essential.[37] Indeed there are important mental operations in which the awareness of the right hemisphere seems more acute and more complete than that of the left. These concern visual and haptic apprehension of form and simultaneous topological geometric relations in the space of potential action. It is of interest in this connection that Einstein thought that his mathematical conceptualization included an important non-verbal component representing experiences of bodily motion.[38] Again these findings accord with the results of neuropsychological tests of patients with lateralized focal brain lesions.[24]

The right hemisphere is superior to the left in discriminating shapes and complex patterns, such as the faces of different persons (Fig. 3), that require a simultaneous analysis of the proportions and positions of features relative to each other.[39] It is also rather more competent than the left in the perception of harmony in complex sounds, including that special kind of harmony which defines voice quality and its modulation to express feeling. Aesthetic understanding of music is definitely stronger in this hemisphere. The right hemisphere understands all grammatical categories of words, but the vocabulary of the non-speaking half of the brain is less than that of the speaking half.[37] A severe defect in logical reasoning shows up in certain tests with the right hemisphere on its own. This highly conscious and knowledgeable hemisphere fails in tests of inference that demand detection of arbitrary, decontextualized elements and formation of equally artificial combinations of them. Mental calculation

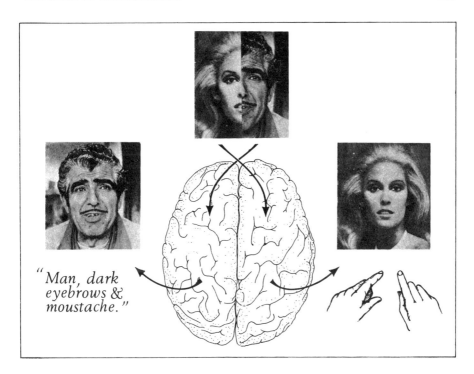

FIG. 3. With chimeric faces, commissurotomy patients used the right hemisphere to match what they had seen, by pointing; either left or right hand may indicate. When asked to say what they saw, they gave elaborate feature list descriptions and used the left hemisphere.[39]

is poor, like that of a little child or an illiterate. A very simple test of language comprehension involving descriptions of how to place and group a few meaningless tokens distinguished by colour, shape and form produces catastrophic failure.

Studies of patients who have lost a cerebral hemisphere when adult show the same kind of hemispheric differences, but they also reveal how much better two disconnected hemispheres are than the combination of two isolated hemispheres. An adult with one hemisphere is severely handicapped. The much less severe effects of hemispherectomy in early childhood confirm that specialization of function takes many years to develop. A person with either hemisphere removed in infancy can develop language and some facility in all other realms of consciousness, though careful measurement reveals deficits and confirms that the hemispheres are unequal in functional potential at birth. Congenital absence of the corpus callosum is associated with symmetry of cerebral function. The hemispheres of the normal person become more different (asymmetrical) during childhood through a process of mutual induction. There are indications that even after commissurotomy in the mid-teens, the brain may partly overcome loss of direct interhemisphere communication, and that the ability to use words for thinking may become distributed in both halves of the brain.

Neuropsychological studies of brain-injured patients indicate that each cortex has regions that contribute different aspects to consciousness.[24] Depending on the locus of a lesion, disorders of the planning of purposive movement may affect only an arm or the eyes, or they may affect the intention to use tools appropriately or to express knowledge and purposes in speech. Awareness may show loss of one cognitive ability such as the ability to see categorical resemblances, or one modality may be severely affected in its cognitive aspects, leaving other modalities intact. Defects of language may affect understanding through hearing or vision, or the execution of speech or writing, or either of the latter may be fluent in detail but without coherent meaning. Some lesions affect learning, motivation or emotional state, leaving perception and voluntary action intact. The memory defects may be obvious in short-term recall over a few minutes, or may affect experiences stored over many years. Defects may be specific for verbal or visual experience. To explain these selective losses neurologists may think in terms of local functional systems. However, most mental disorders result from the break-up of widespread systems of intercommunicating neurons. Many consequences of brain injury are due to loss of connections between structures that normally interact strongly and precisely.

The findings with commissurotomy patients and others with cerebral lesions are strong evidence for the idea that consciousness is a natural, innate property of the human life form, one that is integrated in a precisely structured brain. It is a product of evolution adapted to further the power of action and to permit cooperative intentionality between humans, by language and other forms of intersubjectivity, in the creation of traditions of collective knowledge and understanding. Consciousness emerges as the principal and most unified brain function, which puts it, as Sperry[40] has said, 'in the driving seat', able to subordinate the elementary interneuronal processes to its own integrative states.

BRAIN SYSTEMS OF DISCRIMINATION AND THEIR GROWTH

In primates the precision and speed of neural control for the hands is increased by development of direct connections between cortical motor neurons (large pyramidal cells of the precentral motor cortex) and spinal motor neurons. The distal motor system regulates delicate patterns of prehension, fine exploratory movements of information pick-up for focal awareness in vision, hearing, touch, taste, and articulations of facial expression and speech. It has separate lines of communication from those for trunk movements, being more laterally placed in the brain-stem and spinal cord. All levels of the central nervous system show the separation of efferent tracts on somatotopic lines, proximal systems being more medial, distal more lateral. Taken together, the motor columns form a coherent set. This anatomy may be interpreted as an outcome of embryogenic processes but they reach maturity after birth.

The distal motor functions depend on precise sensory information of a high spatial resolution. The best-known sensory analyser is the striate and parastriate system for vision in carnivores and primates, made famous by the work of Hubel and Wiesel.[41,42] Mountcastle[43] and others have undertaken exploration of the somataesthetic system. This has led to discovery of how the senses of sight and touch are linked within a unitary process of orienting and attending by means of 'commands' that arise in the posterior-parietal association cortex.[21] This is a step towards a description of how proximal and distal systems are integrated together, how the largely unconscious actions of the core motor system and brain-stem reticular formation contribute to the conscious awareness that is essential to the correct deployment of the precise and discriminatory acts governed by the distal system. Relevant is the discovery of intimate reciprocal relations between the brain-stem visual system and the visual association cortex (see Fig. 1).

There are two parallel visual systems informing the cortex.[44] Their convergence in the association cortex would appear to govern the more elaborate and more voluntary aspects of exploratory action. The route via the colliculus is found to be an ancient one. It is closely integrated with the motivation-regulating systems of basal ganglia, hypothalamus and brain-stem. The geniculostriate system has evolved into a separate unimodal component in response to selection for more powerful analysis of visual input for control of consummatory acts, but the visual association cortex, which is greatly enlarged in man and essential to high level visual cognition, evolved first early in the life of vertebrates.

The basic somatotopic plan of sensory-motor coordination in the central nervous system is determined in the embryo, but cerebral cortex and cerebellum are elaborated in the fetal stages.[16] The human brain has a particularly elaborate antenatal phase in which the main groups of neurons differentiate throughout the brain. All the motivational and coordinating systems are present at birth and functioning at least in a rudimentary way. Nevertheless, much of the refined anatomy of the cortex and the reticular integrative networks is incomplete (Fig. 4).

Micro-electrophysiological research and the newly developed tracer techniques of experimental neuroanatomy reveal that cortical grey matter and brain-stem nuclei have a microscopic modular design. The cortex appears to have a regular structure based on columnar units about 0.25 millimetres in diameter and each containing 2500 neurons. These elements were first recognized in cortical sensory systems. In them there is refined anatomical segregation of afferent and efferent components. For example, inputs of the two eyes are meticulously separated, then combined for stereoptic and other types of analysis in micro-columnar units which are arranged in the larger hyper-columns.[42] This anatomical organization in modules may be compared to the segmentation of the body. I believe its discovery will help us to understand the embryogenic determination of elaborately coordinated systems in the brain, including that which is preadapted to the fine differentiations and integrative unity of consciousness. Experimental studies of the visual system indicate that segregation of elements is begun antenatally but that final steps in the formation of intercellular links are assisted by the patterning of stimulation.[46] Most important is the regulation of connections in the nerve network by effects that are under direct control of motor action. Partly differentiated perceptual systems achieve anatomical refinement by being drilled in the coincidences of stimulation that acts of looking and attending may programme.[47] Perhaps the next advance in developmental neurobiology will come in filling the great gap in our understanding of the inner motivations of consciousness as manifested in the formation of selective memory traces. A step in this direction has come from discovery of microanatomical changes in the dendrites of hippocampal neurons that depend upon the coincidence of adequate motivations with repetition of significant stimuli.[45]

It is of great interest that the parts of the nervous system with the longest cycles of epigenetic development, continuing for decades after birth, include the association cortices, the reticular system of the brain-stem and the great interhemispheric commissure (corpus callosum). The two hemispheres are asymmetric in cortical organization from before birth, but the asymmetric

→

Fig. 4. Prenatal and postnatal growth of the human brain.[16, 24]. Myelin deposits on nerve axons show that brain components mature at different stages. Integrative neurons of the cortex, the long association fibres and local neuropil, mature after birth, when cultural skills are acquired. Brains drawn on the same scale show that development of connections in the cortex is accompanied by little increase in brain bulk. The arrow marks the central sulcus, stippled areas are 'association' cortex, richly connected to the other hemisphere. The corpus callosum doubles in size postnatally.

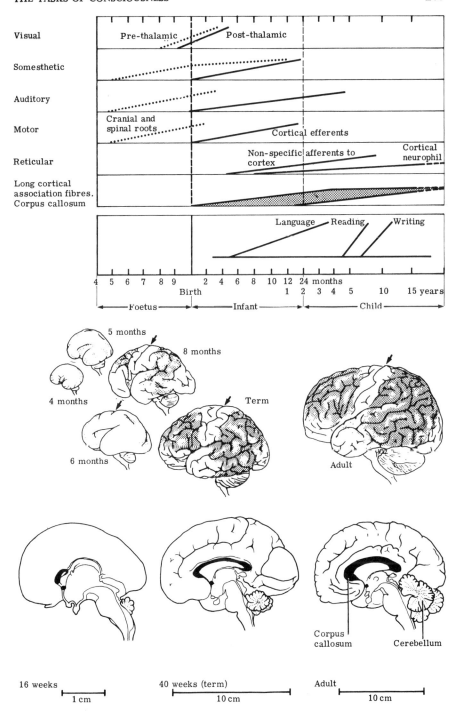

Corpus
callosum   Cerebellum

16 weeks   40 weeks (term)   Adult

1 cm   10 cm   10 cm

tissues of consciousness develop progressively more distinct refinements throughout the first third of life.

CONSCIOUSNESS IN INFANCY

The behaviours of infants reveal a rudimentary human consciousness. A neonate is weak in movements of body and limbs and imprecise in attending. Consciousness is surely present for only brief periods and it must lack discrimination of details and recognition of particular objects. Nevertheless, descriptions and experiments with the movements of infants show that even a neonate may direct the eyes or ears to choose things to perceive. Older infants may suck, shift gaze, move the head or limbs, and use voice and face expression to control the recurrence of events that are interesting. They do much more than simply act to satisfy bodily needs. Most importantly, neonatal babies are highly sensitive to many signs of the presence of persons and they quickly learn to recognize the mother as a particular individual. Response by a newborn to an attentive gentle person is made up from a wide repertoire of facial movements, vocalizations, gestures and posturings.[48] These are acts of expression that are specially adapted for communication with persons and for no other purpose. They are hard to describe because they are highly variable in strength, form and combination. But they are both close enough to adult expressions and sufficiently sensitive to the expressions of others to give rise to a strong impression that the baby has the beginnings of conscious understanding, and some intention to express this to others.

Among the most surprising responses of neonates are imitations of certain exaggerated face and hand movements of adults. These prove that the infant brain obtains a perceptual image of a person's expression and gesture, and that this is linked to an image for corresponding movement of the infant's vocal organs, face and hands (Fig. 5).

By the second month a baby is capable of complex communicative exchange in face-to-face interaction with the mother.[20,48] Now orientation and focalization are more rapid and sure, and the baby spends more time alert and attentive. Visual exploration is particularly lively. Prehension is ineffectual, but the hands make reaching and grasping movements in the direction of objects in motion nearby. Clearly the fields of visual awareness and intending to grasp are integrated to some degree by prenatal morphogenesis of brain systems.

There are now a number of detailed studies of 'protoconversational' exchanges between two-month-old babies and their mothers.[49] These have remarkably complex structure. The mother imitates many of the expressions

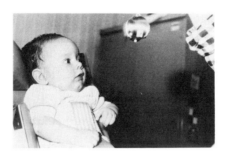

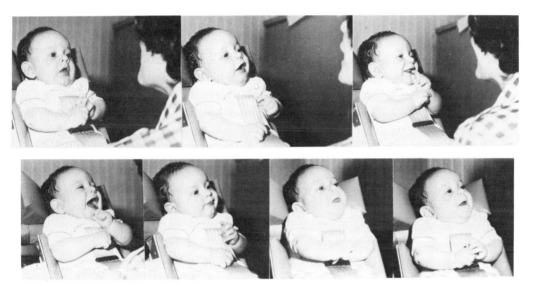

FIG. 5. An eight-week-old infant tracks a bright and colourful ball with attentive expression and the beginnings of a 'reach'. When spoken to by his mother he vocalizes, smiles, grimaces and gestures.[7]

and posturings of her infant, but both are responsive, so between them regular exchanges of 'utterances' are created by mutual adjustment. Infant utterances lack the articulations of speech and their vocalizations are little differentiated. However, there are movements of lips and tongue that closely resemble articulation of speech. Expression of mood and a shifting concentration are sufficiently clear and well-modulated for the baby to be seen to be taking interest, pleasure, displeasure or doubt, and shifts of motivation or emotional reactions to what the mother does may be observed. The mother's 'baby talk', a highly specialized form of speech, with a solicitous manner of gesturing and posturing that facilitates communication with the infant, may include a running commentary on the mother's intuitive conception that the infant is trying to talk to her.

Out of the rich human expressivity and sensitivity to persons that the young infant possesses comes a power to create close affectional relationships or 'attachments'. The patterns of intersubjective exchange between two-month-old babies and their mothers show that conscious sharing and a representation of processes in an I–you relationship are innate in the human brain. Subsequent developments involve the infant in increasingly subtle sharing of awareness with familiars and an increasing wariness with strangers. At four or five months after birth an infant begins to be effective in reaching and grasping an object. Thereafter great interest is shown in exploring objects by handling and mouthing them while looking and listening, smelling and tasting. The interpersonal consciousness also undergoes important changes that encourage playful teasing in companions. Games of intention and excitement cause outbursts of smiling and laughing. Gradually these games come to involve the effects of acting on objects that thus become toys. Our recent observations suggest that solitary or individual playing with objects is a special form of a much richer play with other persons.[50] It seems likely that play is essentially intersubjective (see Fig. 6).

It is not possible to review here the elaborate cognitive and interpersonal mental functions of infants. There has been a revolution in developmental psychology in the past few years. Now the view that infants have to build up concepts, perceptual images and intentions in a formless network of cortical connections from a set of innate reflexes and a general 'need to function' must be revised. Awareness of objects in space and intentions to use them in particular ways now appear to be due to an organization in the infant mind that anticipates experience. I leave aside the evidence that infants know phenomenal objects in a space of action and instead emphasize an ability that an infant may show before the end of the first year to cooperate with others in the use of objects.

About ten months after birth infants appear to achieve a new understanding of the common field of experience.[50] They become eager to share their experiences of objects with other persons. For the first time, they are able to organize their intentions to transmit messages about experiences. That is they begin to make 'acts of meaning'.[8] This is not only the start of true language development. It is the opening of a door to education for participation in a society and for sharing its cultural understanding.[51] The way in which this ability develops suggests that fundamental structures for cooperative understanding of the world, unlike anything in any other species, are innate in the human brain. Psychological research with infants strongly supports the

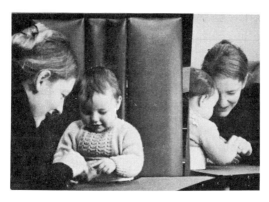

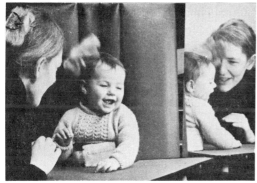 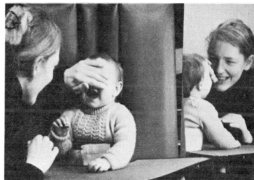

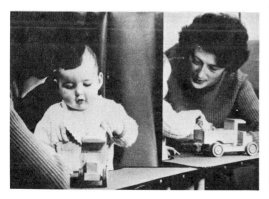 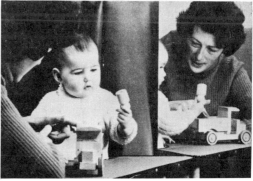

FIG. 6. A nine-month-old (top and middle) enjoys playing games like touching fingers and peek-a-boo.
A one-year old (below) is also capable of attending to instructions and of cooperating in constructive play.[50, 51] (Photographs courtesy of Penelope Hubley)

idea of a natural evolutionary origin for human consciousness, interpersonal mental life and the cooperative intentions that make cultural development possible.

EPILOGUE: CONSCIOUSNESS AND THE CULTURAL HABITAT

I see no reason to look for the mechanism of consciousness anywhere but in the organized processes of brain activity. But, like other organic activities, consciousness requires a facilitating environment. This environment is not passively endured; it is acted upon, moulded, made to impinge on the organism, with increase of advantage to the organism. Thus consciousness depends upon and is developed by an environment of objects and meanings which is inevitably altered by consciousness. Tangible and intangible products of human consciousness come from cooperative action and cooperative understanding over the historical scale of time. They are the customs and artifacts of culture and technology. Individual human consciousnesses are born into a pre-existing pattern of culture, take up its opportunities and automatically contribute to its change.

Historical change, over hundreds of years, is much quicker than evolutionary change. Human history depends on stories, records and constructions that retain elements of past conditions, activities and beliefs. The process is not unfamiliar in nature. It can be compared to biome change, as in the emergence and slow maturation of a forest. Trees make an ecosystem by creating shade, shelter, change of soil, accumulation of leaf mould, etc. This transforms the environment in the scale of decades or centuries. Generations of one kind of tree profit from and add to the beneficial conditions, or alter the conditions so that in the end other species of plants are favoured to take their place. Leaf mould is, for the life of trees, like written texts for the life of human consciousness. Both are equally 'natural', unless one insists on calling all human artifacts unnatural, by definition.

It is as mistaken to attribute human awareness to cultural artifacts, as Popper and Eccles[52] do, as it is to attribute the growth of a tree to the annual fall of leaves. There might be no trees without leaf fall, but there is more to a tree than the dead leaves over its roots. Likewise, human consciousness has generative and self-regulatory potential, a fundamental intentionality or conscious motivation which transcends any particular artificial environment of rituals, texts, buildings, machinery, institutions, etc. This is proved by the ease with which human societies exchange cultural effects, and the ability of individuals to transplant themselves from one stream of cultural history to another, unrelated one.

There are common needs which are met in all human societies. These are the primary dimensions of consciousness as the prime evolutionary adaptation of human kind. They include the deep structures of mental cooperation which allow humans to recognize joint purposes and mutual relationships and to make a milieu of conventional signs and objects of use.

Such structures are doubtless in the brain, with a life history of development related to brain growth, and they are vulnerable to injury of the brain. Trying to understand their organization, the principles of their function and their formation in development constitutes a leading and increasingly important goal of psychology. We shall never complete the job, but if, in trying to explain the human mind, we misrepresent the mind–brain question, or use our fragmentary knowledge of brain mechanisms to mislead more direct enquiry into behaviour and mental processes, the success of an enterprise will be correspondingly diminished.

References

1. GHISELIN, M. T. (1969) *The Triumph of the Darwinian Method*, University of California, Los Angeles
2. JAMES, W. (1890) *The Principles of Psychology*, vol. 2, ch. 28, Henry Holt, New York
3. BERNARD, C. (1957) *An Introduction to the Study of Experimental Medicine* (Greene, H. C., transl.), p. 197, Dover, New York (original French edn, Paris, 1865)
4. MACMURRAY, J. (1961) *Persons in Relation*, Faber & Faber, London
5. BUBER, M. (1970) *I and Thou* (Kaufmann, W., transl.), Charles Scribner's Sons, New York
6. TREVARTHEN, C. (1979) Modes of perceiving and modes of acting, in *Modes of Perceiving and Processing Information* (Pick, H. & Saltzman, E., eds.), pp. 99–136, Erlbaum, Hillsdale, N.J.
7. TREVARTHEN, C. (1979) Communication and cooperation in early infancy. A description of primary intersubjectivity, in *Before Speech: The Beginnings of Human Communication* (Bullowa, M., ed.), pp. 321–347, Cambridge University Press, Cambridge
8. HALLIDAY, M. A. K. (1978) Meaning and the construction of reality in early childhood, in *Modes of Perceiving and Processing Information* (Pick, H. & Saltzman, E., eds.), pp. 67–96, Erlbaum, Hillsdale, N.J.
9. MENZEL, E. W. (1979) A group of young chimpanzees in a one-acre field, in *Behavior of Nonhuman Primates*, vol. 5 (Schrier, A. M. & Stollnitz, F., eds.), pp. 83–153, Academic Press, New York
10. SEARLE, J. R. (1969) *Speech Acts: An Essay in the Philosophy of Language*, Cambridge University Press, London
11. HABERMAS, J. (1972) *Knowledge and Human Interest*, Heinemann, London
12. NEISSER, U. (1976) *Cognition and Reality*, Freeman, San Francisco
12a. MARCEL, A. J. (1979) Conscious and unconscious reading: the effects of visual masking on word perception. *Cognitive Psychol.* in press
12b. MICHOTTE, A. (1962) *Causalité, Permanence et Réalité Phénomenales*. Publications Universitaires, Louvain
13. JOHANSSON, C. (1975) Visual motion perception. *Sci. Am. 232* (6), 76–88
14. LEE, D. N. (1978) The functions of vision, in *Modes of Perceiving and Processing Information* (Pick, H. & Saltzman, E., eds.), pp. 159–170, Erlbaum, Hillsdale, N.J.

15. BERNSTEIN, N. (1967) *The Coordination and Regulation of Movements*, Pergamon, Oxford

16. TREVARTHEN, C. (1979) Neuroembryology and the development of perception, in *Human Growth: A Comprehensive Treatise*, vol. 3 (Falkner, F. & Tanner, J. M., eds.), pp. 3–96, Plenum Press, New York

17. DESMEDT, J. E. (ed.,) (1977) *Attention, Voluntary Contraction and Event-Related Cerebral Potentials*, Karger, Basel

18. GIBSON, J. J. (1966) *The Senses Considered as Perceptual Systems*, Houghton Mifflin, Boston

19. GIBSON, J. J. (1977) The theory of affordances, in *Perceiving, Acting and Knowing* (Shaw, R. & Bransford, I., eds.), Erlbaum, Hillsdale, N.J.

20. TREVARTHEN, C. (1974) The psychobiology of speech development. *Neurosci. Res. Program Bull. 12*, 570–585

21. MOUNTCASTLE, V. B., LYNCH, J. C., GEORGOPOLOUS, A., SAKATA, H. & ACUNA, C. (1975) Posterior parietal association cortex of the rhesus monkey: command functions for operations within extrapersonal space. *J. Neurophysiol. 38*, 871–908

22. WALSH, K. W., (1978) *Neuropsychology: A Clinical Approach*, Churchill Livingstone, Edinburgh

23. DONCHIN, E., MCCARTHY, G. & KUTAS, M. (1977) Electroencephalographic investigations of hemispheric specialization, in *Language and Hemisphere Specialization in Man: Cerebral Event-Related Potentials* (Desmedt, J. E., ed.), pp. 212–242, Karger, Basel

24. TREVARTHEN, C. (1979) Brain growth and the value of infancy, in *Developmental Psychology and Society* (Sants, J., ed.), Macmillan, London, in press

25. SPERRY, R. W. (1967) Mental unity following surgical disconnection of the cerebral hemispheres. *Harvey Lect. 62*, 293–323

26. SPERRY, R. W. (1974) Lateral specialization in the surgically separated hemispheres, in *The Neurosciences: Third Study Program* (Schmitt, F. O. & Worden, F. G., eds.), pp. 5–20, MIT Press, Cambridge, Mass.

27. SPERRY, R. W. (1961) Cerebral organization and behaviour. *Science (Wash. D.C.) 133*, 1749–1757

28. SPERRY, R. W., GAZZANIGA, M. S. & BOGEN, J. E. (1969) Interhemispheric relationships: the neocortical commissures, syndromes of hemisphere deconnection, in *Handbook of Clinical Neurology*, vol. 4 (Vinken, P. J. & Bruyn, G. W., eds.), pp. 273–290, North-Holland, Amsterdam

29. LEVY, J. & TREVARTHEN, C. (1976) Metacontrol of hemisphere function in human split-brain patients. *J. Exp. Psychol. 2*, 299–312

30. PENFIELD, W. (1954) Mechanisms of voluntary movement. *Brain 77*, 1–17

31. TREVARTHEN, C. & SPERRY, R. W. (1973) Perceptual unity of the ambient visual field in human commissurotomy patients. *Brain 96*, 547–570

32. TREVARTHEN, C. (1974) Analysis of cerebral activities that generate and regulate consciousness in commissurotomy patients, in *Hemisphere Function in the Human Brain* (Dimond, S. J. & Beaumont, J. G., eds.), pp. 235–263, Elek Books, London

33. PENFIELD, W. & ROBERTS, L. (1959) *Speech and Brain Mechanisms*, Princeton University Press, Princeton, N.J.

34. LEVY, J. & TREVARTHEN, C. (1977) Perceptual, semantic and phonetic aspects of elementary language processes in split-brain patients. *Brain 100*, 105–118

35. GALABURDA, A. M., LE MAY, M., KEMPER, T. L. & GESCHWIND, N. (1978) Right-left asymmetries in the brain. *Science (Wash. D.C.) 199*, 852–856

36. KIMURA, D. (1979) Neuromotor mechanisms in the evolution of human communication, in *Neurobiology of Social Communication in Primates: An Evolutionary Perspective* (Steklis, H. D. & Raleigh, M. J., eds.), Academic Press, New York, in press

37. ZAIDEL, E. (1977) Auditory language comprehension in the right hemisphere following cerebral commissurotomy and hemispherectomy: a comparison with child language

and aphasia, in *Language Acquisition and Language Breakdown: Parallels and Divergences* (Caramazzo, A. & Zurif, E. B., eds.), pp. 229–275, Johns Hopkins, Baltimore

38. HADAMARD, J. (1945) *The Psychology of Invention in the Mathematical Field*, Princeton University Press, Princeton, N.J.
39. LEVY, J., TREVARTHEN, C. & SPERRY, R. W. (1972) Perception of bilateral chimeric figures following hemispheric deconnection. *Brain 95*, 61–78
40. SPERRY, R. W. (1976) Mental phenomena as causal determinants in brain function, in *Consciousness and the Brain* (Globus, G. G. *et al.*, eds.), Plenum Press, New York
41. HUBEL, D. H. & WIESEL, T. N. (1962) Receptive fields, binocular interaction and functional architecture in the cat's visual cortex. *J. Physiol. (Lond.) 160*, 106–154
42. HUBEL, D. H. & WIESEL, T. N. (1974) Sequence, regularity and geometry of orientation columns in the monkey striate cortex. *J. Comp. Neurol. 158*, 267–294
43. MOUNTCASTLE, V. B. (ed.) (1974) Neural mechanisms in somesthesia, in *Medical Physiology*, 13th edn., vol. 1, pp. 307–347, Mosby, St Louis
44. TREVARTHEN, C. (1968) Two mechanisms of vision in primates. *Psychol. Forsch. 31*, 299–337
45. FIFKOVA, E. & VAN HARREVELD, A. (1977) Long-lasting morphological changes in dendrite spines of dentate granular cells following stimulation of the entorhinal area. *J. Neurocytol. 6*, 211–230
46. HUBEL, D. H., WIESEL, T. N. & LE VAY, S. (1977) Plasticity of ocular dominance columns in monkey striate cortex. *Philos. Trans. R. Soc. Lond. B Biol. Sci. 278*, 131–163
47. WILLSHAW, D. J. & VON DER MALSBURG, C. (1976) How patterned neural connections can be set up by self-organization. *Proc. R. Soc. Lond. B Biol. Sci., 194*, 431 445
48. TREVARTHEN, C. (1977) Descriptive analyses of infant communication behaviour, in *Studies in Mother-Infant Interaction: The Loch Lomond Symposium* (Schaffer, H. R., ed.), pp. 227–270, Academic Press, London
49. SCHAFFER, H. R. (ed.) (1977) *Studies in Mother-Infant Interaction: The Loch Lomond Symposium*, Academic Press, London
50. TREVARTHEN, C. & HUBLEY, P. (1978) Secondary intersubjectivity: confidence, confiding and acts of meaning in the first year, in *Action Gesture and Symbol: The Emergence of Language* (Lock, A., ed.), pp. 183–229, Academic Press, London
51. TREVARTHEN, C. (1979) Instincts for human understanding and for cultural cooperation: their development in infancy, in *Human Ethology* (von Cranach, M. & Aschoff, J., eds.), Cambridge University Press, Cambridge, in press
52. POPPER, K. R. & ECCLES, J. C. (1977) *The Self and Its Brain*, Springer International, Berlin

Neurophysiological mechanisms and consciousness

O. D. CREUTZFELDT

Max-Planck-Institute for Biophysical Chemistry, Department of Neurobiology, Göttingen

Abstract Consciousness may be understood as a behavioural state and thus levels of consciousness may be distinguished. But consciousness as we understand it is an experience. Any critical reasoning about it will lead to a dualistic formula. A neurophysiological mechanism may exist for this.

In the neocortex various aspects of the world and of the physical and social relationships of the individuum to the world are represented through thalamo-cortical projection systems. There is no unified representation of the world in any single cortical area. All neocortical outputs feed into action systems of the brain. The synthesis of the distributed cortical representations of the world is thus realized through the action elicited by their combination. The action systems of the midbrain–cerebellum and the basal ganglia feed back into neo-cortical areas (internal loops). The action itself changes the relationship of the individual to the outside world and thus its representation in the brain (external loops).

The role of the basal ganglia in the normal functioning of processes in consciousness and in the synthesis of cortical representations is described, which further emphasizes the intricate connections between motor performance and consciousness. The function of the reticular substance and related structures is seen as a gating mechanism for the (thalamic) access gates to the cortex and thus to mechanisms of conscious experience.

The basis for the experience of consciousness is the symbolic representation of the world and of the individual to that individual's brain. This self-representation is based on the linguistic competence of the brain in a broad sense and is therefore possible only for brains with such a competence. The symbolic self-representation is called the reflective loop and its conditions are briefly discussed.

THE DUALISTIC EXPERIENCE OF CONSCIOUSNESS

The word consciousness as commonly used has many facets. A definition is therefore needed before the neurophysiological basis of consciousness can be

217

analysed. The term 'levels of consciousness' implies that consciousness is a graded phenomenon. Each level may correspond to a certain functional state of the brain, the highest one allowing the brain to work at the highest level of its competence, the lowest one at 'minimum' performance. In this sense, the term consciousness describes states of behaviour and can thus be applied to and investigated in all animals. The term is also used in medicine, where levels of consciousness are graded from the highest performance level to various levels of unconsciousness.

The emphasis is different if consciousness is defined as awareness or directed attention. Attention can also be tested behaviourally, but again this covers only one aspect of consciousness.

In any neurophysiological hypothesis about brain mechanisms for consciousness we have to remember that we know about consciousness only through our own experience. This experience implies that the self relates itself to the world of objects. However, an experience is not a neurophysiological reality and therefore it cannot be described in neurophysiological terms.[1] On the other hand, consciousness is the condition of all experience; therefore its essence cannot be recognized from this experience.[2] As consciousness involves the experience of a subject (or a brain) of its own actions, such an experience must necessarily alter the state of this brain continuously, since any experience continually adds new information which will be the object of further experiences —and so on, spiralling upwards. Therefore no state of brain activity can be defined as consciousness.

One may, then, define consciousness as an ongoing process rather than a state.[3] Such a process is possible only if the gates of access to the highest mechanisms of the brain are open. Such a state of open gates may be definable in neurophysiological terms.

Conscious experience and consciousness imply an experience of the self and thus a concept of the self. This idea goes back to Descartes and Leibniz, whose thinking about consciousness is basic to modern psychology. It finds its philosophical expression in the synthetic principle of Kant: 'The synthetic sentence, that the various forms of empirical consciousness must be connected in a unified self-consciousness, is the absolutely first and synthetic principle of our thinking'.[4] Also Husserl, in his attempt to analyse the phenomenological aspects of consciousness as a primary experience of our *Lebenswelt*, recognized that the primary experience of the self is the necessary condition of consciousness. On the other hand, Husserl rightly points out that consciousness always means being conscious of something,[5] thus coming close to Spencer's definition.[3]

The very nature of our experience of consciousness makes it possible to talk and think about it only in dualistic terms. As an experience it *is* dualistic, as it implies the experience of the self, and thus will make the self an object of its own experience. Locke's definition of consciousness as 'the perception of what passes in a man's own mind' and Hume's definition of an 'inward sentiment' both recognize this dualistic nature of consciousness, although neither postulates any ego or mind substance, as Descartes and Leibniz do. Any attempt to develop a 'neurophysiological theory' of consciousness is confronted with the mystery of this dualistic formula, which transcends any possible neurobiological theory of consciousness. Bearing witness to this are the conclusions or confessions of great neuroscientists of the last hundred years, from Wundt[6] and Fechner[7] to Penfield[8] and Eccles[9]. We are dealing with two different levels of cognition.[1] Any brain-mind discussion will therefore arrive at this epistemological impasse. But if consciousness can be understood by the experiencing subject only in dualistic terms, we may ask whether this has a neurophysiological basis.

NEUROPHYSIOLOGICAL MECHANISMS NECESSARY FOR CONSCIOUSNESS

Neurology has contributed to the brain-consciousness problem by demonstrating brain functions that might be considered necessary conditions for consciousness, such as perception, cognition, memory, vigilance, attention (orientation) and linguistic capacity. These depend on the functional anatomical structures of the neocortex, the midbrain, the basal ganglia and their connections. Some aspects of these structures as related to our problem will be discussed in this section.

(A) *The cerebral neocortex*

(a) *Diversity of functional representations within the neocortex.* Perception, cognition, memory and language, as we understand them, are dependent on cortical functions. This is known from human pathology and from ablation experiments in animals, and has been elaborated in much detail during the last hundred years. Total destruction of or damage to the neocortex or its afferents and efferents (white substance) leads to a neurological syndrome called the apallic syndrome or global agnosia,[10] defined as complete loss of conscious functions or responses, with alternating states of vigilance (sleep–wakefulness), the periodicity of which is disturbed.

There is a continuing dispute about the extent to which these higher activities are global functions of the whole cortex or specific to certain circumscribed areas.[11] It may suffice here to state some facts about localization of cortical function that are relevant to our considerations: perceptions do not enter consciousness if the so-called primary cortical projection areas of the sense modalities are not functioning; cognition of sensory objects and symbolic understanding, including language, are disturbed if the parieto-temporal cortex is damaged; the expression of conscious experiences through motor patterns (behaviour) or in symbolic terms (e.g. language) is disturbed if the output structures of the central, frontal or parietal cortex are not functioning; language understanding and performance depend critically on the intactness of circumscribed areas of the temporo-parietal and the lower precentral motor cortex, respectively, and these two activities are lateralized in that only one hemisphere, the so-called dominant hemisphere, has complete linguistic competence. Memory is probably a general property of the cortex, and it may be that that part of the cortex which is involved in a certain activity also has a capacity for memory within that functional sphere. In addition, certain temporo-basal neocortical regions are necessary for storage and/or recall of such memories into consciousness.

The neocortex is a sheet of nervous tissue extending over the whole brain. In spite of certain local morphological differences the functional neurophysiological properties are based mainly on identical internal circuitry which transforms the different inputs in the same way.[12,13] The functional specializations of the various cortical fields are specific only in so far as they depend on specific afferent inputs from different thalamic nuclei and thus from different sense organs or intracerebral structures, and on their efferent connections.

The internal topography of the thalamic projection nuclei is laid out on the cortical surface on maps which preserve the neighbourhood relationship of points or cone-like cylinders in the thalamus. In as far as sensory surfaces are laid down topographically in a thalamic nucleus, the cortical map will represent this sensory surface. This is the case in the so-called primary and to some extent secondary and tertiary cortical projection fields. In cortical areas which receive their thalamic input from parts of the thalamus not directly connected to sense organs, the cortical map may still represent a closely related projection of the internal topography of such a thalamic nucleus. This applies to the so-called association nuclei of the thalamus and to the cortical association areas in the frontal, temporal and parietal lobes.

Thus, a complex temporo-spatial activity pattern elicited in a sense organ by a complex sensory environment will lead to an essentially homotopic spatio-temporal activity pattern in the appropriate cortical sensory projection areas. Such representations may be multiple and each may emphasize various aspects of this environment, if appropriate filters in the sensory organs or in the thalamic relay nuclei separate them out (e.g. colour or colourless contours in the visual system). In addition, stimuli are processed through other cerebral systems and different transformations of each stimulus are projected through the association nuclei to the cortical association areas. In this way, various stimulus transformations, each emphasizing different aspects of a stimulus, are represented in different cortical areas, a mechanism often referred to as 'parallel processing'.

But not only are certain physical aspects of stimuli differentially represented but also their relation to the subject. This may be the most important aspect of transformations in the association areas. Such subject–world relations may be in connection with the body scheme, as assumed for the parietal association areas,[14,15] or with internal states (drives) or social context of the subject, as probably represented in the frontal cortex. The transformation of a stimulus into motor responses within the context of a given movement or posture is finally represented by appropriate activity patterns in the motor cortex, which contains, anatomically, a somatotopic map of the peripheral motor system.

(b) *No hierarchical synthesis within the cortex.* These multiple cortical representations of stimuli in their various relationships to the individuum are synthesized into a unity of perception, as experienced in consciousness. How this synthesis is effected appeared as a problem when the functional differentiation of neocortical areas was recognized about a hundred years ago. In correspondence to philosophical models of cognition, a *hierarchical concept* of cortical organization was assumed and presented in the psychology of Wundt and the aphasia model of Wernicke.[11] This concept was revived in more recent times by neurophysiologists. It states that information which reaches a 'primary' projection area of the cortex is processed there and generalizations from this analysis are projected, via association fibres, to secondary cortical regions and so on. One recognizes in this concept the influence of association psychology. It implies that the higher order sensory and the association areas receive their major afferent input from areas that are further down in the hierarchy and eventually from the primary sensory projection areas. This model must imply that the whole information about the stimulus is contained in each transformation. But this is not the case. As stated above, only certain aspects of a stimulus and its cerebral response are represented in each cortical area, and all neocortical areas receive their main excitatory input from a thalamic projection nucleus. The association fibres connecting various cortical areas may modify this thalamic activation, but to what extent we have as yet no idea.[16]

A hierarchy of cortical areas exists only in so far as phylogenetically younger areas, with their respective thalamo-cortical connections, were added to the simple sensory-motor thalamo-cortical systems. These younger areas are the basis for more complex behaviour such as cognition and language or for more degrees of freedom in social behaviour. But they are not the place where aspects of stimuli are synthesized into consciousness, as none of them contains the complete information about a stimulus. In this sense, neither the neocortex as a whole nor any single area can be considered an 'integrative' part of the nervous system, as each area represents reality dissected into various aspects in the different fields.

During the last 20 years there has been some speculation that the unity of perception may be represented in certain higher order neurons or neuron pools which are specifically responsive to complex patterns. Such a concept of a 'pontifical neuron' had already appeared in William James's *Principles of Psychology*[17] in a somewhat different context (free will). James himself refuted such a concept on theoretical grounds and his arguments are still valid. The revival of such a hierarchical concept in the era of neurophysiology has remained mere speculation.

In fact, if the information about sensory objects is contained in the responses of several types of neurons, a higher-order neuron which is excited by lower-order neurons does not increase the available information but rather decreases it. For example, if a stimulus differentially excites four sets of neurons, A–D, the outputs of which excite a higher-order neuron, E, various configurations of activity in A–D may lead to the same activity in E. If the original information contained in the differential response of these four sets of neurons is to be preserved, their output must be represented separately.

(*c*) *Synthesis of perception into action beyond the neocortex.* If one tries to solve the problem of synthesis, one may consider the output organization of the neocortex, since the efferents from the cortex are the only read-out wires for cortical activities. The anatomy of these efferent pathways is known for only a few cortical areas, but one may generalize from these facts to some extent.

Efferent fibres originate from all layers of any cortical area, but strictly speaking only those from layer V can be considered to be output neurons, in that the fibres leave the neocortex. They project downwards into the basal ganglia, the midbrain and/or the spinal cord. The best-known output fibres are those going from the motor cortex through the pyramidal tract to the motor neurons of the medulla and spinal cord. But layer V neurons also project from the sensory cortices into motor systems via the pontine nuclei, and from there into the cerebellum, from where activity is sent back via cerebello-thalamic pathways to the motor cortex. Efferents from the upper part of layer V of the visual cortex (areas 17 and 18) project into the anterior colliculi, i.e. the midbrain tectum, which in this context may be considered a visuomotor interface for directing the gaze and motor system onto a visual target. Some of the collicular output is sent back to so-called higher-order visual areas, such as to area 18 in primates, to area 7, and, maybe, to the temporal cortex via the nucleus posterior thalami and the nuclei of the pulvinar. We call such cortico-fugal systems, which are relayed through other cerebral systems and fed back through thalamic nuclei to other cortical areas, *internal feedback loops*. Internal loops similar to those demonstrated in the visual system probably exist for secondary auditory[18] and somato-sensory cortical areas, although they have not been extensively investigated yet.

A separate set of neurons from the upper Vth layer[19] project into the basal ganglia (neostriatum), mainly from the anterior half of the cortex (motor and frontal). Thus, Vth layer efferents project directly or indirectly into various executive motor systems of the upper and lower brainstem or the spinal cord. The Vth layer outputs from the parietal and frontal association areas feed into the motor system of the neostriatum, the ponto-cerebellar system and the midbrain tectum with their downstream connections, and they also join the internal diencephalo-cortical feedback loops.

Cells from layer VI project down into the thalamic nuclei, from which the same cortical point receives its specific thalamic excitation. Cells from layers II and III project predominantly into other cortical areas via association fibres, and cells from all layers project through the corpus callosum to corresponding cortical fields of the contralateral hemisphere, which represent the same or nearly the same parts of the body or sensory systems (i.e. mainly the midlines of the body representations). Therefore the efferent fibres from layers II, III and VI remain within the cortico-cortical or the respective thalamo-cortical afferent projection systems and should not be included in the cortico-fugal system.

There is abundant evidence to support the assumption that the principle of preservation of the basic topography of cortical areas is maintained in all efferent and feedback connections. That is, the output lines terminate in parallel, although the original cortical topography might become more fuzzy because of divergent and convergent branching of the single fibres. If the efferent cortico-fugal output goes directly to executive motor systems, for example from the motor cortex to the motor neuron system of the spinal cord, it is evident that the temporo-spatial activity patterns elicited in the motor cortex are homologous to the motor action of the system. These patterns result from the cortico-fugal outputs of all other sensory and association areas, with their multiple input transformations, which constitute, via the internal loop, the input to the motor cortex as well as to more direct action systems downstream. *In this way the various representations of the world and the relations of the subject to this world as laid out in the various maps are synthesized and represented in the action they elicit.* In this sense, the action is a transformation of the sensory input.

Since any action changes the relationship of the individuum to the environment, and thus the sensory projection of this environment into its sensory cortical association and motor areas, we can turn this argument around and say that the various aspects of actions are contained in the input to all cortical areas: directly and most completely in the spatio-temporal activation patterns of the motor areas, and as functional transformations in terms of sensory input patterns in the sensory cortices. Therefore, the *unity of perception and the unity of action are two different aspects of the same problem.*[20] We may call this functional connection between input and output of the nervous system through changing relationships between the individuum and the outside world the *external loop.* Through this external loop, input and output are matched continually and the individuum is thus brought into a consistent relationship with the world.[21]

Since what passes through the cortex is synthesized to action programmes and represented as action, the content of any possible conscious experience should be contained in such neuronal action processes. The actions need not necessarily be executed. If they are, the behavioural responses change the relationship of the individuum to the outside world through the external loops, while the internal response states of the different cortical areas are altered through corresponding activities in the *internal feedback loops.* If actions are not executed, a no-go mechanism must prevent execution. This no-go command must be represented by neuronal activities adapted to the input situation as well as to the relation between the individuum and the environment. In this case, alterations in cortical representation are produced only through the internal loop systems, including the no-go command.

One aspect should be emphasized: *Any action evolves over time and so does perception.* This implies that representations of the world in their various transformations from sensory maps into action programmes are changing continually from one moment to the next, and the representations of sensory input signals and of the actions are completed only during the performance of the actions. Therefore, a given state of neuronal activities of the cortex or, in fact, of the whole brain, never represents the material of a perception or the 'programme' of a motor performance completely or in any way sufficiently. The synthesizing integration of transformations of action and sensation patterns of cortical systems also have to take into account the dimension of time, and the integration of the multiple transformations into a unity of perception and action is not only an *integration over space but also over time*. For the temporal integration, the *memory mechanisms* of the neocortex should be mentioned as a necessary mechanism, but we know too little about such mechanisms to justify detailed discussion.

(*d*) *Neocortex and consciousness*. We may conclude, at this point, that consciousness is dependent on the functioning of the afferent–efferent cortical systems, and that all 'What passes through a man's mind' somehow passes through the cerebral cortex. Yet the integrating mechanism is not in the cortex itself but lies in the synthesis of its outputs, over space and time, into action systems and to actions. This mechanism is only the general design of a complex control system by which the organism keeps itself in a consistent and, we may surmise, purposeful relationship with its environment. It is not a mechanism, yet, which could be invoked as a mechanism for consciousness or conscious experience since it need not have consciousness.

(B) *The basal ganglia and their possible role for processes of consciousness*

The basal ganglia are important yet incompletely understood 'integrating' output targets of the cerebral cortex. These phylogenetically old structures in the forebrain receive an orderly projection from all neocortical areas through mono-synaptic connections to the caudate nucleus and the putamen[22,23] (for a review of more general aspects of neo-striatal connections see Ref. 24). Thus the cerebral cortex is topographically represented in the basal ganglia complexes, with a major representation of the anterior (i.e. motor, premotor and frontal) cortex as compared to only a minor representation of the posterior cortical areas. An additional topographic representation of the cortex is found in the claustrum.[23,25] The cortico-fugal activities in the basal ganglia come under inhibitory control from the brainstem through the substantia nigra and then feed into the pallidum, which is the actual efferent interface of the cortico-striatal systems. From here, the activity is distributed to descending pathways which either feed into executive motor command systems, or into specific and non-specific systems of the thalamus and the reticular substance. Pallido-thalamic connections to the ventral anterior and ventromedial parts of the ventral medial nucleus appear to be primarily inhibitory[26], so that activity of pallido-thalamic efferents could lead to a blockade of the thalamic, i.e. the specific excitatory, drive to the motor cortex.

Experimental findings as well as clinical observations emphasize the importance of the basal ganglia for motor control, the traditional restricted view of these structures. For our purpose it is important to emphasize that these ganglia, in their output to the thalamus and the midbrain, appear to integrate cortical output activities to a large extent. They feed not only into the executive systems but also back into the cortex through pallido-thalamic and pallido-reticular pathways, although possibly they act mainly through inhibition, in a specific topographical as well as in a more diffuse 'non-specific' manner. The arrest reaction elicited by electrical stimulation of the striate might well be related to the no-go mechanism that we postulated as a mechanism that cancels the execution of action commands and thus enables the system to run idle, without motor responses.

Striatal activities need to be under inhibitory control if the execution of motor commands from the cerebral cortex is not to be blocked. This inhibitory control is exerted by the inhibitory nigro-striatal pathway. If this is not functioning, as in Parkinson's disease, motor expressions of what goes on in the neocortex are suppressed (akinesia) and voluntary motor acts cannot be started immediately and then run slower (bradykinesia). Correspondingly, thinking is slowed down too and needs specific efforts (bradyphrenia). Consciousness in the clinical sense is not disturbed, but the processes that constitute consciousness in its action and perception aspects are slowed down accordingly. In this sense, normal functioning of the basal ganglia and their connections may be considered a necessary mechanism for normal processes in consciousness.

(C) *Midbrain systems as gating mechanisms for conscious perception and action*

The role of midbrain structures in the maintenance of consciousness in clinical terms has been known for a long time and its relation to the sleep–wakefulness cycle was recognized by von Economo when he was analysing the effects of encephalitis epidemica.[27] Later, the role of the 'reticular substance' in the maintenance of wakefulness and in clinical consciousness was further elaborated, based on clinical and neurophysiological observations in epileptic patients,[28] and by experimental observations after electrical stimulation and lesions in the reticular formation[29] (for reviews see Refs. 30, 31).

Midbrain lesions, today a frequently occurring sequel of brain trauma and hypoxia due to post-traumatic brain oedema and tentorial infarction, further emphasize the importance of structures in these regions for the maintenance of clinical consciousness. The control of the sleep–wakefulness cycle through the serotoninergic neurons of the nucleus coeruleus is now well established.[32] These and other observations suggested that the integrating function of consciousness might be related to the structures concerned. But in the light of the preceding considerations and of experimental findings a somewhat different picture emerges.

Electrical stimulation of the reticular substance leads to an overall change of thalamo-cortical activity into what is generally called an arousal pattern (flattened EEG record with fast, low voltage activity), which is related to behavioural arousal. Cortical neurons may be transiently activated during electrical reticular stimulation, but during physiologically appearing arousal states and after electrical reticular stimulation their firing rate may even be decreased. During wakefulness in the physiological sleep–wakefulness cycle, the average spontaneous discharge rate of cortical neurons is little changed, with some neurons discharging faster, others slower, than during sleep.[33,34]

Lesions of the reticular substance[29] and transection of the mesencephalon at the precollicular level (*cerveau isolé*[35]) lead, like sleep and metabolically induced coma (e.g. hypoglycaemia), to large slow waves in the EEG, which are associated with grouped synchronous discharges of large cortical neuron populations. An intermediate state of clinical consciousness, i.e. lowered vigilance with closed or even open eyes, is characterized, as in the chronic *cerveau isolé* preparation, by regular waves around 10/second (α rhythm), which is accompanied by synchronous slow depolarizations and related discharges or bursts of activity of cortical neurons. Thus, the pattern of spontaneous cortical activity is different during the different states of vigilance and during comatose states (for reviews see Refs. 31, 36, 37).

The spontaneous cortical activity is generated by the thalamo-cortical afferents and thus represents, essentially, activity states of specific and non-specific thalamic nuclei. Thalamo-cortical relay cells are continually excited by their specific afferents (from the sense organs) or through internal loops. They are connected with each other through recurrent inhibitory pathways which induce inhibitory pauses after excitation. In the resting state, these excitatory–inhibitory sequences lead to regular thalamic discharge bursts in the α-frequency range (10/second).[37,38] This internuclear recurrent thalamic inhibition can be inhibited by stimulation of the reticular formation so that reticular excitation induces intrathalamic disinhibition.[39,40] As a consequence, no rhythmical burst activity is produced during states of increased reticulo-thalamic activation and transmission of specific excitatory activity through these thalamic relays is enhanced. In addition, there is good evidence that reticular activation also has a direct influence on cortical cell activity and thus on cortical threshold, although the pathways are not known.[41] Thus the reticular substance or related midbrain structures play an important role in opening or closing the gates of sensory inputs to the cortex and the gates of the internal thalamo-cortical loops.[42]

We need to know more about the control mechanisms which activate these non-specific mesencephalic gating mechanisms and incorporate them into the intracerebral loop systems. It may suffice to mention here their multisensory input, which indicates that they may be switched on by outside stimuli which make it necessary to alert the nervous system, and their excitatory input from internal structures such as the pallidum, which makes this general gating mechanism accessible from inside the nervous system. It is interesting to note, in this context, that to some extent such non-specific activations may be restricted to certain subsystems such as the visual system during visual attention or the motor system during movements;[43] it should also be noted that reticular neurons feed downwards into the executive motor command systems via the reticulo-spinal tract.[24]

THE INSUFFICIENCY OF BRAIN MECHANISMS TO EXPLAIN THE PHENOMENOLOGY OF CONSCIOUSNESS

Our discussion of three different cerebral systems has offered various mechanisms which may be considered necessary for consciousness. They may even explain various aspects of consciousness, as pointed out at various times and in different intellectual contexts. We are reminded, for example, of Spencer's observation that consciousness is a continuous orderly succession of changes; absolute quiescence in consciousness is cessation of consciousness, and 'if the changes are altogether at random, no consciousness, properly so called, exists'.[3] Indeed, there is no stable representation of the world in the cortex or in any part of the nervous system, due to the continuous change in the various representations induced by the internal and external loops. And the changes brought about do not follow each other at random but induce and depend on each other. Our conclusion that perception and action condition each other through the external loop is reminiscent of Victor von Weizsäcker's *Gestaltkreis*,[44] in which he points out that perception is in fact a continuous interaction between the individual and the environment. And one is, of course, also thinking of Piaget's emphasis on the action aspect in cognitive development.

Our conclusion that the synthesis of cortical representations of the world is accomplished in the synthesis of the cortico-fugal output lines into action systems comes, indeed, very close to Kant's definition: 'With synthesis I mean, in its broadest sense, the *act* of bringing together various ideas and to comprehend their manyfold into a cognition'.[4] This is meant with reference to cognition, but the essential point—that cognitive synthesis is in fact an act—is more than a trivial allusion to the processes we discussed in relation to the neurophysiological mechanisms of synthesis of the manifold representations and transformations of the world in the cortex into action systems and thus action.

One is reminded of the role that intentionality (and therefore activity) plays in the constitution of conscious cognition in Brentano's thinking, and also of Husserl's emphasis on the active comprehension in mental activities (aktives Erfassen bei der 'geistigen' Aktivität, die die synthetische Leistung vollbringt) (e.g. Ref. 5, § 38).

But the actual confrontation of the Ego with the world, with action and perception, which we called the dualistic aspect of consciousness, is not at all contained in the mechanisms discussed so far: how does the subject perceive what passes in his or her own mind? The 19th century monistic materialists such as Maudsley, Fischer, Büchner or Haeckel[45] have, probably unintentionally, admitted the insufficiency of such mechanisms by considering consciousness a secondary phenomenon or even an epiphenomenon. This view may explain consciousness sufficiently as a behavioural state, but rather avoids discussing it as a human phenomenon.

SELF-REPRESENTATION THROUGH THE REFLECTIVE LOOP

The dualistic aspect of consciousness, which is our experience, needs a mode by which the brain is able to confront itself with its own action and perception, with its past history and with its expectations. It is proposed here that the ability of the brain to synthesize its inputs (perception) and outputs (actions) to symbols, and to represent them to itself and to others, provides such a mode. This ability to represent symbolically what goes on in an individual's mind, and thus also in that person's world, I call the linguistic ability. Language is a representation of the world, of our relation to it and of ourselves in symbols. In that sense, our considerations may be generalized to any symbolical representation of the world and of the self, including sign language, gesture and even facial expressions. Such linguistic ability is achieved only by brains at the top of the evolutionary scale, and in its full development only in humans.

Language is dependent on certain cortical structures, although once it has developed it involves more than just the major cortical speech systems acquired late in evolution. Its development is restricted to one cerebral hemisphere, in spite of there being non-significant anatomical differences between the two hemispheres. It cannot be learnt by the non-dominant hemisphere once the brain is too old and its circuits too rigidly fixed. This indicates that for the full elaboration of language all the functional cortico-subcortical circuits of one hemisphere are involved and need to be moulded accordingly. Linguistic and symbolic competence is therefore not a symmetrical function of the forebrain, as are all other sensation–action processes. In fact, the structure of language is not a representation of the world in physical dimensions and can therefore not be split into two complementary halves.

Language or symbolic expressions are, like all actions, output activities of the cortex which involve orderly sequences of motor activities. Language is related to cognitive functions of the brain, as clinical and neuropsychological observations indicate. This confirms again the intricate relationship and in fact indistinguishable identity between afferent and efferent activities of the cortex, i.e. between sensation, perception and action. We may also apply to the neuronal language systems the same rules about internal loops as we apply to the other cortico-fugal output systems. Thus, efferent activities from virtually the whole cortex are integrated in language performance. Like any motor action language is affected by lesions of so-called motor-control systems such as the cerebellum, the neostriatum, the thalamus or the appropriate cortical representation fields of language-related motor systems (Broca's area). Clinical evidence for this is ample.

Through the symbolical presentation of the world and of the subject's relation to it the brain transcends its own activity, i.e. sensations and actions, by translating its activities into symbols and by representing these symbols back to itself. This activity we may call reflection and we may therefore introduce the term 'reflective loop' for this function of symbolic self-representation. This transcending reflection on what goes on in the brain in symbolic terms is a primary experience. It cannot be divided into its constituents by introspective exploration, although the signal is produced by the subject's brain. The transcendental reflection on the conditions of this primary experience necessarily leads to Kant's synthetic sentence, quoted above, or to a phenomenological definition of a transcendental consciousness. It is the basis for the primary experience of Descartes' 'Cogito ergo sum' and finds its symbolic expression in the monad of Leibniz. That means it is the condition of the dualistic experience of ourselves.

The reflective loop is not only a necessary but also a sufficient mechanism for the experience of consciousness, in that it constitutes this experience. Just as action as the outflow of sensation alters the activity of the nervous system and thus the representation of the world by distributed neuronal activity patterns, so does the symbolic self-representation lead to a continuous alteration of the subject's transcending reflection. This brings about new sequences of activities, and these in turn bring about new symbolic representations. The nature of such a system is that it is never the same and never closed or at rest. It asks questions about its world and about itself which it cannot answer, because it changes continually (cf. Kant's Introduction to the *Critique of Pure Reason*).

Having reached this point, that we may conceive of a neuronal mechanism for the understanding of consciousness through the reflective loop, although this has not been analysed in detail, we might finally ask whether through such an understanding of brain mechanisms we can in fact understand our own consciousness or that of others. The answer must be no, since the symbols in which we experience ourselves are not identical with the real world outside and inside our brain, and therefore can never represent this world in its physical reality. The symbols develop into an independent symbolical world, which we call the *world of mind, die Welt des Geistes.* It contains in symbols of increasingly broader significance the experience of our being in this world. Although this world of mind may have no substance of itself, it is to our consciousness as real as the physical world that surrounds us, since both depend on a representation in our brain. We therefore may believe in it as we believe in the physical reality. We relate ourselves to it in everchanging reflection, just as we continually change our relation to the physical world. But the knowledge of the brain mechanisms that lead to the consciousness that creates this world of symbols can explain neither consciousness nor the symbols in which it presents itself, since the brain mechanisms are not the symbols. This is the reason—or one may even say the brain mechanism—of the dualistic aspects of consciousness to which any critical reasoning about consciousness leads. The symbolic self-representation is the basis of the dualistic experience of the self, and in that sense dualism is, in fact, the nature of our experience of consciousness.

References

1. CREUTZFELDT, O. D. & RAGER, G. (1978) Brain mechanisms and the phenomenology of conscious experience, in *Cerebral Correlates of Conscious Experience* (Buser, P. & Rongeul-Buser, A., ed.), pp. 311–318, Elsevier North-Holland Biomedical Press, Amsterdam
2. WUNDT, W. (1874) *Grundzüge der physiologischen Psychologie,* Engelmann, Leipzig
3. SPENCER, H. (1855) *The Principles of Psychology,* Williams & Nargate, London
4. KANT, E. (1787) *Kritik der reinen Vernunft,* 2nd edn., J. F. Hartknoch, Riga
5. HUSSERL, E. (1950) *Cartesianische Meditationen* (Husserliana, vol. 1), Martinus Nijhoff, Den Haag
6. WUNDT, W. (1906) Gehirn und Seele, in *Essays,* 2nd edn., Wilhelm Engelmann, Leipzig
7. FECHNER, G. T. (1861) *Über die Seelenfrage,* Joh. Abrosius Barth, Leipzig.
8. PENFIELD, W. (1975) *The Mystery of the Mind,* Princeton University Press, Princeton
9. POPPER, K. R. & ECCLES, J. C. (1977) *The Self and its Brain,* Springer International, Berlin
10. KRETSCHMER, E. (1940) Das apallische Syndrom. *Z. Gesamte Neurol. Psychiatr. 169,* 576–579
11. CREUTZFELDT, O. (1975) Some problems of cortical organisation in the light of ideas of the classical 'Hirnpathologie' and of modern neurophysiology. An essay, in *Cerebral Localization* (Zülch, K. J. et al., eds.), pp. 217–226, Springer, Berlin

12. CREUTZFELDT, O. (1977) Generality of the functional structure of the neocortex. *Naturwissenschaften 64*, 507–517
13. EDELMANN, G. M. & MOUNTCASTLE, V. B. (1978) *The Mindful Brain*, MIT Press, Cambridge, Mass.
14. HYVÄRINEN, J. & PORANEN, A. (1974) Function of the parietal associative area 7 as revealed from cellular discharges in alert monkeys. *Brain 97*, 673–692
15. MOUNTCASTLE, V. B., LYNCH, J. C., GEORGOPOULOS, A., SAKATA, H. & ACUNA, A. (1975) Posterior parietal association cortex of the monkey: command functions for operations within extrapersonal space. *J. Neurophysiol. 39*, 871–908
16. MANZONI, T., CAMINITI, R., SPIDALIERI, G. & MORELLI, E. (1979) Anatomical and functional aspects of the associative projections from somatic area SI to SII. *Exp. Brain Res. 34*, 453–470
17. JAMES, W. (1890) *The Principles of Psychology*, Henry Holt, Toronto
18. DIAMOND, I. I., JONES, E. G. & POWELL, T. P. S. (1969) The projection of the auditory cortex upon the diencephalon and brain stem in the cat. *Brain Res. 15*, 305–340
19. JONES, E. G., COULTER, J. D., BURTON, H. & PORTER, R. (1977) Cells of origin and terminal distribution of corticostriatal fibers arising in the sensory-motor cortex of monkeys. *J. Comp. Neurol. 173*, 53–80
20. CREUTZFELDT, O. D. & NOTHDURFT, H. C. (1978) Representation of complex visual stimuli in the brain. *Naturwissenschaften 65*, 307–318
21. CREUTZFELDT, O. (1976) The brain as a functional unity. *Prog. Brain Res. 45*, 451–462
22. GOLDMANN, P. S. & NAUTA, W. J. H. (1977) An intricately patterned prefontocaudate projection in the rhesus monkey. *J. Comp. Neurol. 171*, 369–386
23. KÜNZLE, H. (1975) Bilateral projections from precentral motor cortex to basal ganglia. An autoradiographic study in *Macaca fascicularis*. *Brain Res. 88*, 195–209
24. HASSLER, R. (1978) Striatal control of locomotion, intentional actions and of integrating and perceptive activity. *J. Neurol. Sci. 36*, 187–224
25. SANIDES, D. & BUCHHOLTZ, C. S. (1978) Identification of the projection from the visual cortex to the claustrum by anterograde axonal transport in the cat. *Exp. Brain Res. 34*, 197–200
26. UNO, M., OZAWA, N. & YOSHIIDA, M. (1978) The mode of pallido-thalamic transmission investigated with intracellular recording from cat thalamus. *Exp. Brain Res. 33*, 493–507
27. VON ECONOMO, C. (1929) Schlaftheorie. *Ergeb. Physiol. Biol. Chem. Exp. Pharmakol. 28*, 312–339
28. PENFIELD, W. & JASPER, H. (1954) *Epilepsy and the Functional Anatomy of the Brain*, Little, Brown, Boston
29. FRENCH, J. D. & MAGOUN, H. W. (1952) Effects of chronic lesions in central cephalic brain stem of monkeys. *Arch. Neurol. Psychiatr. 68*, 591–604
30. MAGOUN, H. W. (1958) *The Waking Brain*, Charles C. Thomas, Springfield, Ill.
31. SCHLAG, J. (1974) Reticular influences on thalamo-cortical activity, in *Handbook for Electroencephalography and Clinical Neurophysiology* (Rémond, A., ed), pp. 119–134, Elsevier, Amsterdam
32. JOUVET, M. (1969) Coma and other disorders of consciousness, in *Handbook of Clinical Neurology*, vol. 3 (Vinken, P. J. & Bruyn, G. W., eds.), pp. 62–79, North-Holland, Amsterdam
33. CREUTZFELDT, O. & JUNG, R. (1961) Neuronal discharge in the cat's motor cortex during sleep and arousal, in *The Nature of Sleep (Ciba Found. Symp.)*, pp. 131–170, Churchill, London
34. EVARTS, E. V. (1961) Effects of sleep and waking on activity of single units in the unrestrained cat, in *The Nature of Sleep (Ciba Found. Symp.)*, pp. 171–182, Churchill, London
35. BREMER, F. (1935) Cerveau isolé et physiologie du sommeil. *C.R. Séanc. Soc. Biol. 118*, 1235–1241

36. CREUTZFELDT, O. (1975) Neurophysiological correlates of different functional states of the brain, in *Brain Work (Alfred Benzon Symp. 8)* (Ingvar, D. M. & Lassen, N A.,. eds.), pp. 21–46, Munksgaard, Copenhagen.

37. CREUTZFELDT, O. & HOUCHIN, J. (1974) Neuronal basis of EEG-waves, in *Handbook of Electroencephalography and Clinical Neurophysiology*, vol. 2, part C (Rémond, A., ed.), pp. 5–55, Elsevier, Amsterdam

38. ANDERSEN, P. & ANDERSSON, S. A. (1974) Thalamic origin of cortical rhythmic activity, in *Handbook of Electroencephalography and Clinical Neurophysiology*, vol. 2, part C (Rémond, A., ed.), pp. 90–118, Elsevier, Amsterdam

39. PURPURA, D. P. & SHOFER, R. J. (1963) Intracellular recording from thalamic neurons during reticulo cortical activation. *J. Neurophysiol. 26*, 494–505

40. SINGER, W. & DRÄGER, U. (1972) Postsynaptic potentials in relay neurons of the cat lateral geniculate nucleus after stimulation of the mesencephalic reticular formation. *Brain Res. 41*, 214–220

41. CREUTZFELDT, O., SPEHLMANN, R. & LEHMANN, D. (1961) Veränderung der Neuronaktivität des visuellen Cortex durch Reizung der Substantia reticularis mesencephali, in *Neurophysiologie und Psychophysik des visuellen Systems* (Jung, R. & Kornhuber, H., eds.), pp. 351–363, Springer, Berlin

42. CREUTZFELDT, O. (1977) Physiological conditions of consciousness, in *11th Wld. Congr. Neurol.* (Den Hartog Jager, W. A. *et al.*, eds.), I.C.S. No. 434, 194–208, Excerpta Medica, Amsterdam

43. ROUGEUL-BUSER, A., BOUYER, J. J. & BUSER, P. (1975) From attentiveness to sleep. A topographical analysis of localized 'synchronized' activities on the cortex of normal cat and monkey. *Acta Neurobiol. Exp. (Warsaw) 35*, 805–819

44. VON WEIZSÄCKER, V. (1940) *Der Gestaltkreis*, Springer, Berlin

45. MAUDSLEY, H. (1876) *Physiology of Mind*; FISCHER, J. L., *Das Bewusstsein*; BÜCHNER, L., *Kraft und Stoff*; HAECKEL, E., *Welträtsel*; RIBOT, T. A., *Les Maladies de la Volonté*

Three types of consciousness [Commentary]

D. M. ARMSTRONG

Department of Traditional and Modern Philosophy, University of Sydney, New South Wales

Abstract   It is useful to distinguish three senses of the word 'consciousness'. 'Minimal' consciousness is the occurrence of any mental activity, whether or not the subject is aware of this activity. 'Perceptual' consciousness is perceptual activity. Minimal and perceptual consciousness may be present, yet 'introspective' consciousness be lacking.

Introspective consciousness is conceived as it was by Locke and Kant: as perception-like awareness of the subject's own current mental states and activities. It includes introspective consciousness of introspective consciousness itself. A useful model for demystifying and naturalizing introspective consciousness is the subject's proprioceptive awareness of bodily states and activities.

Introspective consciousness may be further subdivided into 'reflex' introspective consciousness and 'introspection proper'. The distinction is one of degree: the degree of attention involved.

We attach a quite special importance to introspective consciousness and are particularly unwilling to identify it with a purely physical process in the brain. It is suggested, however, that this springs from (a) the fact that what is introspected is taken to be a state or activity of a single thing, the self; and (b) the fact that event-memory is generally only possible if the event remembered was the object of introspective consciousness at the time. Without introspective consciousness, therefore, awareness of a self and the past history of that self is lacking.

Consciousness is a dizzying phenomenon. It is not even clear that those who use the word always refer to the same thing. I shall distinguish a number of different things that could be meant by the word. I shall speak of 'minimal', 'perceptual' and 'introspective' consciousness.

MINIMAL CONSCIOUSNESS

In order to understand what is meant by 'minimal' consciousness, it is helpful to consider the case where even this sort of consciousness is lacking:

the person who is totally unconscious. Someone in sound dreamless sleep approaches this condition, although here we do not need to decide whether total unconsciousness is or is not a mere theoretical limit, approached but never actually reached.

The totally unconscious person still has a mind. This mind, moreover, may be credited with various states. The person will have knowledge, memories and beliefs. They will have skills, for instance an aptitude for mental arithmetic. They may be credited with likes and dislikes, attitudes and emotions, desires, aims and purposes. They may be said to be in certain moods: 'She has been depressed all this week'.

There is nothing hypothetical about such states. One may point to an unconscious person and attribute current possession of such states. Given what we know, it is natural to conceive of these states as physical states of the brain. A memory, for instance, will be a continuing trace in the brain. A natural analogy is the storage of information and instructions in a computer, a storage which may be unaffected by the fact that the computer is not currently operating.

We may say of the mental states of a totally unconscious person (and also of the states of a computer which is not operating) that they are *causally quiescent*. Nothing, of course, is causally quiescent *absolutely*. But the mental states will not be producing any *mental* effect in the person. (Similarly, the states of the computer will not be producing any *computational* effect.) If the mental states do have mental effects, then we may rule that the person is not *totally* unconscious.

Let us now consider what the totally unconscious person lacks mentally. Such a person does not perceive, and lacks any sensations, feelings or pangs of desire. They cannot think, contemplate or engage in deliberation. They cannot be engaged in carrying out any purpose. For these are all mental *activities* and, by definition, the totally unconscious person is incapable of mental activity. During unconsciousness there are mental states, but no mental life.

We are now in a position to define 'minimal' consciousness. There is minimal consciousness if and only if there is mental activity, if the mind is not completely 'stopped'. If there is dreaming, for instance, there is minimal consciousness.

It is alleged that it sometimes occurs that someone wakes up knowing the solution to, say, a mathematical problem which they did not know when they went to sleep. If we rule out magical explanations, then there must have been mental activity during sleep. To that extent, there was minimal consciousness. This is compatible with the completest 'unconsciousness' in a sense still to be identified.

PERCEPTUAL CONSCIOUSNESS

Among mental activities, there appears to be a special link between *perception* and consciousness. There is an important sense in which, if a person is perceiving, then they are conscious; but if they are not perceiving, then they are not conscious. Suppose that they are dreaming. Dreaming is a mental activity, so they are minimally conscious. Yet is there not an obvious sense in which they lack consciousness? Now suppose that they start to perceive (whether veridically or non-veridically) their environment and bodily state. Are they not now conscious in a way that they were not before? Let us say, therefore, that they have regained 'perceptual' consciousness.

Perceptual consciousness involves mental activity and so is a form of minimal consciousness. But, as indicated, there can be minimal consciousness without perceptual consciousness: mental activity without any awareness of the physical world.

INTROSPECTIVE CONSCIOUSNESS

We now suppose that there is mental activity going on in a person's mind and that this activity includes perception. There is minimal consciousness and perceptual consciousness. Nevertheless, such a person may still 'lack consciousness' in the most interesting sense of the word.

Consider the case of the long-distance truck-driver. After driving for long periods of time in monotonous conditions, for instance at night, it is possible to 'come to' and realize that one has been driving without being aware of what one was doing. It is natural to say that during that time the driver 'lacked consciousness'. It seems clear, however, that minimal consciousness, and, in particular, perceptual consciousness, was present. For how can a truck or car be driven for many miles along a road without perception of that road? What is lacking, then, is something more than minimal and perceptual consciousness.

Some people are tempted to argue at this point that what go on in the brain of the long-distance truck-driver are physiological processes which are the same as, or very similar to, the physiological processes which go on when actual perception occurs; but that in this case actual *perception* does not occur. I agree that we have no reason to believe that there is anything more going on in the truck-driver than purely physiological processes in his brain. But the moral I draw is that these processes *are* his perceptions.

What does the long-distance truck-driver lack? I think that it is a further mental activity which resembles perception. But, unlike *sense*-perception, it is not directed towards the perceiver's current environment and current bodily state. Instead, it is awareness of the mental: awareness of current mental states and activities. Such 'inner perception' is traditionally called 'introspection' or 'introspective awareness'. So let us call this third sort of consciousness 'introspective' consciousness.

Kant spoke of sense-perception as 'outer sense'. Following Locke, he spoke of introspection as 'inner sense', and it is the Locke–Kant view that I am following here. Among the possible objects of inner sense will be current sense-perception, and, of course (an interesting complication), current introspective awareness itself.

One particular form of outer sense has a close formal resemblance to introspection. This is *proprioception*, or perception of one's own current bodily states. In the case of sight, sound, touch, taste and smell it is possible for different perceivers all to perceive numerically the same thing. Compare, this, however, with kinaesthetic perception, which is a particular mode of proprioception. Each person is confined to kinaesthetic awareness of the motion of her or his own limbs. This serves as a model for the fact that, in introspection, each person is confined to awareness of current states in, and activities of, her or his *own* mind.

The chief value, in my view, of the proprioceptive model for introspection is that it *demystifies* and *naturalizes* the latter. The fact that each of us, in introspection, is cognitively locked within our own mind seems far less portentous when we notice that in proprioception we are similarly locked within our own body. We easily apprehend, also, that our proprioceptive powers are limited—we are not proprioceptively aware of *all* our current bodily states and activities—and that, on occasion, we may be subject to proprioceptive illusion. This makes it easy to accept, as the psychological evidence makes it clear that we should accept, that we are not introspectively aware of all our current mental states and activities, and that we may be subject to introspective illusion. Introspection is a human faculty with human limitations.

I speak of introspection as a human faculty. The case of the long-distance truck-driver presents itself to us as a special and spectacular one. But in evolutionary terms it appears to be regression to a relatively primitive level of mental functioning. It is natural to surmise that the other animals are always, or at least normally, in the state into which the long-distance truck-driver has got himself temporarily. If there are exceptions to this, they will be among the primates and other higher mammals. Introspection is a late evolutionary development.

It is not difficult to see the evolutionary value of the development of introspective powers. Increased sophistication of behaviour demands increased sophistication in the mental processes which give rise to behaviour. Increased sophistication in mental processes demands greatly increased and greatly sophisticated parallel processing. Such parallel processing, however, cannot proceed in an 'anarchistic' manner: there must be a careful coordination of what is going on. Nor can it proceed in the way that a 'command economy' is supposed to proceed: the mere obeying of instructions from above will not yield sufficient flexibility. Coordination of sophisticated parallel processes will be best achieved if the coordinating processes are made continuously aware of the current states and activities which have to be coordinated. The mind will therefore need to perceive itself as well as perceiving its body and its environment. It is an as yet unproved, but plausible, assumption that this perception of the mind by itself is a purely physical process within the central nervous system.

TYPES OF INTROSPECTIVE CONSCIOUSNESS

There seems a need for further distinctions. A distinction can be drawn between mere 'reflex' consciousness, normally always present while we are awake (but temporarily lost by the long-distance truck-driver), and consciousness of a more explicit, self-conscious, sort—the sort of thing which is present when we deliberately gaze within ourselves.

I suggest that this difference is parallel to the difference between mere 'reflex' seeing, which is always going on while we are awake and our eyes are open, and the careful *scrutinizing* of the visual environment which may be undertaken in the interest of some purpose which we have. The eyes have a watching brief at all times that we are awake and have our eyes open; in special circumstances, they are used in a more attentive manner. (In close scrutiny by human beings introspective consciousness is often also called into play. We not only give the object more attention but have a heightened awareness of so doing. But, presumably, in lower animals such attentive scrutiny does not have this accompaniment.) Similarly, introspective consciousness normally has only a watching brief with respect to our mental states. Only sometimes do we carefully scrutinize our own current state of mind. We can mark the distinction by speaking of 'reflex' introspective awareness and opposing it to 'introspection proper'. It is a plausible hypothesis that the latter will involve, not simply introspective awareness of mental states and activities, but also introspective awareness of that introspective awareness. It is in any case a peculiarly sophisticated sort of mental process.

WHAT IS SO SPECIAL ABOUT INTROSPECTIVE CONSCIOUSNESS?

There remains the feeling that there is something quite special about introspective consciousness. There is an important sense, we think, in which the long-distance truck-driver does not have any experiences, is hardly a person, during his period of introspective unconsciousness. Some have thought that introspective consciousness is so special that no materialist or physicalist account of it could possibly be given. It is, furthermore, an important part of any intellectual position to explain plausibly why others should think the position implausible. Can a naturalist and physicalist explain why introspective consciousness seems unique?

The first point to notice is that introspective consciousness is bound up in a quite special way with consciousness of self. I do not mean that the self is one of the particular objects of introspective awareness. Rather, it is the case that human beings, or at any rate reasonably adult and socialized human beings, take the states and activities which they are introspectively aware of as states and activities of a single, continuing, thing. There is a certain amount of theory in this. A comparison may be made, once again, to proprioception, where it is a considerable, if early accomplished, theoretical achievement to refer the states and activities proprioceptively perceived to a single, continuing, physical object: the body.

What the nature of this self is, mere introspection does not inform us. We do not learn whether it is immaterial or material, and, if material, just how the self stands to the body. But we do learn, or at any rate we assume, that it is a unitary thing. *Pace* Kant, there is nothing necessary about the assumption. It may even be denied on occasion. Less sophisticated people than ourselves, on becoming aware of a murderous impulse springing up, may attribute it not to a hitherto unacknowledged and even dissociated part of themselves but to a devil who has entered them. Dickens' Mrs Gradgrind, when dying, says that there seems to be a pain in the room, but she is not prepared to say that it is *she* that has got it. Normally, however, the assumption is not denied, and there is good reason for not denying it: the different parts, tendencies, etc., in the one mind form, in normal circumstances, a tightly organized and interlocking system. This is what is meant by a unitary thing.

It seems, second, that there is a special connection between introspective consciousness and event-memory. When the long-distance truck-driver recovers introspective consciousness, he has no memory of what happened during unconsciousness. One sort of memory processing cannot have failed him. His successful navigation of his vehicle depended upon him being able to *recognize* various things for what they were and treat them accordingly. He must have been able to recognize a certain degree of pressure on the accelerator, a certain degree of curve in the road, for what they were. But the things which happened to him during unconsciousness were not stored in his event-memory. He lived solely in the present.

It is tempting to suppose, therefore, that unless whatever happens in our mind (including our perceptions) is monitored by introspective consciousness, then it is not remembered to have occurred, or at least it is very unlikely that it will be remembered. It is obvious that introspective consciousness is not sufficient for event-memory, but perhaps it is necessary, or at least generally necessary. It is notoriously difficult, for instance, to remember dreams, and it is clear that, in almost all dreaming, introspective consciousness is either absent or is at a low ebb.

So, given that introspective consciousness is a consciousness of self, and further that without introspective consciousness there would be little or no event-memory and so no memory of the past of the self, the apparent utterly special character of what is revealed by introspective consciousness is explained. Without introspective consciousness we would not be aware that we existed— the self would not be self to itself. Nor would we be aware of what the particular history of that self had been, even its very recent history. No wonder it seems that introspective consciousness is like a light switched on that lights up utter darkness. No wonder it seems that with introspective consciousness a wholly new thing has entered the universe.

Discussion: Consciousness

Bennett: Seeing the split-brain phenomenon as suggesting two centres of consciousness was described as something that philosophers are prone to do and shouldn't do. I don't know about philosophers generally, but I plead guilty. However, it seems to me that with someone who has undergone a commissurotomy, who is in the special kind of situation that Colwyn Trevarthen and his colleagues have created, there *is* a problem about counting how many people are involved. You have not made it clear to me why it is so wrong to think that there are two minds here. Their information is different. As I understand it, one of them may perform tasks, with any failures being noted by the other, though the other is not in a position to help. A lot of inter-relationships of this sort seem very like relationships between different people.

Trevarthen: Nothing we know about the commissurotomy patients suggests to me that there is a double agency, but there are certainly two conscious awarenesses. The geographics of the word centre is such that only the left hemisphere can speak and there are problems and paradoxes about the reasoning power and creative awareness of the mute right hemisphere, which has its own mental abilities. But as a free agent the commissurotomy patient has an intrinsic unity. All the information we have shows that the person who is looking at half of a chimera with one half of the brain and the other half of the chimera with the other half of the brain has two coincident experiences at one place. The person can recall enough afterwards to show that both parts of the brain were aware and each perceived a whole figure. You can say that there are two completely different images and they could be in categorical or prospective conflict, so long as there is no actual conflict of purpose. For the subject ready to act in the world, the two experiences are, I believe, in the same place.

I think that this dual awareness of the commissurotomy patient is not totally different from the kinds of awareness we may have when tired, especially in rapid and confusing activity. It is significant that the cortical awareness machinery is not simply divided into left and right halves. It is fed by a number of satellite systems which have equivalents in experience: we can hear a word, we can see it and we can spell it out in writing, and for short periods we can do several such things at once. That does not make us feel we have a divided self. We just feel we have different agents working for us. I think we may have occasionally overstated the separation or division of agency in the commissurotomy patient. The subjects who give evidence of divided awareness had been asked to sit and fixate a point, but when allowed more freedom of action they seem to quickly reconcile images in their two hemispheres. By controlling orienting one can deliberately trick them into paradoxical states and can cause the two consciousnesses to fall apart. This is an essential step in observation of their mental processes. But the subjects might lose confidence in their experience if made acutely aware of contradictions in their actions. We do not allow that to happen, of course. Occasionally very bizarre states of consciousness with elements of double intentionality can be obtained when the subject has been working very hard with consistent concentration on a task for one hemisphere. Conflicting movements of manipulation by the two hands have been seen, but it is probable that these are due to cerebral damage besides the disconnection. Other happenings appear to be more directly due to bisection of the cerebral motor system. One subject's left hand floated into the air from the table when she was working hard with the left hemisphere; and she looked at me, surprised, and pulled it down with her right hand. Evidently her right hemisphere was in a trance-like state, or its antigravitation mechanism was disturbed.

Searle: So your answer to Jonathan Bennett is that although there are two centres of awareness there is only one centre of intentionality, in your sense of that word?

Trevarthen: There are two realms of awareness but one generator of intention to act.

Wikler: I still agree with Jonathan. It is true that sometimes we collect information from different sources without the collection process being particularly integrated in our experience; but this occurs only when we are not really thinking about the different sources. What we don't have is the sensation of focusing our attention on one clear stimulus and not knowing it. Yet, in a sense, that is what would be happening if you regarded these two awarenesses as belonging to the same person. Consider the following *gedanken*-experiment. A surgeon removes my (whole) brain from my body; hooks me up to a part of someone else's efferent nervous system and perceptual apparatus; cuts nerves to make that part inaccessible to the other person's brain; and makes sure that I cannot send out active orders. There would be two centres of awareness, and one centre of intention to action. Would I and my host cease to be distinct individuals? I can certainly imagine my own consciousness proceeding through this surgery, and being very upset about it, but still being myself. I don't think you would want to say that I and the person I was spliced into were now the same person just because I was incapable of affecting his behaviour. The existence of two different centres of awareness, one of which can be completely ignorant of even the strongest and most clearly felt stimuli in the other, is enough to suggest that there are two different persons there. This is so whether the two consciousnesses are the result of a 'fusion' by splicing together two nervous systems—as in my example—or of a 'fission' such as is encountered in the split-brain phenomenon.

Trevarthen: I do not think you need to do that experiment. We have firm evidence of double awareness. If you put emphasis on conscious awareness and call that the conscious person, what you say is true, but I do not wish to do that. I feel we must realize that active effective people, even those who have trained themselves to reflect a lot or to think hard about what they are perceiving, can feel conflicts and their resolution between different states of consciousness going on inside the head—at least that is my own experience. I do not know what the final answer is about the simultaneity of awareness in the commissurotomy patient. It is still possible that these subjects don't have two awarenesses precisely at the same time, but that they can change between two alternative images very quickly, each leaving a record that may be recalled.

Fried: The unity of the person which it is our instinct to see, split brain or no, is a complex unity rather in the domain of symbolization that Otto Creutzfeldt put forward—although the symbolization of a person with a split brain is perhaps more difficult than the symbolization of a normal person. Nevertheless a man with a split brain symbolizes himself and his proprioception as belonging to one person, and that makes him one person. In contrast we would hesitate a long time before deciding to execute a man without a split brain but who is crazy and symbolizes himself as two people. That goes to show that it is the symbolization which makes one or two people rather than the anatomy.

Trevarthen: You have slightly shaken my argument about intentionality in commissurotomy patients by causing me to think of culpability. The philosophers are perhaps justified in thinking that the commissurotomy patients have two selves if we consider cases where irresponsible acts are admitted to be not intended by one hemisphere. One of the patients obtained a dishwashing job in a hospital and one day found that his left hand was throwing the dishes on the floor—not dropping, throwing. He was so ashamed that he ran away. So, it can happen that one of these people will do something they in part do not mean to do. However, this man has, we know, lesions in the hemisphere that are likely to be responsible for apraxic movements of his right hand. Perhaps the brain system that made those unwanted thoughtless acts was like the long-distance truck-driver. We do not use this patient for many experiments because he is likely to do automatic movements which cannot be shut out, but other commissurotomy patients have their motor control uncomplicated by such things. From their behaviour one would conclude that disconnection does not divide responsibility for action.

Cooper: I would be very cautious about interpreting the split-brain data as having anything to do with the subject of this meeting. Even if not all the patients are epileptic, they all have a pre-existing disease affecting consciousness. They are performing automatic activities, throwing dishes and having fits. So how can you fail to think that this might affect the validity of the study of their conscious awareness?

Trevarthen: This particular objection to the commissurotomy studies has been made very often, but it is mistaken. We are very careful to select out those behaviours that could be due to pathological states separate from commissurotomy. The claims that we make are based upon behaviours that would be highly improbable as a consequence of other pathological states. We are using entirely the opposite logic. This is dealt with very carefully in our publications.

I want to correct one point relating to Dr Creutzfeldt's comments. Sperry believes that it is terribly important that the state of the disconnected right hemisphere is not subsidiary unconsciousness. It has its own mode of awareness. He thinks that division of the elaborate mental states of man into two consciousnesses demonstrates the reality and the power of consciousness in brain function.

It is very important to him, and to me, that one of these consciousnesses does not seem to mediate its representations verbally. It does not seem to be using language or language-like processes for its conscious states, its self-awareness or communication with other people, and so on. I suspect that this is very relevant to the question of the nature of self-awareness, and how it arises.

Marsden: I am sure that the greatest care is taken to exclude the impact of epilepsy in the observations that you make, but the commonest cause of someone throwing away a plate, if they are epileptic, is that they have had a fit. You can't exclude the possibility that that man had had a motor seizure arising in the opposite hemisphere.

Trevarthen: If that is the explanation we would not have to consider that brain bisection had made two wills. If all the patients behaved like the dishwashing man it would be very different. In that particular case, is that man culpable?

Plum: The argument against epileptic activity causing the behaviour you have observed is that all your subjects behave essentially the same. Therefore to a degree you have eliminated the random or individual factor by obtaining essentially reproducible stimulus-response curves. I have examined patients with commissurotomy and have little doubt that you are looking at the existing non-epileptic function in those hemispheres. But if those right hemispheres had evolved in isolation, would they possess the verbally related functions, in particular, which they learned from the left hemisphere during development?

Trevarthen: I don't think we know the final answer to this. The initial impact of these findings and the subsequent exploration, which has been greatly advanced by Zaidel's work,[1] have enormously enriched our knowledge of the mental processes of the right hemisphere. It must be taken into consideration that a mental realm of awareness and of thinking can exist which is apparently incapable of creating phonological images of words.[2]

What happens in the development of hemispheric functional specialization we do not know, entirely, but it is relevant that babies, whose brains are anatomically asymmetric in language-related areas before birth, have a considerable semantic capacity before they speak any words. The nine to ten months' transition to secondary intersubjectivity which leads to what we describe as the development of cooperative understanding in performance of a task is the same point in development at which Halliday[3] said protolanguage begins. As a linguist Halliday describes protolanguage as linguistic behaviour, acts of meaning, without words. The psychological process that manifests itself then may fundamentally derive from morphogenesis and from changes going on in the baby's brain, not from experience, although experience is needed too. The mechanism for cooperative understanding is probably bigger than that for language and essential to it.

The course of hemisphere development, including the structures inter-connected by the corpus callosum, is so complex that the hemispheres may change places several times in the regulation of a psychological function such as communication. You are absolutely right that we mustn't forget we are dealing with adult patients. The boy who was operated on at the age of 14 has somewhat different kinds of mental processing in his hemispheres from those of the woman operated on in her 30s. Maybe his language functions were still becoming lateralized when his brain was divided.

Putnam: Creutzfeldt has answered no to the question of whether there is any specific correlation between the physical performance of the brain and an act or state of mind, and Armstrong answered yes. I would suggest that there is a third answer: yes and no.

To illustrate why a simple yes or no won't do, let me use an analogy. Frege discovered that the *numbers* 0, 1, 2, 3, . . . can be identified with *sets*. Today, following von Neumann rather than Frege and Russell, we identify zero with the empty set (as opposed to the singleton of the empty set), one with the singleton of the empty set (as opposed to the set of all singletons of the appropriate type), and so on (so each number is the set of all smaller numbers). But one can also identify 0, 1, 2, 3, . . . with still other sequences of sets. Call a theory which postulates natural numbers as distinct from sets (i.e. a theory which says numbers are not sets) a theory of *unreduced* numbers. Does a theory of the kind that Frege and von Neumann constructed, a theory which omits the *unreduced* numbers, a theory whose ontology consists merely of sets, 'leave something out'? If not, does this mean that 'numbers are really sets'? *Are* numbers *really* sets? And if numbers are really sets, is there a fact of the matter *which* set the number zero is really identical with?

What we have just given is an example of two theories which are both 'true' (or adequate to the purposes they are supposed to serve)—set theory with unreduced numbers, and 'two sorted' mathematics, with both sets *and* unreduced numbers—but which do not possess a unique translation. *Numbers can be identified with sets.* That is a 'fact'. But there is no fact as to which set a given number 'really is'.

I think this is a general phenomenon in language, not just one that pops up in mathematics. Mind talk and brain talk are two theories which arose in response to different needs and which subserve different interests; there need not be a fact of the matter (a fact independent of every trace of legislation or convention) as to *which* brain state a given mental state 'really is'.

To motivate this, observe that one can have *observationally indistinguishable identity theories* in the area of brain–mind identity. For example, in the split-brain case, the theory that the right lobe is only simulating consciousness (it is 'dark' in the right lobe—Eccles' theory) and the theory that both lobes are separate loci of consciousness (Blakemore?) lead to the same predictions (if properly worked out) with respect to the experience of all observers with unsplit brains. So any scientific theory that ever decides this question will have to be accepted, if at all, on wholly non-empirical ('methodological') grounds. Of course, a diehard realist could still maintain that there is a fact of the matter as to which is right, even when our choice is based on *a priori* preferences; but must there always be such a fact of the matter? Or is this an illusion? I am inclined to think it is an illusion; but in any case, the question is a philosophical one, and not a scientific one.

Bunge The *Leitmotiv* of Professor Creutzfeldt's presentation seems to be that 'there is no way of describing conscious experience in neurophysiological terms'. My question is: now or never? *Ignoramus* or also *ignorabimus?* If you mean 'never' you could be accused of prophesying the future or rather the non-future of science.

Secondly, you have been criticizing materialism of the eliminative type but neither Armstrong nor I are materialists of this kind. We both admit that there are conscious states that are brain states peculiar to human beings. Would you allow the hypothesis that conscious states are states of subsystems of the brain that monitor the activity of other systems of the same brain?

Thirdly, if you identify, as you apparently have done, consciousness with the ability to speak a particular language, you are denying that subhuman primates, and also deaf people, have the capacity for having conscious states. This seems to derive from regarding speech as an indicator of consciousness, but it is a very different matter to identify consciousness with the ability to symbolize.

Fourthly, I understood you to say that the somatotopic representations we have are neighbourhood-preserving (i.e. topological) maps. But the homunculi don't seem to be like that at all. Apparently some adjacent regions of the body are represented in distant parts of the brain, and conversely. Of course they are maps but they are not neighbourhood-preserving or topological maps.

Searle: One of those questions seemed to be based on a misunderstanding. Dr Creutzfeldt did not say, as I recall, that consciousness was based on language but rather that the unity of consciousness had to do with action and symbolization.

Creutzfeldt: Yes, that is true. As to somatotopic maps, I restricted myself to the topographic representation of thalamic projection nuclei in the respective cortical areas, where there is good anatomical evidence that neighbouring points in the thalamus are also adjacent in the cortex (with some scatter and overlap). There may be some topological problems in bringing the three-dimensional volume of thalamic structures onto the two-dimensional cortical surface. There are further problems in the two-dimensional representation of the three-dimensional surfaces of the body and even of the retina (which is a hemisphere). I realize these problems but think it would be irrelevant to discuss them further in this context. More important are the transformations of sensory maps into functional maps in the non-primary and the so-called association areas. But here too the thalamo-cortical neighbourhood relation of adjacent points is supported by anatomy. This would lead to the conclusion that these transformations are present already in the respective thalamic nuclei, for which some evidence exists.

As to whether I mean *ignoramus* or *ignorabimus*, I hesitate to expose myself to the accusation of prophesying the future of science in either direction. For myself, I admit: *ignorabo*. Even if a description of consciousness would in principle be possible in neural terms, such a description may be so complex and lengthy that it would be useless. John von Neumann[4] realized this long ago, when he was referring to a much simpler problem of cognition: 'It is, therefore, not at all unlikely that it is futile to look for a precise logical concept, that is, for a precise verbal description, of 'visual analogy' [the example he has chosen]. It is possible that the connection pattern of the visual brain itself is the simplest logical expression or definition of this principle'. Relating this statement to our problem of consciousness would mean that even if we could in principle describe neural processes the functioning of which would imply consciousness, we would not have described experience of consciousness since the mechanisms and terms of such a model are not accessible to and are not part of that very experience.

Bunge: The question is not whether we have not understood up to now but whether we shall ever be able to understand.

Creutzfeldt: This is not a question of understanding or not, but a problem of two different ways of describing and analysing a process which is not the same phenomenon for the two analysers. To use David Armstrong's example: I can describe a painting or the world for you in every detail, but this is not the same painting or the world as you experience it. If I describe the chemical composition and physical dimensions of a lump of iron, this may enable you to build a model of it or to imagine it. This is one way of experiencing it. But your experience will be quite a different one if you inadvertently stumble over that lump. I would find it strange to be confronted by philosophers who refuse to recognize these principally different approaches to reality.

Blakemore: But one's personal experience, however convincing, does not necessarily and inherently provide the appropriate terminology by which to describe any phenomenon, just as observing the processes of burning, oxidation and so on didn't make the phlogiston theory right even though it provided an internally consistent way of describing the phenomena.

Creutzfeldt: Yes, but it could be internally consistent with what you believe, and you believe in the phenomena produced by the brain. You see the world in the context of the references of your beliefs.

Trevarthen: There is something remarkable about the interest of babies in the products of other people's actions. They are also exceedingly interested by one year of age in artifacts that are presented to them as toys. We are beginning cross-cultural studies of this. We think that, presented as they are in play with different aspects of cultures, infants are already beginning to be adapted to their culture's aims at one year of age. They actively seek to join the culture and cooperate with it. It is already innate in them to be cultural, which may seem a bizarre notion. Yet, there is something very good about the idea that the products of minds are natural food for the young mind in human culture.

Wall: I said earlier that the powerful evidence for the existence of maps in these systems is to a certain extent a diversion from what one might hope to have found. Dr Creutzfeldt offered a solution by suggesting that the maps must undergo topological transformations. This is obviously true but it is easier said than done. The pyramidal tract was suggested by Dr Creutzfeldt as a source of orders linked to movement and perhaps to such transformations. Unfortunately it has been shown that it is possible to change pyramidal tract firing without influence on skilled motor behaviour. So even when you seem to be deep in the system, with beautifully locked correlations, you can frequently disturb them and destroy the correlation. More interestingly, the sensory systems which provide input for these maps obviously have the necessary cells for transporting information from the detectors into the brain. Every single sensory cell is under enormously powerful descending control. This is not at all an automatic transmission device but one in which the brain is itself somehow deciding which sensory world it wishes to live in. This comes towards your point of the active ordered brain. The sensory brain is active not only in terms of what action is impending but of what it needs to know in order to carry out the action.

Young: And of what it wants to know in the light of its past experience.

Searle: Otto Creutzfeldt made the extremely strong claim that the problem of the unity of the mappings, the problem of the unity of the experience, is solved or explained by an agency which engages in symbolic action. But I don't see the neurophysiological basis for showing how that solves the problem. It appears to be inconsistent with Colwyn Trevarthen's view that the question of the unity of our experience is morphogenetic.

Trevarthen: Yes, I feel it is a great pity that no one here has talked about embryological causality If we are talking about phenomena in the universe the brain is ontogenetically unique. The brain is the only organ in the human body that has unfinished embryogenesis. According to the anatomists it goes on differentiating and changing until it collapses, and even then it has not finished. Yet at all stages it has a morphogenetically created unity of organization.

Searle: So we have two rival neurophysiological answers to one of the oldest questions in philosophy. I hope we will come back to that.

Delgado: I have three questions about the basis of consciousness. First, do we accept consciousness as an intrinsic property of the brain in the same way as, say, oxygen consumption? Secondly, is consciousness really innate, that is determined exclusively by genetic factors that will appear only through maturation? Thirdly, could consciousness (a) originate and (b) be maintained in the absence of external or internal sensory inputs? My own answers would be 'no' to each of the three questions. I think that consciousness is a dynamic phenomenon related to transaction of information through the neurons. The brain, by itself, is not enough to maintain consciousness. When we discuss anatomy we are only considering the supporting mechanisms, without really dealing with consciousness itself. In my opinion, consciousness may be described as the outside world going through the inside framework of the brain. In the absence of either element, consciousness is not possible.

Creutzfeldt: I may have been misunderstood on some points and I shall try to clarify them. In response to Pat Wall, I thought I had specifically stated that neither the somatotopic maps nor their functional transformations in the neocortex explain the unity of consciousness, and I fully agree with you in this respect. This does not exclude the possibility that cortical mechanisms as yet unknown exist for this purpose. But what we know is that the unification is accomplished in organized action. This 'agent' is not contradictory to a morphogenetic concept, since action programs also have a morphological basis. This action, I also said, does not explain consciousness either. It is for this very reason that I introduced the additional mechanism of the external loop of symbolical self-representation. Here, I agree with David Armstrong about introspection proper. What I do not understand is how materialists as they understand themselves can say anything about the reality of our mental and spiritual world. They can't. I personally believe in the *reality* of what can be said only in poetry and music, and in aesthetic values like beauty.

Bunge: So do we!

Creutzfeldt: But the materialistic view hasn't explained these things.

Bunge: Nor have you. Now you say they cannot be explained, which is worse.

Creutzfeldt: I am saying that they cannot be explained in materialistic terms.

Trevarthen: No organism has any existence outside its own kind of environment. In evolution reciprocal relationships must exist between organism and environment, habit and habitat. I never used the word genes or genetic factors, by the way. One of the problems in talking here about mechanisms of poetry, music, moral sense and so forth, is that there are not enough psychologists at this meeting. The philosophers may have a right to talk about everything, but psychologists have a way of looking at these things systematically which is different from the viewpoint of a neurobiologist. Babies, it seems to me, have a fairly comprehensive though little differentiated outline of what it would require to be human in a complete sense, including humour, poetry and so on. In the second year of life infants have a delight in fantasy play. We have to try to understand innateness for such things in the proper biological sense of being actively there at birth or built into the life history. To say they are genetically determined adds not clarity but obscurity. That is quite a different level of structural analysis.

References

1. ZAIDEL, E. (1977) Auditory language comprehension in the right hemisphere following cerebral commissurotomy and hemispherectomy: a comparison with child language and aphasia, in *Language Acquisition and Language Breakdown: Parallels and Divergences* (Caramazzo, A. & Zurif, E. B., eds.), pp. 229–275, Johns Hopkins, Baltimore
2. LEVY, J. & TREVARTHEN, C. (1977) Perceptual, semantic and phonetic aspects of elementary language processes in split-brain patients. *Brain 100*, 105–118
3. HALLIDAY, M. A. K. (1978) Meaning and the construction of reality in early childhood, in *Modes of Perceiving and Processing Information* (Pick, H. & Saltzmann, E., eds.), Erlbaum, Hillsdale, N.J./distributed by Halsted [Wiley], New York
4. VON NEUMANN, J. (1951) in *Hixon Symposium on Cerebral Mechanisms in Behaviour* (Jeffres, L. A., ed.), pp. 23–24, Hafner Publishing, New York (2nd printing 1967)

Clinical, physiological and philosophical implications of innovative brain surgery in humans

IRVING S. COOPER

Center for Physiologic Neurosurgery, Westchester County Medical Center, New York Medical College, Valhalla, NY

Abstract Abnormal states of motor behaviour can be reversed by interruption of facilitating mechanisms and augmentation of inhibitory mechanisms. Similarly, psychological and emotional behaviours which were abnormal due to disinhibition, such as screaming, repetitive speech and aggressive violent behaviour, have been favourably affected from a clinical and sociological standpoint.

The mechanisms of the facilitatory and inhibitory systems which modulate motor behaviour also modify psychological and emotional behaviour. The findings of our studies in experimental neurosurgery may help to provide new insights into mechanisms of mental capacity and behaviour.

During the past twenty-five years I have been engaged in an investigation of the neurosurgical treatment of involuntary movement disorders in human beings. This ongoing study has involved the introduction of both surgical methods and hypotheses which could be tested and utilized therapeutically only in a long-range programme of experimental surgery in humans. It is the purpose of this report to summarize the principal observations of this study up to the present. Based on these observations, I shall present some conclusions and generalizations which pertain not only to our understanding of movement and its disorders but which also embody implications of physiological mechanisms contributing to mental function and behaviour.

It is my concept that involuntary movement disorders are motor manifestations of disorders of sensory communications. The basic abnormality underlying involuntary movements and abnormal postures of neurological origin is essentially an abnormality in data processing in the central nervous system which affects mechanisms responsible for control of muscle length. This is ultimately a function of the complex reflex arc of the spinal cord. However, the role of the motor neuron as the final common pathway is defined

255

by the processing of sensory data by virtually the entire central nervous system. The principal pathways and systems involved are illustrated in Fig. 1.

The principal afferent pathways carrying sensory information from muscle ascend to the cerebellum via dorsal and ventral spinocerebellar and spino-olivary tracts. From the cerebellar cortex all outflow is via Purkinje cells and is entirely inhibitory. Cerebello-fugal sensory data are carried upstream

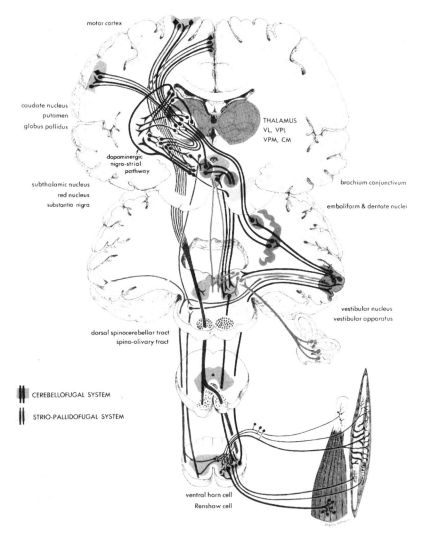

FIG. 1. Diagram of the major pathways of the basal ganglia showing the two principal systems of modulating motor cortex activity. (From Cooper.[2])

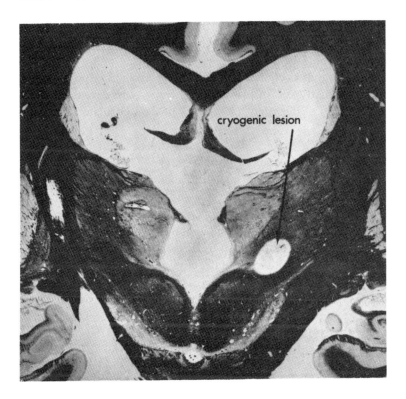

FIG. 2. Cryogenic lesion in ventrolateral nucleus of thalamus. The lesion interrupts abnormal sensory data from cerebellum and basal ganglia. (From Cooper[2].)

via the brachium conjunctivum to the thalamus and caudate, or downstream via the fastigial nucleus to the brain-stem and thence via vestibulospinal and reticulospinal pathways into the spinal cord. The classical basal ganglia system which receives sensory information via the caudate nucleus from the entire cerebral cortex passes these data through the pallidofugal pathway to the thalamus, where pallidofugal and cerebellofugal pathways terminate and overlap.

Our studies demonstrated that a lesion of the posterior half of the ventrolateral nucleus of the thalamus (Fig. 2), which prevents abnormal sensory information from the cerebellar and basal ganglia systems from reaching the cerebral cortex, can consistently abolish Parkinsonian tremor and rigidity without inflicting neurological, intellectual or psychological abnormalities upon the individual.[1,2] This conclusion was contrary to the reports of Bucy[3] and others that abolition of tremor required sacrifice of motor power, and to the report of Hassler[4] that motor weakness and/or psychological abnormalities accompanied complete relief of tremor. If this were the case, the pathological mechanism would have to involve motor rather than sensory systems. Thus the fact that tremor could be abolished without sacrificing motor power had basic physiological as well as clinical implications. Principles of physiological surgery essential to this type of neurosurgical therapy were developed which facilitated confirmation of the safety and efficacy of the ventrolateral thalamic lesion.

These principles, which enabled us to extend experimental techniques of physiological neurosurgery to other syndromes, are:

(1) The patient must be awake and cooperative during the procedure.

(2) The operation must, therefore, be rapid so that the patient can tolerate the procedure while remaining alert and cooperative for psychological, physical and physiological testing while the thalamic lesion is being created.

(3) Lesion creation should be preceded by a reversible functional inhibition of the target zone or some other absolute physiological verification of the correct lesion site for that particular patient. The clinical result is determined not only by the surgical lesion and specific symptoms, but also by the degree of physiological ageing of the brain, the presence or absence of widespread brain disease and individual anatomical and physiological variations. Flexibility of judgement and technique is essential in each instance.

(4) The lesion should be induced incrementally to increase both the safety and the efficacy of the procedure.

The fact that this relatively large lesion can be placed in a major intracerebral structure without observable abnormal neurological or psychological behavioural changes must affect our concept of how the thalamus functions. Since the thalamus is a major information processor of the brain, and since we cannot yet define the mechanisms which compensate for this lesion, new questions are raised concerning integrated actions of the brain, and many previous conceptions must be reconsidered.

Further studies demonstrated that familial tremors, the postural and intention tremor of multiple sclerosis, the flapping movements of Wilson's disease, the purposeless movements of chorea, and the violent limb-flinging movements of hemiballismus could, in most properly selected patients, be alleviated by thalamic surgery (Figs. 3A, B).

Virtually the same lesion can reverse severe incapacitating dystonic syndromes, which are characterized by simultaneous contraction of antagonistic muscles (Figs. 4 and 5). Consideration of the syndrome of dystonia musculorum deformans[5,6,7] is particularly germane to the subject of this symposium. One group of patients suffering this genetically induced malady demonstrate a measurably significant intellectual superiority compared with control subjects of the same age and cultural background. Many children with this syndrome have been subjected to two to six thalamic operations, with maintenance of their intellectual capacity. Most have pursued higher education, some to the

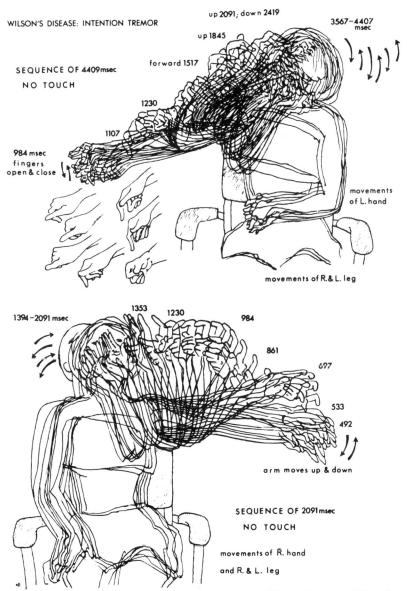

FIG. 3. A: Serial tracings from cinematographic record illustrating severe bilateral intention tremor during finger-to-nose test. (From Cooper.[2])

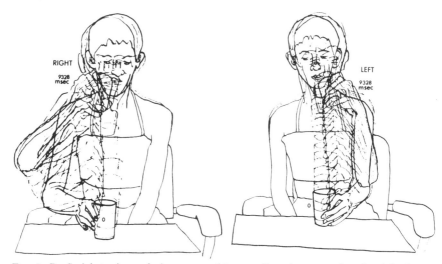

FIG. 3. B: Serial tracings of cinematographic recording three months after left chemo-thalamectomy. (From Cooper.[2])

doctoral level, despite multiple surgical interventions in the thalamus. The same multiple procedures might have produced at least temporary confusion, intellectual fall-off and memory deficits in elderly patients or those in whom cerebral cortical atrophy or early organic mental disease was present. The

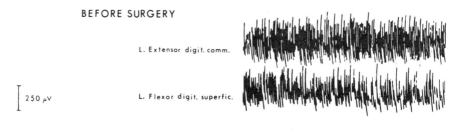

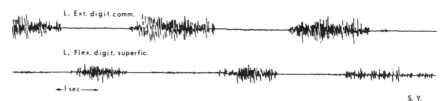

FIG. 4. Electromyogram in a dystonic limb before and after cryothalamectomy. (From Cooper.[2])

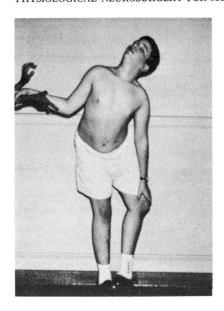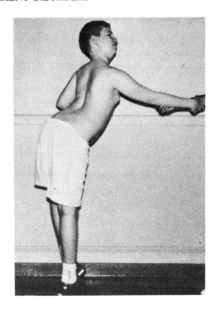

Fig. 5. A: Photographs demonstrating preoperative status.

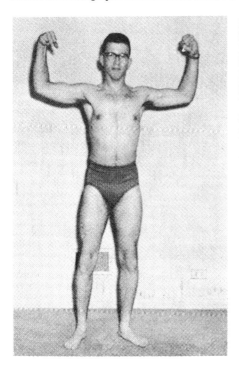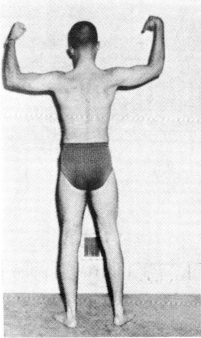

Fig. 5. B: Photographs of same patient as in A, ten years after bilateral chemothalamectomy. (From Cooper.[2])

role of the thalamus in mental processes and behaviour is variable and this variability is dependent upon the overall condition and conditioning of the particular individual brain in question.

We have learnt that a lesion of the pulvinar, the largest and phylogenetically most recently developed nucleus of the thalamus (Fig. 6), may sometimes have a profound effect on dystonic–spastic syndromes. The pulvinar is a poly-sensory structure. Although the results of pulvinar surgery at first appeared to us to be capricious, a pattern is emerging which is exemplified by the case report given below. This case is presented because of its relevance to our inquiry into mental capacity and behaviour.

D.M., a 43-year-old female, suffered a severe hemiplegic dystonia as a result

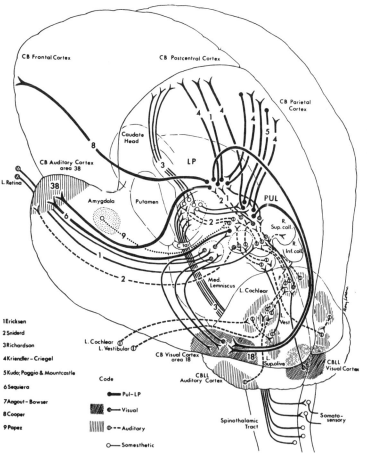

FIG. 6. Diagram showing the neuroanatomical connections of the pulvinar (PUL). (From Cooper et al.[9])

of embolic infarction of the midbrain. The fixed posture of her left arm and hand and of her left leg and foot was so severe that no voluntary motion was possible (Fig. 7A). Moreover, passive movement of the limbs was also virtually impossible because of the extreme muscular contractions. Surgery of the dentate nucleus, ventrolateral nucleus of the thalamus and pulvinar alleviated these dystonic manifestations, so that the patient regained useful voluntary motion of the left limbs, with abolition of the severe fixed dystonic deformity of the left foot and ankle (Fig. 7B).

Before the neurosurgical procedure there was also a marked behavioural abnormality manifested by screaming, high-pitched, repetitive speech. For example, when someone entered the patient's room, she would invariably scream, 'Know you./Know you./Know you'. When asked her name she would scream it over and over, but could not reply to more complex questions. After the third operation, at which time a lesion was placed in the right pulvinar, speech immediately became almost normal, as demonstrated by pre- and postoperative recordings of her speech. When the patient was asked why

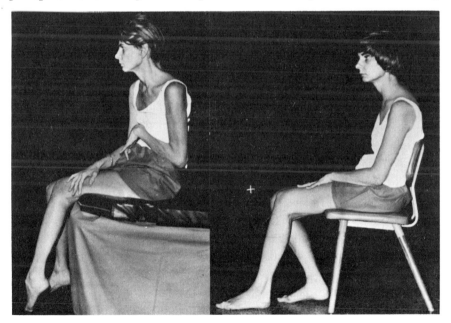

A   B

FIG. 7   A: Hemiplegic dystonia after a cerebrovascular accident involving the midbrain. Clinically, the patient appeared as though she had a spastic hemiplegia.
B: Reversal of dystonia, including the severe postural abnormalities of the hand and foot, after destruction of the ipsilateral dentate nucleus, and placement of cryogenic lesions in the contralateral ventrolateral nucleus of the thalamus and pulvinar. (From Cooper.[2])

she had been screaming repetitively previously, she replied that she had been unable to stop it—it had just run away once she initiated it. The patient was actually saying that her speech, similarly to her contracted muscles, had been disinhibited.

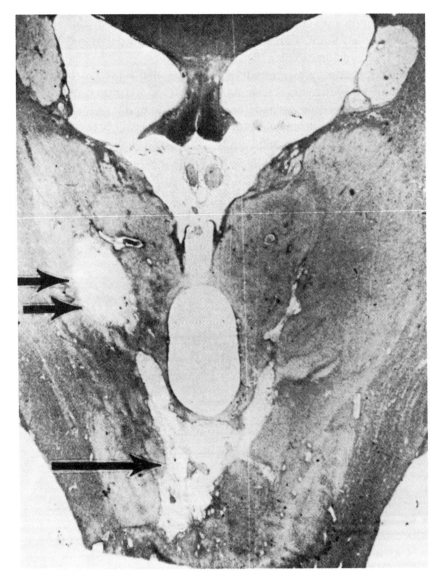

FIG. 8. Infarct of midbrain in patient D.M. indicated by single arrow. Double arrow indicates cryogenic thalamic lesion. (From Cooper.[6])

The severe fixed postures, simulating a total spastic hemiplegia, were abolished in D.M. to the extent that she became ambulatory, independent and capable of maintaining a household for 18 months, at which time she died as a result of acute bacterial endocarditis.

The pathological and surgical lesions can be summarized. Her dystonic hemiplegia, so severe as to result in total abolition of movement, was caused by a rather circumscribed lesion of the midbrain (Fig. 8), involving the red nucleus and reticular substance, but completely sparing the cerebral peduncle. Destruction of the left dentate nucleus of the cerebellum resulted in a temporary decrease of muscular hypertonia, with a full recurrence of symptoms within two weeks. A cryogenic lesion of the ventrolateral nucleus of the right thalamus abolished the tremor (3/second) of the left upper and lower limbs. The fixed posture of the left foot and ankle, however, remained unchanged. A cryogenic lesion of the right pulvinar resulted in an instantaneous restoration of useful voluntary motor function of the left extremities. By the fifth postoperative week, the severe fixed posture of the left foot and ankle was totally reversed.

The fact that a circumscribed lesion of reticular substance of the red nucleus could result in a totally incapacitating dystonic hemiplegia, as well as speech and behavioural abnormalities, is noteworthy. The additional fact that super-imposition of lesions of the left dentate nucleus of the cerebellum, the ventro-lateral nucleus of the right thalamus and the right pulvinar progressively contributed to a reversal of dystonia in this patient emphasizes the complexity of dystonia and of compensatory brain mechanisms in each individual patient. In patient D.M. intellectual function, speech, and behaviour were also markedly improved after the pulvinar lesion.

During the past five years of this study, we have also investigated the possibility of prosthetically mobilizing mechanisms which are primarily inhi-bitory in nature to modify various disorders of disinhibition. The technique used has been chronic stimulation of cerebellar cortex by platinum electrodes placed on the surface of the anterior and posterior lobes of the cerebellum. The electrodes are activated from an external power source using a radio frequency stimulus via transcutaneous induction.

Fig. 9 summarizes the clinical neurophysiological effects of chronic cerebellar stimulation in humans. This procedure inhibits somatosensory and visual cortical evoked responses. Responses attributable to thalamic structures are reduced in amplitude, while midbrain reticular responses, presumably repres-enting inhibitory reticular substance, are often increased. At the spinal cord level H reflexes as well as V_1 and V_2 reflexes are usually depressed. In some epileptic patients there is a statistically significant reduction in the number and duration of paroxysmal discharges recorded by the electroencephalograph,

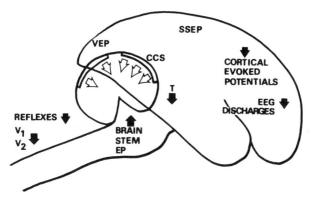

Fig. 9. Diagnostic illustration of neurophysiological effects of cerebellar cortex stimulation in humans. Spinal reflexes and evoked potentials in thalamus and cerebral cortex are inhibited. Inhibiting reticular substance of midbrain is facilitated. (From Cooper & Upton.[8])

with rebound exacerbation of these discharges when the stimulation is interrupted.[8]

Favourable clinical responses to this technique of prosthetic augmentation of inhibitory mechanisms have been reported in the treatment of spasticity of cerebral palsy, intractable epilepsy and the aggressive behaviour of some epileptic syndromes and violent behaviour in schizophrenia. No adverse neurological, psychological or intellectual effects have occurred in about 1000 reported cases of chronic cerebellar stimulation.

References

1. COOPER, I. S. (1953) Surgical occlusion of the anterior choroidal artery in parkinsonism. *Psychiatr. Q. 27*, 317–319
2. COOPER, I. S. (1968) *Involuntary Movement Disorders*, Harper & Row, New York
3. BUCY, P. C. & CASE, J. T. (1939) Surgical relief of tremor at rest. *Arch. Neurol. Psychiatr. 41*, 721–726
4. HASSLER, R. (1955) Pathological basis of tremor and Parkinsonism, in *2nd Int. Congr. Neuropathol., London, 1955*, I.C.S. No. 7, p. 769 (abstr.), Excerpta Medica, Amsterdam
5. COOPER, I. S., CULLINAN, T. & RIKLAN, M. (1976) The natural history of dystonia. *Adv. Neurol. 14*, 157–169
6. COOPER, I. S. (1976) Dystonia: surgical approaches to treatment and physiologic implications, in *The Basal Ganglia* (Yahr, M. D., ed.), pp. 369–383, Raven Press, New York
7. COOPER, I. S. (1976) Twenty year followup study of the neurosurgical treatment of dystonia musculorum deformans. *Adv. Neurol. 14*, 423–452
8. COOPER, I. S. & UPTON, A. R. M. (1978) Use of chronic cerebellar stimulation for disorders of disinhibition. *Lancet 1*, 595–599
9. COOPER, I. S., RIKLAN, M. & RAKIC, P. (1974) *The Pulvinar-LP Complex*, Thomas, Springfield, Ill.

Outcome from severe neurological illness; should it influence medical decisions?

FRED PLUM and DAVID E. LEVY

Department of Neurology, New York Hospital–Cornell Medical Center, New York, NY

Abstract Most persons now accept the concept that when brain is dead, self is dead, and are willing to act accordingly. Much more difficult is to decide what to do when illness irreparably deprives the brain of cognitive functions. To facilitate less impassioned discussion of this question, 500 consecutive patients in coma from non-traumatic causes have been studied in the USA and Europe and the outcome has been compared against carefully selected early neurological signs. Medical coma was itself a dangerous sign, with only 15% of patients recovering independence within the first month. Within the first six hours, when most medical decisions are made about applying intensive care, neurological signs predicted with 95% confidence between the extremes of favourable and unfavourable outcomes in as many as a quarter of the patients. Only 5% of patients who failed to regain cognition by the end of one week regained any independence. Other more detailed guidelines were equally informative. If prognostic signs that confidently separate potentially favourable from unfavourable outcomes can be identified in severe neurological illness, perhaps society can more easily help medicine in reaching difficult ethical decisions.

Among educated Western people one nowadays finds essentially no major dissent from the view that mind and brain are one, the question being not whether but how the identity is generated. As a corollary, almost all agree that brain and self are united, so that if, by some miracle of surgery, this skull-encased 1.5 kilograms of jellified fat and protein could be moved from one body to another and correctly wired in, the brain would regard its 'self' as having a body transplant rather than the other way around.

Acceptance of the brain–self identity, once it was pointed out, has meant that most people also rapidly accepted the concept that when the brain is dead, *we* are dead, no matter how much vitality may endure in our peripheral organs.[1] The result is that in the face of unequivocal brain death, only occasional controversies or resistances surround the practice of salvaging viable organs which can be transplanted so that others may live, after which support of the donor's heart and lungs may be discontinued.

But the diagnosis of brain death and the medical decisions that follow upon it are relatively easy ethical matters. It is much more difficult for both doctors and lay people to come to terms with what one should do when, in the course of severe illness or injury, the brain, although not dead, becomes irreparably deprived of its cognitive functions. Most of us would undoubtedly like to die with our boots on and we find it abhorrent to anticipate some illness or injury that would force upon us prolonged survival deprived of mind, speech and movement. Yet such vegetative or severely disabled survivals do occur, and reports in the medical and public press suggest that their frequency is increasing.

Advances in emergency resuscitation and intensive care give critically ill patients improved chances for recovery yet concurrently increase the risk that some will be spared only to undergo indefinite survival with hopelessly damaged brains. The wide differences in potential outcome from what begins as humane, even heroic, medical efforts have stimulated extensive discussion and debate. People concerned with maintaining and delivering resources for health care fear the impact that disabled survivors of new and expensive medical treatments may have on the 'medical commons'—the necessarily limited public economic preserve of any community on which the total requirements of health and welfare must feed.[2] By contrast, many practising physicians see their primary obligations to the patient as requiring that they apply every possible treatment until death or recovery decides the issue; any concern for public considerations is beside the point. The resulting tension in views has generated considerable debate, some highly emotional in tone, over how much care to initiate for patients with severe brain damage and how long to continue it.

But in medicine, as in many other things, the most strident differences of opinion centre on issues where a minimum number of well-documented facts intrude upon the argument. Whenever we have discussed the care of the severely brain-injured with either colleagues or lay people, it has quickly become clear that strongly opposing opinions about how much acute care to provide more often reflect a lack of knowledge of what to expect than any necessarily deep divisions in personal philosophy. Many, perhaps most, people agreed that excessively active medical efforts that doomed the bodies of physically helpless and badly demented patients to prolonged, mindless survival were inhumane and medically unethical. But nearly all to whom we spoke raised the questions, 'How do you know? How can you predict early enough during illness who will do well and who badly? Isn't it playing God to make life and death decisions when you might make a mistake and overlook someone who could recover, given the proper, extraordinary treatment?' Appropriate answers to these difficult points could only be found by seeking more and better information. If we know that specific medical findings can say, with a strong probability, who will recover and who will not, then society can decide how to act. Decisions about who shall live and who shall die cannot be left to doctors alone.

Although prognosis represents a classic cornerstone of medicine, it has rarely been elevated above art into the exactness of science. Physicians traditionally have taken the appearance of an altered state of consciousness in almost any illness as a 'grave sign'. Little or no evidence, however, has quantified its gravity, and until about a decade ago practically no evidence existed to indicate exactly *which* illnesses portended a favourable or unfavourable outcome. As such matters often do, the deficiencies on this important subject struck more than one mind at about the same time. A chance discussion in 1970 between Bryan Jennett, Professor of Neurosurgery at Glasgow, and one of us (Plum) brought out that Jennett had been struck by the same uncertainty about precisely what would happen to patients with head injury as had troubled us in trying to make prognoses for patients with non-traumatic coma. In characteristically effective and energetic fashion, Jennett had begun collecting quantitative information on the subject in 1968, somewhat before the Cornell group started plotting early clinical findings against neurological outcome in patients with cardiac arrest at New York Hospital. Our first discussions with Jennett led to many more and eventually, with still other investigators, we entered into collaboration to study prospectively patients in seven different medical centres in three countries. Information about patients unconscious after head injury was obtained in neurosurgical and neurological centres in Glasgow, Rotterdam, Groningen and Los Angeles, while observations on patients with non-traumatic coma came from The New York Hospital, the Royal Victoria Infirmary, Newcastle upon Tyne, and later the San Francisco General Hospital.* The clinical data from all the patients were stored in a computer and analysed by statisticians and computer experts at Glasgow and, now, New York.

The neurosurgeons have already completed observations on over 1000 patients with severe head injuries and have published several papers describing

---

*The principal individuals concerned in the trauma studies were B. Jennett, G. Teasdale and M. Bond in Glasgow, J. Minderhoud and R. Braakman in the Netherlands, and T. Kurze in Los Angeles. Our medical colleagues have been Drs David Shaw, Nial Cartlidge and David Bates in Newcastle, and John Caronna in San Francisco. Dr Robin Knill-Jones has provided the main assistance in the statistical analyses.

their results.[3,4] Without going into details, one can say that the correlation between early clinical signs and outcome is remarkably similar among the different neurosurgical centres, despite some substantial differences in approaches to laboratory diagnosis and management. Furthermore, at least in broad terms, it looks as though many of the indicators that can predict outcome from head injury are similar or identical to those that foretell the future course of patients in coma from non-traumatic disease. As might be expected, however, patients with medical illness are older and have a higher incidence of medical complications, which means that as a total group they have a lower overall survival rate than do the younger group of subjects with head injury. Since our own studies have focused on the patients with non-traumatic coma, the rest of this discussion will concentrate on those results.

Certain major questions defined our purposes:

(1) What was the natural history of coma in medical illness as treated by the best available methods?

(2) Could one identify, on the basis of early clinical or laboratory findings, those patients most likely to survive? If so, did any specific findings predict the quality of survival, and how accurately?

(3) Could one identify signs or findings during the early hours of coma which indicated little chance of cognitive survival? If so, in what percentage of patients and with what kind of accuracy?

(4) In any given illness, did early clinical changes predict a specific outcome sufficiently accurately to provide a benchmark of natural history against which the effects of future therapy could be measured?

(5) By quantifying information that influenced ethical decisions, did those decisions become easier to make?

So far we have studied 500 patients with non-traumatic coma admitted between September 1973 and June 1977 (225 patients at the Royal Victoria Infirmary, Newcastle, 208 at The New York Hospital, and 67 at the San Francisco General Hospital). All patients underwent full medical and neurological clinical examination. Coma was defined in strict terms (Table 1). The neurological profile consisted of previously described and reproducible signs of forebrain and brain-stem dysfunction.[5] These signs included verbal responses, eye opening, pupillary size and reaction to light, spontaneous eye movements, oculocephalic (doll's eyes) and oculovestibular (caloric) responses, corneal responses, extremity motor responses, deep tendon reflexes, skeletal muscle tone, and respiratory pattern. Demographic and laboratory data were also encoded. A five-point scale of functional outcome was used in assessing the potential for neurological recovery; this included *no recovery* (persistent coma or death without awakening), *the vegetative state* (Table 1), *severe*

TABLE 1

Definitions

Coma: A sleep-like state of eyes-closed, unarousable unresponsiveness, without evident psychological awareness of self or environment.

Vegetative state: A state of being awake but not aware. The eyes open spontaneously or in response to auditory stimuli and sleep–wake cycles exist. Subjects utter no comprehensible words and obey no commands. Autonomic functions (temperature, blood pressure, gastrointestinal function, breathing, etc.) remain intact.

Locked-in state: Wakeful awareness of self and environment remain but paralysis of speech and limbs prevents communication except by eye movement.

---

disability (conscious but dependent), *moderate disability* (independent but disabled), and *good recovery* (return to previous function).[6,7]   The clinical examination was performed at admission to the study and daily thereafter, and the best responses were encoded at the following times: at admission, 24 hours, one to three days, four to seven days, eight to fourteen days, and fifteen to twenty-eight days. The cause of coma was determined on the basis of all available clinical and laboratory information including, when done, the results of post-mortem examination. Of the 500 patients, 210 had diffuse hypoxia–ischaemia, mostly from cardiac arrest, 143 had focal cerebral vascular disease, 38 had subarachnoid haemorrhage, 51 had hepatic coma, and 58 had miscellaneous other, mostly metabolic, disorders. Patients with drug or alcohol poisoning were excluded because it is already known that they do well with proper therapy. Outcome was assessed at the end of one, three, six and twelve months; in addition, the best outcome achieved between each of these observations was recorded. Preliminary results have appeared elsewhere.[8] Results given in the following paragraphs describe the best level of recovery achieved within the first month.

Recovery from coma was determined by at least two major factors. One was the extent of the initial neurological damage as reflected by clinical signs of dysfunction, and the other was the nature of the disease process causing these signs. Recovery was apparently not influenced by age or sex, by the geographical origin of the patients, or by the general approach to their treatment. Table 2 gives the specific best outcomes of patients in the various diagnostic categories. (Best outcome, which reflects *capacity* for neurological recovery, was better than actual outcome, which reflects the patients' total medical problem, including complications and recurrences.) Most patients (61%) remained in coma and died; of the remainder, about one-third (12%) improved only to the vegetative state, and another 12% were left severely

TABLE 2

Outcome from coma in 500 patients

Cause of coma[a]	Best 1-month outcome (%)				
	NR	VS	SD	MD	GR
Hypoxic–ischaemia (210)	68	20	11	3	8
Focal cerebrovascular disease (143)	74	7	11	4	4
Subarachnoid haemorrhage (38)	74	5	13	5	3
Hepatic encephalopathy (51)	49	2	16	10	23
Miscellaneous (58)	45	10	14	5	26

[a]No. of patients given in parentheses.
NR: no recovery; VS: vegetative state; SD: severe disability; MD: moderate disability; GR: good recovery.

disabled. Even after one month, the serious nature of the underlying illnesses was apparent, so that total mortality by the end of a month was 75%. Fully independent activity was achieved by only 8% of patients with stroke and subarachnoid haemorrhage, by about 11% of those with hypoxic ischaemia, and by about 32% of patients with hepatic and miscellaneous metabolic disorders.

In estimating the predictive value of individual clinical signs, we should emphasize that at this stage of our analysis only the most glaring associations

TABLE 3

Signs associated with poor outcome (less than half as good as group as a whole)

% Favourable outcome in entire series	Vascular 8%	Hypoxic–ischaemia 11%	Other 33%
Admission			
No motor response		+	
Pupils non-reactive		+	
Absent OV or OC reflex	+	+	+
Absent corneal response		+	
24 hours		Same plus	
Motor worse than withdrawal	+	+	+
No eye opening	+	+	
No verbal response	+	+	
Pupils non-reactive	+	+	+
Absent corneal response	+	+	+
3 days		Same plus	
No verbal	+	+	+

OV, OC: oculovestibular, oculocephalic.

TABLE 4

Cumulative favourable signs (twice as good as group as a whole)

% Favourable outcome in entire series	Vascular 8%	Hypoxic–ischaemia 11%	Other 33%
Admission			
Some oculovestibular response	+		
Roving spontaneous eye movement	+	+	
24 Hours	Same plus		
Motor of withdrawal or better		+	
Any eye opening	+	+	
Any verbal	+	+	
3 Days	Same plus		
Any verbal	+	+	+
Reactive pupils	+		
Any OV or OC	+		
Corneals present	+	+	

Note that since 33% of all patients with 'other' disorders had a good outcome, signs indicating twice that chance were hard to find when patients were still in coma.

stand out. We have not finished analysing either possible cross-correlations between the relative value of two independent signs or the predictive accuracy of certain combinations of signs taken together. Table 3 lists signs in various disease groups which were associated with an outcome less than half as favourable as that for the group as a whole, while Table 4 indicates early signs that were associated with an outcome twice as favourable as for the group as a whole. It will be noted that of 253 patients without spontaneous eye movements on admission, only 21 subsequently regained independence, and only 10 out of 162 patients with absent motor responses on admission achieved a similarly desirable recovery. The chances for regaining independent activity were even worse for patients with absent corneal responses (6 out of 144), absent oculovestibular responses (4 of 122), and absent pupillary reactions (2 of 134). No patients whose corneal reflexes were absent throughout the first day subsequently achieved as much as a moderate disability or good recovery. Furthermore, except for one patient with no pupillary reactions and another without spontaneous eye movements, no patients regained independent activity if they remained throughout the first three days without any of the five responses (spontaneous eye movements, motor responses, corneal responses, oculovestibular responses and pupillary reaction). Even though they had spontaneously opened their eyes, none of 25 patients with motor responses of withdrawal or worse at three days achieved eventual independence. In contrast to these unfavourable signs, 23 of the 57 patients who made any sounds at all on admission achieved independence later, as did 59 of the 277 who showed full tonic eye movements in response to head movement or caloric stimulation on admission. Of patients who within three days regained normal eye movements and normal motor responses, over half regained function either to the level of moderate disability or good recovery.

As noted, although recovery from coma was closely related to the severity of clinical signs, differences in outcome also depended on whether these signs were caused by metabolic or by structural diseases. Patients with hepatic and miscellaneous causes of coma had the greatest chances of regaining independence and they also enjoyed a consistently low frequency of unfavourable clinical signs. Similarly, absence of pupillary reactions and caloric responses were noted more commonly on admission in the patients with vascular disease who, as a group, had the worst prognosis. By contrast, however, comparison between the hypoxic–ischaemic group and the vascular group showed that although hypoxic–ischaemic patients showed absent motor responses twice as often as the vascular group, and included nearly 50% more subjects without spontaneous eye movement, they had a somewhat better overall prognosis.

Individual signs strongly associated ($P < 0.01$) with outcome from coma emerged most often in hypoxic–ischaemic patients. Fifty-two hypoxic–ischaemic patients had no pupillary reactions on admission, and none regained independent activity. Only 4% of hypoxic–ischaemic patients who had no motor responses on admission regained independence, whereas the presence of any movement at all increased the future likelihood of independent activity to 18%. Among hypoxic–ischaemic patients who had no spontaneous eye movements on admission, only 7% recovered independence, whereas a full 30% of those with roving conjugate eye movements on admission recovered independent activity.

Accurate analysis of data from a large clinically changing population presents considerable difficulties and pitfalls even when computer assistance is available. We will need time to digest and interpret all our findings. To draw conclusions prematurely would be irresponsible and potentially dangerous. The above results, however, already indicate that in as many as 25% of patients with certain diseases one can predict with a confidence of better than 20:1 between the extremes of favourable and unfavourable outcomes within six hours of the time of onset of coma. Furthermore, the figures indicate that if patients regained no cognitive function by the end of one week, none recovered fully and only 5% achieved any independence at all. Although limited, these numbers may begin to provide the kind of information that physicians and families seek to guide their actions during the critical period of acute care after severe brain illness.

The most terrifying prospect in severe brain injury is that the patient will be left either in a 'locked-in' state or to undergo a chronic vegetative existence (Table 1). Locked-in patients suffer a selective injury to descending motor pathways in the lower brain-stem, with the lesion sparing other parts of the brain as well as the more dorsally placed reticular grey matter of the brain-stem itself.[9] Most such lesions are the consequence of irreversible strokes. The result is a person condemned to live with paralysis of the muscles of speech and of all four limbs but apparently capable of self-aware thinking, and of retaining peripheral and special sensory stimuli, including vision and hearing. Fortunately, the disorder is rare, but once it occurs with vascular lesions it usually remains until death, which may not occur for weeks or months if the care is 'too good.' Recognition is possible early and doctors should act accordingly.

The persistent or chronic vegetative state functionally reflects a total loss of cognitive activities of the cerebral hemispheres combined with retention of the primitive and autonomic functions that emanate from the hypothalamus and the brain-stem (Table 1). Primitive sleep–wake functions are governed by brain-stem mechanisms, and since mere survival requires that most of the brain-stem be preserved, sleep–wake cycles return within a few days or weeks to almost all patients in coma. (The only exceptions here are a few permanently asleep patients with restricted lesions of the posterior hypothalamus.) Once unconscious patients open their eyes, they can no longer be considered in coma, creating the operational definition of vegetative existence as one in which none but autonomic functions proceed in normal fashion. The unfortunate Karen Quinlan, whose illness received so much public attention, is a typical example of a chronic vegetative patient.[10]

Vegetative states that last as long as a month nearly always follow cardiac arrests, stroke or severe head trauma and represent about 5% of the coma population. As can be imagined, the longer the physician waits after the onset of severe brain damage to make the decision not to treat vigorously, the more difficult that decision becomes to carry out. Unfortunately, in the persistent vegetative state, we have been unable thus far to identify with any confidence either single signs or combinations of signs that would accurately predict such an outcome soon after the onset of coma. Among patients who were vegetative or in coma at one week, 57% never improved beyond that point, but that is a confidence level far too low to guide early management. At one month, however, the future course became clearly defined. Among 25 survivors who were vegetative at one month, not a single one ever followed commands or regained even a measure of independence. Higashi et al.[11] report a similarly poor outcome among patients vegetative at one month. But at 30 days the sometimes merciful ravages of intercurrent infection and other complications have generally passed; for most physicians, allowing such patients to die by withholding care is an extremely difficult task.

Thoughtful persons are increasingly aware that the meaning in their lives is directly proportional to the functional capacities of their brains. We live at a time when extraordinary advances in preventive and applied medicine have stretched the lifespan, both in years and in resistance to particular illnesses that would once have been fatal. No one wishes to abandon these advances, or the days of pleasure they bring to most persons, but few discussions thus far have addressed themselves rigorously to the problems created by the growing number of badly brain-limited individuals who emerge as by-products of this century's revolution in medical care. This conference seems a suitable place for philosophy and science to begin jointly to examine the problem.

We recognize that our efforts to predict the outcome of coma at an early time, when medical decisions can be made less emotionally than during later convalescence, are just a beginning and leave many questions still unanswered. Nevertheless, the initial results begin to provide a baseline against which the possible effects of future therapy can be measured. It is hoped that the results will also begin to answer questions about whether some critically ill patients are being prematurely denied the care they need, while others are being exposed to the indignity involved in valiantly resisting death only to survive with hopelessly damaged brains. If this goal is fulfilled, then perhaps the approach described here can serve as a model of how to generate accurate epidemiological facts about the outcome for the brain after severe illness, so that philosophers can then more dispassionately help doctors to consider the implications of their decisions.

ACKNOWLEDGEMENT

The research studies described herein were supported by the National Institutes of Health, contract NO1-NS-42328.

References

1. VEITH, F. J., FEIN, J. M., TENDLER, M. M., VEATCH, R. M., KLEIMAN, M. A. & KALKINES, G. (1977) Brain death. *J. Am. Med. Assoc. 238*, 1651–1655, 1744–1748
2. HIATT, H. H. (1975) Protecting the medical commons: who is responsible? *N. Engl. J. Med. 293*, 235–238

3. JENNETT, B., TEASDALE, G., BRAAKMAN, R., MINDERHOUD, J. & KNILL-JONES, R. P. (1976) Predicting outcome in individual patients after severe head injury. *Lancet 1*, 1031–1034

4. JENNETT, B., TEASDALE, G., GALBRAITH, S., PICKARD, J., GRANT, H., BRAAKMAN, R., AVEZAAT, C., MAAS, A., MINDERHOUD, J., VECHT, C. J., HEIDEN, J., SEWALL, R. & KURZE, T. (1977) Severe head injuries in three countries. *J. Neurol. Neurosurg. Psychiatry 40*, 291–298

5. BATES, D., CARONNA, J. J., CARTLIDGE, N. E. F., KNILL-JONES, R. P., LEVY, D. E., SHAW, D. A. & PLUM, F. (1977) A prospective study of nontraumatic coma: methods and results in 310 patients. *Ann. Neurol. 2*, 211–220

6. JENNETT, B. & BOND, M. (1975) Assessment of outcome after severe brain damage: a practical scale. *Lancet 1*, 480–484

7. PLUM, F. & CARONNA, J. J. (1975) Can one predict outcome of medical coma, in *Outcome of Severe Damage to the Central Nervous System (Ciba Found. Symp. 34)*, pp. 121–139, Elsevier/Excerpta Medica/North-Holland, Amsterdam

8. LEVY, D. E., BATES, J. J., CARONNA, J. J., CARTLIDGE, N. E. F., KNILL-JONES, R. P., SHAW, D. A. & PLUM, F. (1978) Recovery from nontraumatic coma. *Ann. Neurol. 4*, 169

9. PLUM, F. & POSNER, J. B. (1980) *Diagnosis and Prognosis of Stupor and Coma*, 3rd edn., Davis, Philadelphia

10. BERESFORD, H. R. (1977) The Quinlan decision: problems and legislative alternatives. *Ann. Neurol. 2*, 74–81

11. HIGASHI, K., SAKATA, Y., HATANO, M., ABIKO, S., IHARA, K., KATAYAMA, S., WAKUTA, Y., OKAMUR, T., UEDA, H., ZENKE, M. & AOKI, H. (1977) Epidemiological studies on patients with a persistent vegetative state. *J. Neurol. Neurosurg. Psychiatry 40*, 876–885

Experimental surgery, and predictions of outcome from severe neurological illness: legal and ethical implications [Commentary]

CHARLES FRIED

Harvard Law School, Cambridge, Massachusetts

I am asked to discuss the ethical and legal implications of two very different papers. Professor Cooper offers some extraordinarily optimistic proposals regarding treatment for a number of previously intractable neurological illnesses. This treatment involves brain surgery of a type which would probably be regarded as experimental or innovative. I am, of course, in no position at all to comment on the validity of Professor Cooper's science. The ethical and legal issues which his thesis raises are common to any kind of experimental medicine: what hope of benefit justifies what risk of harm even with a fully informed, consenting patient? And where circumstances such as infancy or incapacity (including an incapacity arising from the very condition sought to be treated) preclude a reasonable approximation to informed consent, what ratio of risk to benefit justifies the surgeon in proceeding? Professor Cooper does not purport to enlighten us on these standard questions, as it was not part of his assignment to do so.

There are, perhaps, special problems regarding this kind of experimental medicine which Professor Cooper proposes. The recently completed work of the National Commission for the Protection of Human Subjects gave distinct attention to the subject of brain surgery. There have been a number of legal decisions and legislative forays dealing specifically with that kind of issue. I refer, of course, to the raging debate concerning psychosurgery.[1,2] To some extent that debate has proceeded on the erroneous assumption that psycho-surgery is radically different from all other experimental medical procedures. What is troublesome about psychosurgery is that:

the claims that are made for it are highly controversial;
the subjects are often incapable of giving an understanding consent, and

often particularly because of the very condition which is involved; that is, the disorders are disorders of cognition and volition, disorders which vitiate the individual's judgement in acceding to the operation;

many of the subjects are confined in penal or other institutions and their consent is further clouded by the fact that they are thought to be subject to undue pressures or an undue desire to be released from such institutions;

the effects of the procedure are grave and irreversible;

the procedure is intended to and is likely to affect behaviour and personality, and thus in a particularly disturbing way to suggest human intervention with the core of the self—a kind of intervention which makes many persons uneasy.

Of course, many forms of psychosurgery do not display all of these features, and many other kinds of intervention than psychosurgery do display them. For instance, certain kinds of drug therapies have all of these features, including the aspect of irreversibility. Incidentally, many treatments not directed to brain function at all may have all of these features, including the effect on personality and behaviour. Indeed, this is where one may quibble with the easy equation of mind and brain. I would suppose that certain interferences with sexual functioning, with movement or with sensory capacities would also have radical effects on behaviour, and therefore personality and therefore mind. Now Professor Cooper's techniques differ from some of the more drastic and well-publicized forms of psychosurgery in that they are directed at motor rather than at personality disorders. The National Commission defines psychosurgery as follows:

The term 'psychosurgery', as used in this report, means (except as stated below): brain surgery, implantation of electrodes, destruction or direct stimulation of brain tissue by any means (e.g., ultra-sound, laser beams), or the direct application of substances to the brain when any of these procedures is performed either (1) on normal brain tissue of a person, for the purpose of changing or controlling the behavior or emotions of such person, or (2) on diseased brain tissue of a person, if the primary purpose of performing the procedure is to control, change, or affect any behavioral or emotional disturbance of such person. Such term does not include (a) electric shock treatments, (b) surgery or other invasions of the brain designed to cure or ameliorate the effects of movement disorders (e.g., epilepsy, parkinsonism), and (c) excision of brain tumors. With respect to relief of pain, surgical or other invasions of the brain which interrupt the transmission of pain along sensory pathways are not within the definition of psychosurgery; however, when such procedures are designed to relieve the emotional response to pain (without affecting the sensation of pain) they fall within the definition of psychosurgery.[3]

Thus I assume that Professor Cooper's techniques are excluded from the strictures of those recommendations. Since the techniques are experimental, however, they do fall into the domain where scrutiny of institutional review boards is generally required in the United States. I say generally, because a surgeon not affiliated with a government-aided institution is free even of these strictures, and then falls into the residual regulation of the common law generally. And the common law requires only informed consent and reasonable care, as determined after the fact in a trial court.[4] Nevertheless it would be imprudent and I think unethical for any surgeon not to subject his experimental techniques voluntarily to some prior scrutiny. The history of medicine is full of tragedies caused by overzealous innovators with a good idea, which could not withstand searching enquiry from scientific colleagues.

Professor Cooper is lucky that his techniques do *not* fall under the special strictures of the National Commission, for what they propose in that domain is restrictive indeed, particularly as regards prisoners and institutionalized persons.[5] Some of this seems to me to be seriously overdone. I believe that prisoners are capable of giving informed consent to experimental procedures, and if the risk/benefit ratio is appropriate and that consent has been obtained, then it should be valid in this as in other areas without procedures so elaborate as to make the matter impracticable. To be sure, those with cognitive and judgemental disorders are not able to give such consent. But that is also true of a number of other more or less experimental therapies, and I see no reason to propose a separate, distinct regime in this domain. If experimental surgery offers some hope of relieving the distress (physical or psychological) of incarcerated or institutionalized individuals I would not wish to deprive them of the opportunity to experience that relief, any more than I would deprive such people of the relief they might expect from an experimental cancer therapy.

Professor Plum and Dr Levy raise a wholly different set of problems. They offer statistical methods for determining the prognosis in certain kinds of neurological illness—particularly injuries to the brain and other causes of coma. The legal and ethical issues which their analyses raise have to do with the measure of certainty which is required before certain steps may properly be taken or omitted. In this regard, the most significant recent development has been the growing acceptance of the so-called Harvard criteria of brain death as a criterion of death *tout court*. In many jurisdictions for many purposes a person who is brain-dead is dead.[6,7,8] If the brain death has been brought about through the wrongful act of another person, that person is liable for murder,[9] and if the organs are removed for transplant purposes from such a brain-dead person, the original perpetrator, not the surgeon, is thought of as the agent of that donor's death. What is significant about the so-called Harvard criteria is that they are virtually certain and inexorable. Persons who are brain-dead have *never* been known to regain consciousness. Indeed, not only are the probabilities for an amelioration of this state non-existent when the Harvard criteria are met, but the end-point itself, the conditions to which the criteria apply, are drastic: a total absence of all mental functions and a flat EEG.

When, however, the end-point is less drastic—from the still extreme situation of the vegetative state, as in Karen Quinlan in whom only certain automatic responses are present, through the mysteries of the locked-in syndrome, to the much more mild end-point of impaired mental functioning and consciousness —the relevance of the Plum–Levy statistics becomes much more problematic. When people are brain-dead we may treat them as dead. But what may we do when a person is in an irreversible (with a certainty approaching one) vegetative state? May we remove that person's heart, liver, kidney, etc., for purposes of transplant? The law has certainly not moved anywhere near that proposition. The most one can say is that the absence of any hope for sapient existence, for consciousness, makes it appropriate to withhold certain life-sustaining measures, allowing the natural processes to take their course. The Supreme Court of the State of New Jersey in reaching this decision in the *Quinlan* case did so on an interpretation of the presumed wishes of the patient herself.[10,11,12] The action was not authorized on the grounds that to sustain the life of a person in that condition was wasteful of scarce resources. Perhaps the same reasoning would apply to the 'locked-in' syndrome, but there are subtle differences. After all, can we be sure that all modes of communication have been exhausted, and that therefore we may guess that the patient would desire life support to be terminated? And as the end-points become less drastic or the probability of a drastic end-point no longer approaches certainty, altogether different considerations arise. Where the predictors predict, let us say, with only 90% certainty, the fact that we are dealing with neurological illness rather than other kinds of illness seems irrelevant. Indeed, the fact of coma in the neurological cases makes the decision more difficult, since we cannot even comfort ourselves with the thought that by allowing the patient to die we are alleviating present suffering. Yet Plum and Levy obviously believe that their statistics are significant even where they do not present sufficient conditions for a drastic outcome—that is, sufficient conditions for a prediction that there can be no return to consciousness.

I suspect that one important conclusion we might draw from such statistics relates not to the rationality of treatment in individual cases (where traditional obligations to the patient may continue to dictate that one should do one's utmost), but rather to what facilities, routines and the like should be made available on a systematic basis for what categories of cases. Thus, though we may not remove from life-support systems any person with only a 10% chance of return to sapiency, we might very well decide not to make sufficient life-support systems available for such patients to be placed on them at all. The decision, then, is an impersonal one, made at one remove, when no particular patient is involved.[3,13,14] When the patient enters the hospital presenting the stated clinical signs, it is not decided for that patient that it is best to allow him or her to die; rather an abstract and impersonal decision has been made to make only a certain amount of facilities available, with the result that not enough facilities exist to put that patient on them in the first place. The dilemma arises, of course, when in particular circumstances the intensive care unit happens to be underutilized and a patient with a poor prognosis arrives at the unit. Can one then withhold resources which *are* available? I would suppose not, but nothing prevents that patient being removed from these life-support systems so that another more hopeful patient can be accommodated who might arrive later when there is no longer any slack in the facilities.[15]

Thus, what Plum and Levy do for us is to illustrate how much better we might predict from early signs ultimate outcomes. The interest of the conclusions should not lead us to assume that there is any one-to-one relation between public or medical policy and the probability of recovery. Rather, our response will display the complexities and structure which I have suggested.

References

1. U.S. National Commission for the Protection of Human Subjects of Medical and Behavioral Research (1977) DHEW publication No. (OS)77–0001, Washington, D.C.
2. Symposium (1974) *Boston Univ. Law Rev. 54*, 217
3. See Ref. 1, p. 57
4. FRIED, C. (1974) *Medical Experimentation: Personal Integrity and Social Policy*, North-Holland, Amsterdam and New York
5. See Ref. 1, p. 64
6. CHARRON, W. C. (1975) Death: a philosophical perspective on legal definitions. *Wash. Univ. Law Rev. 979*
7. SKEGG, P. D. G. (1974) Irreversibly comatose individuals: 'alive' or 'dead'. *Cambr. Law J. 33*, 130
8. VAN TILL-D'ALUNIS DE BOUROUILL, H. A. H. (1976) Diagnosis of death in comatose patients under resuscitation treatment: a critical review of the Harvard report. *Am. J. Law Med. 2*, 1–40

  9. Anonymous (1975) Comment: The law of homicide: does it require a definition of death? *Wake Forest Law Rev. 11*, 253
 10. COBURN, D. R. (1977) In re Quinlan, a practical overview. *Arkansas Law Rev. 31*, 59
 11. SMITH, W. F. (1976) In re Quinlan, defining the basis for terminating life support under the right of privacy. *Tulsa Law J. 12*, 150
 12. Symposium (1977) *Rutgers Law Rev. 30*, 243
 13. FRIED, C. (1978) *Right and Wrong*, Harvard University Press, Cambridge, MA
 14. CALABRESI, G. (1977) *Tragic Choices*, Norton, New York
 15. SKILLMAN, J. J. (1974) Ethical dilemmas in the care of the critically ill. *Lancet 2*, 634–637

Discussion: Experimental surgery and clinical neurology

Crown: Dr Cooper's modesty stopped him from telling us more about his contributions to work on brain function as a whole. Some years ago he was involved, as I was, with another team over here at the National Hospital, Queen Square, in stereotactic operations on the basal ganglia for Parkinson's disease. Dr Cooper and his psychologist colleague Riklan in New York published a large series of cases. We had a much smaller series of 30 patients whom we also studied from a psychological, psychiatric and neurosurgical point of view.[1] The results of the two studies were in broad agreement and two points are relevant to our discussion here: the cognitive aspect of consciousness and the emotional aspects.

On the cognitive aspect, it was interesting that there were differences between left- and right-side operations on the basal ganglia. On the left one tended to get verbal deficits and on the right visual–spatial deficits. These results were very similar in terms of cerebral function to what was found some years earlier after the original operations on the temporal lobe for epilepsy, when the same kind of lateralized deficit was found on cognitive testing.

On the emotive side the effect of Parkinsonism on the mental state and the resulting interactions are fascinating. The common occurrence of depression in Parkinsonism and its relationship with tremor is one example; the relationship of motivation for the operation to how people fare afterwards is another. Most of our patients had unilateral signs. We might get a very good post-operative result neurologically but, in unmotivated patients, some weeks later they might develop a tremor on the non-operated side.

Creutzfeldt: Parkinsonian patients have a slowing down of their speech performance and accordingly a slowing down of their thought processes. Here we have another good example of the interrelation of identity between action and thinking.

Medawar: Both Dr Fried and Dr Plum implied that the degree of disablement can be quantified without assessing the value of a variable which cannot in fact be measured. The kind of disability that a peasant could put up with easily might be a major disability for a concert pianist. How can the degree of disability be properly quantified?

Fried: If the physician knows the patient that point will be taken into account, whereas the bureaucrat who has a rather global picture would have to run all those things together.

285

Plum: We lump moderate disability with recovery, the only criterion being the capacity for independence. The peasant who didn't require total external support would qualify for moderate disability, as would the concert pianist.

Medawar: People who have recovered will almost always say they are grateful because people have a very great preference for being alive over being dead, so isn't their judgement absolutely unreliable?

Plum: Patients who recover sufficiently to be grateful would almost always be classified as having moderate disability, Sir Peter. No vegetative patient possesses either the capacity to say anything or, as best we can tell, to think it. The severely disabled are little better off—they may gropingly make contact with the environment, but severe disability after central nervous system injury or illness almost always means extensive paralysis of three or four limbs plus substantial dementia.

Bennett: I grant that the notion of the value of a life isn't measurable in a scalar way, but is made up of a very large number of things. Charles Fried seemed to be saying that the central question is a counter-factual one about what the patients themselves would prefer if they were in a position to express a preference. I don't see that that is worthless, as Sir Peter Medawar implies it is. Another point: 'What would the patient say if presented with this situation in advance and asked what he wants?' is a significantly different question from 'If he recovers will he be glad to have recovered?' I know a quadriplegic who is now on the whole glad to be alive but who spent all his waking hours for three years wishing to be dead. Asked the question in advance, he would have chosen not to be given his survival. That is not cancelled or disqualified by the fact that he has now worked himself through to being, on the whole, glad to be alive. Although glad to be alive, he could—and I suspect that he does—think that the price he has paid was too high.

Trevarthen: I have wondered about the relationship between the law and psychology and medicine, for example in connection with baby bashing. I have also thought about the justification for the brain operation on epileptics with whom I have been closely associated. When you mentioned the spectrum of decision-making processes, Dr Fried, you gave the doctor a central role and I can see that all you say is justified. When you referred to bureaucratic decision-making processes I thought that we could get a better, more objective, understanding of the problem and responsibility from research on social psychology and from the psychological study of family life. This ought to produce a much stronger, more differentiated set of predictions about the human consequences of a given course of action. I would not like to go on trusting bureaucrats or doctors for ever. That is not a criticism of either of those professions. What do you feel as a lawyer about the future of more direct knowledge about these human interpersonal factors?

Fried: There is no problem about that. The doctor who is making the decision, as well as the bureaucrat, must make it on the fullest range of knowledge possible.

Trevarthen: But it is very tragic that in spite of efforts to find people with sufficient objective experience and knowledge to make confident statements about the chances of happiness, social workers have tended to be ignored. Social workers have low status compared with doctors or lawyers and so forth, yet in many cases they know more about what is going on.

Marsden: I warmly agreed with your whole argument, Dr Fried, until your last point. The dilemma there was that doctors were doing what Hippocrates told them to do—the best for their patients—and the bureaucrats decided how to apportion resources. Unfortunately, in a country like ours, with limited resources, the bureaucrats now turn to the doctors and say 'we haven't got the facilities or the knowledge to distribute the resources—you the doctors must do that'.

Plum: Don't they make the decisions anteriorly? Don't they simply provide a certain number of intensive care beds, so that in a kind of triage system, at about the eighth or tenth day, doctors have to decide to move people who are showing no improvement into general beds, where they quickly succumb? What makes one uneasy is that in many instances such decisions are being made not on medical–neurological grounds of what *can* be the outcome but on transient indications that worsen illness, such as the presence of treatable intercurrent infections. We started this work on the positive side, to see who could most benefit from intensive care if resources were scarce. If resources are limited, who is going to tell people this—the doctor or the bureaucrat?

Wall: I match you in your dislike of bureaucrats in this connection but there is one important exception. In committing people to a lunatic asylum the doctor remains in relation to the patient and the relatives. It is then good to have a distant third party who is responsible for the decision.

Wikler: It is all very well to say that the physician should look after the interests of the patients and let other people worry about the other questions. But can one realistically expect this to happen? Recent sociological data[2] indicate that the people with the best chance of having physicians acting in their interests are the patients who can communicate best with the physicians or with others and who are in a position to influence the physicians. Physicians are most likely to spend more energy saving those who have excellent communicative abilities or who have ties with others who can communicate with the doctors. The ones who can't communicate generally are not treated as well. If that is true, then with all the best intentions in the world the physician may still be under the same kind of social pressures that cause us to act differently towards different kinds of people. In law courts those unable to communicate are represented by lawyers able to communicate and their rights are more likely to be honoured. Even with your division of labour between doctors and bureaucrats there still seems to be room for the court.

Young: You mean it is better to be advised by a lawyer than by your doctor?

Wikler: No; it is better to have a lawyer pleading your case on the spot.

Fried: Studies on courts and lawyers would probably show that, like doctors, they favour those who can communicate with them, so rather than get into that endless regress of who is going to watch the guardians, I would be happier just to leave the judgement to the person who is responsible at the beginning of the line.

Bunge: The major problem in this area is: what figure for recovery probability is reasonable? If we had an instrument that enabled us to compute and measure this probability, we could adopt the following decision rule: terminate the life-support apparatus if, and only if, that recovery probability is lower than or equal to the experimental error. But we don't seem to have either theories or instruments capable of computing or measuring probability and error. At present our decisions are only semi-rational, only semi-fair and only semi-moral.

Dr Plum, when you hesitatingly equated the vegetative state to being awake but not aware I didn't understand, and I don't think you like it either. How can anyone be awake without being aware of his or her surroundings and of the events going on in the body?

Plum: Waking and sleeping comprise a vegetative function which originates from nuclei in the lower level of the brain-stem and requires no contribution from the cerebral hemispheres.[3] As far as anyone can judge, this primitive wakefulness has nothing directly to do with cognitive activity, although cognition can only occur during wakefulness. Animals with brain-stems sectioned at the supracollicular level develop waking and sleeping responses in the isolated forebrain segment. There is even some evidence that the spinal cord shows circadian variations in its physiological rhythms, although not to the degree seen in waking and sleeping. Neurologists care for many badly brain-damaged patients, who simply lie with their eyes open, go to sleep at night and wake up the next morning, without ever demonstrating any evidence of cognitive mentation. Furthermore, such mindless states can last for years.

Young: That is fine when there is a lesion but how do you know whether someone is awake but not aware or awake and aware?

Plum: We agonize over that. One only has behavioural criteria to go on, plus laboratory and clinical evidence of the existence of extensive brain damage.

Creutzfeldt: The ethical aspects of interfering with brain activity in motor or sensory diseases produce few doubts now. But if we accept the materialistic view that what a person is, thinks and does are due to activities of the brain, thus seeing the brain as a machine, the question is whether there are any moral limitations to interfering with brain activities which disturb this person. Certain operations which brought about personality changes led to great moral arguments. The people who did these operations thought they were doing them for the good of the patient and of society. But on what do we base our ethical or moral judgement if we think of the brain as a machine, as we might feel obliged to do as biologists? Where is the system of values based in such a system, and—in short—the moral or legal implications of such brain operations?

Searle: From all we know, the brain, though a machine, is the machine on which everything we value depends. That is why we are worried about it.

Dunstan: We have started asking ethical questions—who maintains what sort of life, and when, and so on. I support all Dr Fried's positive statements, particularly in his preferring the judgement of doctors to the judgement of courts. The practice in England is that doctors come before courts only when they misbehave very badly or have very bad luck. I hope that will continue. But my question is, do we set limits to what doctors may decide? Are there limits beyond which decisions are not possible? This question occurred to me because I thought I detected a slight confusion either in Dr Fried's presentation or more probably in my hearing of it. As I understand it, 'Harvard death' refers to a state in which there is 'life' only because of organ support, and the question arises, when may that support be removed? But a lot of Dr Plum's presentation concerned life *without* support, and this is where some of the major ethical issues lie. There seems to be a world of difference between the decisions open to the doctor in the two cases.

Plum: It depends on the level of support that you talk about. In most societies, through most of man's history, feeding, washing, cleansing, covering and heating would have been considered as support in the same way that using a ventilator and using an intravenous drip are considered as support now. With brain death, no dilemma exists because what life goes on is an artifact of machines. With overwhelming brain damage and a vegetative existence, life can go on without machines but not without enormous amounts of sustained attention. We think it would be an advantage to know when the avoidance of heroic treatment would also result in avoiding a prolonged, meaningless existence.

Dunstan: I would distinguish between the ordinary support (washing, feeding etc.) due to people because they are human beings and the extra-ordinary support that they receive when you buy time with the machine. There is a radical difference in the decisions that have to be made in the two cases.

Fried: You spoke about removing life support or even terminating the life of people who are not Harvard-dead but let us say Yale-dead, Professor Dunstan. I would accept the consequence for what I am saying that where there is no conscious life it would be a considerable advance if we treated that person as dead and, for instance, proceeded to transplant organs from that patient.

Wall: You made gentle, witty references to surgeons as freebooters, Dr Fried. We haven't yet had an answer to questions about the conditions under which surgical operations might or might not be carried out. Professor Cooper, you spoke here of sensory and motor systems but these words are not used by physiologists. People say that afferent equals sensory and efferent equals motor in the peripheral nervous system but in the central nervous system nobody makes this differentiation any longer. In talking about stimulation of the cerebellum, which is far less destructive than what you were talking about, you used the physiology of Sherrington without quoting the counter-results of Dow and Snider. What was the basic justification, before the operation, for the series of lesions which you made in the lady whose condition improved so dramatically?

Cooper: I should like to address the physiological question first. I believe I was saying—or trying to—precisely what you have just stated, Professor Wall, namely that not only afferents in the nervous system but virtually all efferents are sensory, in that they are communicating data. I do not see any discrepancy in our viewpoints in that regard.

Many neuroscientists still refer to the so-called extrapyramidal motor system. All I am saying is that such a motor system doesn't exist. Everything going on in the basal ganglia, as far as I know, is sensory communication or data processing.

I am somewhat puzzled by your request for a justification for alleviating the total incapacitation of Mrs M, whose case I presented. I am a doctor. It is my legal and moral responsibility to try to make sick people well, or make the disabled able, without allowing them to take undue risks. In the case of Mrs M I did precisely that. Before I operated upon her she could not move her left limbs, she could not speak intelligibly. She was totally helpless. After surgery she could speak, recovered the use of her limbs, and became independent. As a doctor I helped her to become well. What other conceivable justification could there be?

Before that my colleagues and I had operated on 8000 to 10 000 patients with Parkinsonism and related movement disorders. There was ample reason to believe that Mrs M's tremor and rigidity could be relieved, and the risk–benefit ratio was entirely in the patient's favour.[4] Your reference to Dow and Snider is incorrect. Before their notable investigations Sherrington[5] stimulated the anterior cerebellum and decreased cerebrate rigidity. In the same year (1897) the same findings were reported independently by Lowenthal and Horsley.[6] It has been confirmed many times since then.[7]

Snider, to whom you referred, has been one of my co-workers, and has carried out physiological monitoring upon several of my patients during precisely the type of operation I have reported here today. Dow and Snider have stated that the rationale underlying my clinical investigations was supported by their earlier work. Each has been my co-author in monographs on the cerebellum.[8,9] Perhaps you were thinking of two different people.

The reason for placing a lesion in the pulvinar was somewhat empirical. Speech arrest had been achieved by stimulation of the pulvinar.[10] Based on that study I received permission from our hospital human research committee to attempt to stimulate and/or make a lesion in the pulvinar of totally aphasic patients. The first patient on whom we operated obtained relief of spasticity but no change in speech. That relief of spasticity provided the lead that initiated my study of the pulvinar.[11] I have dealt with the moral justification for such investigative surgery as diligently as with the clinical aspects. They are inseparable. In 1974 I presented a lecture on this subject in the room in which we are now assembled (I. S. Cooper, unpublished work). I have just come from a four-day meeting which I organized under the title 'What Should We Do?' Both Reverend Joseph Fletcher and C. P. Snow, who took part in the meeting, agreed that this is THE ethical question. It is an integral part of the fabric of every clinician's daily life.

As early as 1967 I published a plea for multidisciplinary consideration of the moral dilemma involved in the institution of new therapies—or even the continuation of long-used procedures of questionable value.[12] Other published references to my own moral stance are available.[13,14]

The moral questions always remain open and must be continually re-examined. Defining 'Harvard death' is, in my opinion, far less complex than dealing with the living who are locked into their own bodies and who cry out to be released. For those who accept the responsibility of caring for desperately ill humans such questions must be constantly agonized over.

On the other hand, to return to the scientific implications of Dr Wall's question, I would like to state the following. I have for many years refused to apologize for the therapeutic benefit of these operations simply because the results could not immediately be explained by laboratory or clinical scientists on the basis of existing physiological ideas—ideas which ultimately were demonstrably incorrect. If I may quote a remark Sir Peter Medawar made to me early in this meeting: 'It is a doctor's job to do good. It is the scientist's job to explain the facts'. By operating on the cerebellum, pulvinar and ventrolateral thalamus of Mrs M I fulfilled my obligation to do her good—immeasurable good. I have also tried to explain these results, but that is secondary to my responsibility to the patient. I invite Dr Wall, as a scientist, to examine the unprecedented facts emerging from this experience and explain them. If the facts do not fit his present concepts, then he will have to rethink the concepts, because the facts will not change.

Fried: I want to reiterate my sincerely meant expression of admiration for the freebooter. Freebooters get into trouble but they also do great things. Working on an empirical basis sometimes does great good and I would be very unhappy if everything was so neat and bureaucratized that none of this kind of enterprise was going on. But it does involve risks.

References

1. Asso, D., Crown, S., Russell, J. A. & Logue, V. (1969) Psychological aspects of the stereotactic treatment of Parkinsonism. *Br. J. Psychiatry 115*, 541–543
2. Crane, D. (1975) *The Sanctity of Social Life: Physician's Treatment of Critically Ill Patients*, Russell Sage, New York
3. Plum, F. & Posner, J. B. (1980) *Diagnosis and Prognosis of Stupor and Coma*, 3rd edn., Davis, PA.
4. Cooper, I. S. (1969) *Involuntary Movement Disorders*, Harper & Row, New York
5. Sherrington, C. S. (1897) Double (antidrome) conduction in the central nervous system. *Proc. R. Soc. Lond. 61*, 243–246
6. Lowenthal, M. & Horsley, V. (1897) On the relations between the cerebellar and other centers, namely cerebral and spinal, with special reference to the action of antagonistic muscles. *Proc. R. Soc. Lond. 61*, 20–25
7. Moruzzi, G. (1950) *Problems in Cerebellar Physiology*, Thomas, Springfield, Ill.
8. Cooper, I. S., Riklan, M. & Snider, R. S. (1974) *The Cerebellum, Epilepsy and Behaviour*, Plenum, New York
9. Dow, R. S. (1978) Summary and evaluation of chronic cerebellar stimulation in man, in *Cerebellar Stimulation in Man* (Cooper, I. S., ed.), pp. 207–212, Raven Press, New York
10. Ojemann, G. A., Fedio, P. & Van Buren, J. M. (1968) Anomia from pulvinar and subcortical parietal stimulation. *Brain 91*, 99–116
11. Cooper, I. S., Amin, I., Chandra, R. & Waltz, J. M. (1973) A surgical investigation of the clinical physiology of the LP-Pulvinar complex in man. *J. Neurol. Sci. 18*, 89–110
12. Cooper, I. S. (1967) Medicine of the absurd. *Mayo Alumnus 3*, 1–5
13. Cooper, I. S. (1973) *The Victim Is Always the Same*, Harper & Row, New York
14. Cooper, I. S. (1977) *It's Hard to Leave While the Music's Playing*, Norton, New York

Three phases of evil:
the relation of injury to pain

PATRICK D. WALL

Cerebral Functions Research Group, Department of Anatomy, University College London

Abstract It is proposed that injury may be followed by three phases of behaviour in human beings and animals. In the immediate phase, pain may not occur and other activities take precedence. Even when the victims are fully aware of their injury, these other activities may include fighting, escaping and obtaining safety and aid. Once relative safety from the source of injury has been achieved, a new form of behaviour related to allowing recovery begins. This is the acute stage. The need for the initiation of this behaviour is signalled by pain. In the transition stage from injury to the beginning of recovery, anxiety is a cardinal feature. The anxiety is directed at assuring safety from the original damage, at assuring the best conditions for the initiation of treatment and recovery, and at the possible future consequences of the damage. This phase merges with the third period, during which quiet inactivity is the optimal tactic to encourage cure and recovery. This third stage associated with pain and depression may appear prolonged far beyond the necessary period for recovery. It is proposed here that pain is associated with the search for treatment and optimal conditions for recovery.

Proust has written 'Illness is the doctor to whom we pay the most heed: to kindness to knowledge we make promises only: pain we obey'. What could be this curious condition which takes command of a man who flatters himself with his talk of free will, of voluntary behaviour, of options, decisions and control? If we open a textbook of medical physiology, the chapter on pain begins with an apparently direct straightforward statement: 'Pain is that sensory experience evoked by stimuli that injure.'[1] The simplicity of the sentence is initially attractive and immediately suggests a tactic for the analysis of pain mechanisms. One has only to observe an injury and then to detect the nervous signals generated by the injury and to follow their course through the nervous system. The sentence says that injury generates pain and pain implies injury. Given such a strongly linked chain of causal events, the scientist should be capable of dissecting out the chain in terms of nervous events from stimulus to response and have finished with the problem. On second thoughts, I begin to realize that the simplicity is illusory because I do not fully understand the meaning of any of the words other than 'injure'. Furthermore, my professional and personal experience makes me doubt the inevitability of the link and its straightforward simplicity. Therefore let us set aside the introspective conclusion that pain signals injury and ask what are the observed consequences of injury.

THREE ANECDOTES ABOUT THE SENSORY BEHAVIOURAL CONSEQUENCES OF INJURY

It will be my contention that animals and the human species share a common sequence of phases of reaction to injury. To support this view I shall first use three anecdotes without apology. The anecdote is not conclusive evidence but if it seems to fit the reader's experience, it deserves the honour of attention and investigation. Later I will support the conclusions of the anecdotes by more usual evidence. My reason for introducing animal behaviour when it is possible to ask human beings about their own experiences is to suggest that if a common pattern exists, we may later look for a common biological significance of this behaviour. Of course we shall encounter species-specific and socially tailored behaviour but this should not allow us to miss the general syndrome if such exists.

A. Deer

For fifteen years, I spent every weekend in a wooded area of New England. Family groups of deer ranged freely, grazing mainly at dawn and dusk, resting and ruminating in quiet cover in the night and in full day. Once a year this pastoral scene was disturbed by the hunting season. The skill of these hunters was shown statistically by the fact that the number of deer killed only slightly exceeded the number of hunters killed. Domestic cattle were shot in enclosed fields. Dead fallen trees whose branches reminded the boozy sportsmen of antlers were repeatedly blasted with bullets. Under these circumstances, it is not surprising that many deer received substantial non-lethal bullet wounds. I often saw these unfortunate beasts soon after hearing the shooting. They would run in spite of obvious wounds. I wish to emphasize that this was no blind frenzied activity. The animals ran at very high speed through dense cover, leaping and swerving with extraordinary skill and power. If one visited the usual deer resting places over the next few days, one was likely to encounter survivors. They lay quietly curled up. Repeated visits showed that they did not move for hours. The wound was licked but the coat was untended. Their threshold for disturbance was markedly raised, so it was possible to approach closely before they moved off. Movement was slow, lacking energy and skill. They were solitary and did not react in the usual way to movements of the herd. Here I wish to stress only two of the phases of response to injury. In the early stage, it is difficult to see that the wounded animal behaved in any way different from an alarmed escaping unwounded animal. At a later stage, one observed a solitary inert animal with marked changes of its eating, escape and social behaviour.

B. Dogs

For a period of some ten years, I had the honour to be adopted by a dog of the streets. One of the civic duties he had taken upon himself was to sweep the district clear of other dogs. On hearing a squealing in the street one day, I went out to find him shaking a cocker spaniel by the scruff of the neck like a rag duster. I grabbed my dog and started to throttle him. The spaniel's owner came over with a garden spade and with a single blow hit the dog's skull. The scalp was opened and the blade went through the insertion of the temporal muscle to periosteum and arterial blood spurted from the wound. I could detect no change in the dog's behaviour; jaw closure, head shaking and growling were uninterrupted. I eventually separated the wounded dog from his lightweight victim and took him into the house. Now began the second phase. The animal was agitated, barking and highly active. I began to examine the head injury and the dog promptly bit me. The animal followed this by licking the hand he had just bitten. This phase is well known to veterinary surgeons who, wiser than I, always tie the jaws of any injured dog before attempting an examination.

The dog was anaesthetized, the muscle and skin were sutured, and he was returned home and entered the third phase. The dog's movements were reduced to a minimum and sleep was very prolonged. The usual pattern of dog sleep where the animal shifts position every half-hour or so was absent. Approach and a kind word evoked the minimal signal of one or two tail wags. Attempts to move the animal evoked growling. Tit-bits of food were refused and drinking was minimal. Examination showed no local or spreading infection and a cleanly resolving wound. Over the next week, the dog slowly returned to its normal behaviour with only his duelling scar of honour left as evidence of the episode. In summary, this dog showed three phases of behaviour after injury: first no immediate signs of injury, second a period of agitation and unusual 'irrational' behaviour, and third a stage of inactivity.

C. Man

Three years ago, in another country, I attended a riot out of that curiosity which is not only known to kill the cat but on occasions the man. I was a passive observer. The situation was calm except for some shouted insults. A mob blocked one part of the street, then there was a clear gap of some 40 metres and then armed paratroops were lined up across the road. I stood on the pavement between the two groups, well to one side, talking with a friend who is a reporter. Suddenly I felt and heard a dull thud on my forehead. Later examination showed that a glancing hit had ripped a jagged 4 centimetre long slit in the forehead and had torn through the frontalis muscle to skull. My first intimation of injury was feeling blood stream over eye and face. I took off my spectacles and pressed a handkerchief to the wound. Immediately a police car drove up and took me to a first-aid post. After a brief inspection there, I was driven to hospital and after an hour the injured area was locally anaesthetized, cleaned and sutured. Let me summarize what seem to be the essential features of this minor episode. I did not have clouding of consciousness for even a second. For at least an hour, the injury was totally painless. The area of the wound was not anaesthetic since I could feel touch and pressure. My first reactions were surprise and then anger that one side or the other should hit a passive bystander. In the police car I realized that, against all sense and expectation, this injury did not hurt at all, even on palpation. At the aid station, I inspected the wound in a mirror so that I could help decide what treatment was suitable. It still did not produce pain in any sense. I did not feel faint, I had rational actions such as asking the police to drive more slowly since this was not a serious wound. I was not in any sense in shock having lost at most 10 to 20 millilitres of blood. I began to worry that my family would be worried if they heard that I was injured and later the thought crossed my mind that infection might result. At this stage, I began to feel a minor deep dull headache. This first phase ended with the introduction of local anaesthetic.

By next morning, deep and superficial pain and tenderness were very obviously present, distressing and disturbing. This died down day by day as the wound healed cleanly without problems. In spite of this obviously impending successful end to the episode, and in spite of good company and interesting work and in spite of taking no drugs, I found myself unusually listless, sleepy, irritable, unable to concentrate, shunning food and company. This also disappeared over a period of seven to ten days.

I have described three examples of injury where there seemed to be three periods of response.

THE PHASES OF RESPONSE

(1) *Immediate*

I wish to propose that the immediate phase after injury is more commonly painless than has been previously recognized. Clearly this phenomenon represents a challenge to the proposal that injury equals pain. Therefore, there has been the tendency to dismiss such episodes as anecdotal or to give them special *ad hoc* explanations. The most famous investigation is that of H. K. Beecher[2] who surveyed wounded men without head injuries admitted to the US field hospital on the Anzio beachhead and compared them with a matched group of men in a civil hospital. He writes 'In a comparative study of wound pain, a group of male civilian patients undergoing major surgery was asked the same questions as those put to wounded soldiers. Of the wounded soldiers, about one third wanted medication to relieve their pain and two thirds did not. Of the civilians suffering from far less trauma, four fifths wanted medication to relieve their pain and one-fifth did not. Thus the figures are reversed'. He goes on to make his interpretation of these crucial findings: 'The important difference in the two groups seems to lie in their responses to the wounds. In the wounded soldier it was relief, thankfulness for his escape alive from the battlefield, even euphoria (his wound was a good thing); to the civilian his major surgery even though essential, was a depressing, calamitous event'. On this one point I disagree with Beecher who was one of the great innovators in our present understanding of pain. I believe Beecher was misled by the desperate shambles of the Anzio situation. As part of an ongoing study of Israeli soldiers who had suffered traumatic amputations during the Yom Kippur war, we asked about their initial reactions.[3] Confirming Beecher, the majority spoke of their initial injury as painless and used neutral terms such as bang, thump, blow, etc. to describe their first feeling and often volunteered their surprise that it did not hurt. On enquiry about the actual circumstances, some told of being in the same type of desperate situation as at Anzio but some injuries were caused by accidents, sometimes of their own making. Far from relief and euphoria, some spoke in their pain-free state of feeling guilt at letting down their comrades, annoyance at allowing the injury to occur, and misery about the future consequences. Furthermore, 24 hours later all were in considerable pain, no matter what the circumstances of their injury—heroism, blundering or being a passive inactive victim. It is quite apparent that the pain-free period after injury can occur in situations where the wound has no survival advantage. What are those situations?

Pain-free injury is not the monopoly of the battlefield. The sports field also frequently produces the effect although there are those who consider this arena as only a socially permissible analogy to military combat. Purely civilian home, road or industrial accidents may also surprise the victim or the inexperienced casualty officer in producing no complaints of pain. Again, enquiry shows the full awareness of the patient. A young lady with a leg amputated by an explosion said 'Who is going to marry me now?' A machine-shop foreman with an amputated foot said 'What a fool they will say I am to let this happen'. These patients were free of pain but a long way from Anzio and euphoria. Such patients are often not believed and are given narcotics on the grounds that they obviously must be in pain, no matter what they say. Furthermore, the period is cut short by anaesthesia and surgery with pre-medication which clouds the memory for preceding events.

If we are finding difficulty in defining the circumstances under which injury occurs with pain, we should perhaps turn for help to the equally clear episode where injury and pain seem almost coincident. An obvious example is accidentally hitting one's own thumb with a hammer. Everyone has done it and no one doubts that it hurts instantly. In what way does this injury differ from a painless equal or far more severe injury under other circumstances? My interpretation is that the episode is entirely self-contained. Attention was fully concentrated on the hammer and target and not on other goals. The only possible relevant biological action is to nurse and treat the injured tissue. This action takes precedence over all other possible actions in the victim's repertoire. The victim fully understands and controls the causes of the injury. There is no escape needed, there are no known unexpected dangers and repetition will not occur. Attention and behaviour are now completely monopolized by caring for the injury, with one odd exception. The hammer is often thrown to the ground and cursed. Here is a curious piece of anger and aggression directed at a totally passive innocent object. What sort of nonsense behaviour is that for a rational person who ought to be tending the injury? Could this be a remnant of the one possible conflicting form of behaviour—attacking or escaping the agent of the injury?

The other situation in which injury and pain are coincident is in medical treatment such as an injection or in dental care such as drilling or even in pain suffered by the volunteer in an experimental situation. Here, in a sense, the injury is self-inflicted, albeit indirectly. Training, learning, decision and social conditioning have to some degree suppressed the tendency to withdraw, escape or hit the doctor. However powerful the intention may be to submit to injury for some eventual benefit, this does not hide the fact that damage has occurred which itself requires attention, care and the need for recovery.

In summary, it is proposed that injury may be followed by circumstances in which treatment of the injury does not have the highest biological priority.

Pain does not occur in this phase. The two obvious high priority behaviours are fighting and escaping. Injured people, like injured animals, may be more than normally aggressive. Escape in humans includes calling or even screaming for help and it includes organizing help. As the necessity or possibility of destroying or avoiding the cause of injury subsides, the second phase after injury begins.

Before discussing the acute phase, I wish to include an addendum. We must face the undoubted and common existence of a state of injury without pain, the placebo reaction. At least a third of American or European adults suffering from the painful effects of accidental injury or from surgery or from cancer respond to the administration of an inert substance which they and the therapist believe will relieve their pain. The response is highly socially conditioned. It does not work in young children. The effect is more common and powerful with intravenous injections than with intramuscular injections, which in turn are more effective than tablets. The period of relief mimics that produced by narcotic injection. The effect fades if repeated injections are given without reinforcement with active drugs. Somehow the placebo reaction and the much less frequent effects of acupuncture and hypnosis must be included in any general theory of the nature of pain.

(2) *Acute*

A man is in pain and indicates that some part of his body is damaged and he is anxious. What does he mean when he says something hurts? The traditional explanation of the word takes it to be one of our possible sensory experiences and in the same class of personal observations as seeing a light or hearing a note or feeling a touch. A sensory experience in this sense refers to a representation in terms of nerve impulses of the existence of a real event whose existence can be checked by other devices and by other observers. The existence of phase 1, where injury occurs without pain, already casts doubt on the classification of the word pain as a sensation, since the man may be aware in detail of the existence and nature of his injury through the use of his visual and tactile senses and yet feel no pain. As the patient enters the second and third phases he feels pain, but the relation between the amount of injury and the amount of pain varies in one patient from time to time. Furthermore, the relation of the amount of pain and amount of damage varies over a huge range between individuals. No such variability occurs in the normal population if one considers the ability to report on intensities of lights, sounds, pressures, tastes and smells.

There exists a different class of feelings which are not included in the classical

Aristotelian five senses. These feelings include hunger, thirst and asphyxia. They differ from the classical senses in a number of ways. They reflect something of the internal state of the person rather than events on the surface of the body or in the outer world. However, the most sophisticated quantitative measures of the actual state of the internal milieu show that the intensity of the feelings varies wildly, with only a mild correlation with the actual state of the body. Furthermore the existence of these feelings is strongly correlated with predictable behaviour. The detection of light, sound, pressure, taste and smell has no predictable behavioural consequence in human beings or animals. A declaration of hunger predicts a search for food. The stronger the feeling, the more the behaviour will be monopolized. This observation of the monopolization of behaviour to achieve a certain direction has led to the concept of 'drives'. The person or animal seems driven to achieve certain goals: to eat to abolish hunger; to drink to abolish thirst.

How then shall we classify the feeling of pain? It fits none of the criteria we expect of the classical senses. It fits all of the criteria of the feelings about body state. There is however one serious problem if we accept that pain should be classed with such feelings as hunger and thirst. What is the drive and what is the goal to be achieved? It is not true to say that pain allows the avoidance of injury, although this statement is often made. It is patently obvious that in most situations the primary damage is done by the time the pain is experienced. It is quite true that the experience of pain is a powerful concomitant of learning to avoid a repetition of the stimulus which evoked the pain. The same is true for hunger and thirst. It is also quite true that if a stimulus very slowly increases there may be time to take avoiding action, but these situations are more common in the experimental laboratory than in the real world. Furthermore, the obvious avoidance responses such as the flexor reflex long precede the feeling of pain. Pain is a poor protector in cases of sudden injury and is perhaps even worse where damage slowly intrudes. With the steady destruction produced by diseases such as cancer, tuberculosis, leprosy, etc., pain more often signals the arrival of the undertaker than some useful action.

Could it be that pain does not simply announce the presence of damaged tissue but rather announces the need to enter a mode of behaviour best suited to treat and cure the damage? Then the drive would be to permit recovery from damage and the fulfilment of that drive would be cure. Let us follow this idea by looking at the rare situation of congenital analgesia in its pure form, where intelligence is normal and there are no other defects.[4] These patients are recognized early and the patients and their parents learn to avoid injury by the many clues of danger other than pain and by careful intellectual analysis of permitted and dangerous situations. However, the commonest and often fatal complaint reported is of serious joint disorder, seen in denervated joints and first described by Charcot. No gross injury has occurred but small sprains and strains are not followed by the period of guarding and immobility which normal people carry out after minor injuries. Without this splinting and protection by immobility, the injured joint is moved and the damage is increased. The joint surfaces erode and disappear and eventually osteomyelitis may develop as a fatal disease. My suggestion here is that the important deficit of these patients is that they fail to initiate and maintain the behaviour necessary for repair.

Let us return to an examination of the characteristics of the acute phase which are the combination of tissue damage, pain and anxiety. It is a transition stage between coping with the cause of the injury and preparing for recovery. The rapidly moving transitional nature of the phase is shown by the direction of the anxiety after injury. Anxiety occurs in a spectrum from specific to free-floating. The specific anxieties are directed in three directions: to the past, the present and the future. The past and completed act which caused the injury may be highly defined but the reaction is prolonged and diffuses. For the wounded soldier, the person who fired the shot is the specific object of fear and threat but the victim is alerted to a more and more general awareness of the threatening nature of the world. The slamming of the hatch of the helicopter which signals the beginning of the journey to safety and care is taken as an ambiguous event which might signal another assault. Step by step the possible origin and nature of threat diffuses until everything and nothing is threatening. Drugs or sleep which cloud consciousness produce abreaction in which the diffusing process is reversed and the original situation with its specific threat reappears.

Present anxieties relate to treatment in progress. Here in particular there is a demonstration of private suffering and public display. The balance between these two is immensely subject to personality and social factors. The citizens of Oslo and of Naples have learnt in their different ways about socially accepted and expected behaviour and about the nature of authority and about acceptable quality of medical care. Patients call for help with words and actions in their personal and national languages. I went up to the bedside of a British injured soldier who was surrounded by French-speaking staff in a French hospital. The man was shouting, swearing and struggling. 'What's up mate?' I said. My three words translated him from an unknown unknowing world to the familiar and he became the classical stolid tough stereotype. Mixed in with anxiety about the past and present, there is the obvious fear of future consequences. Death or prolonged suffering are possibilities. The assessment of this threat and therefore the degree of anxiety will depend on personality, experience, knowledge, information, religion and trust. While the backward-directed anxiety represents a diversion from the injury, the present and future-directed anxieties concentrate on the damage. Acute pain and acute anxiety of the latter types are completely coupled. The treatment of one is the treatment of the other. There is no justification for considering the two states as independent variables. They appear as two aspects of the same phenomenon, both triggered by damage to tissue but more related to treatment and recovery processes than to the injury itself. The acute stage of injury in animals shows some of the same aspects as those seen in humans. Arousal, agitation and aggressiveness suggest an irrational continuation of the actual fight–flight period and a diffusing of assessment of threat. The helping hand is bitten and the familiar home becomes a threatening prison from which escape is mandatory. Normally effective low doses of tranquillizers or narcotics provoke a recurrence of wild escape and fighting behaviour.

(3) Chronic

Patients with chronic pain show a syndrome which differs radically from the acute stage. We are indebted to R. A. Sternbach[4,5] for the recognition and description of this miserable condition. The behaviour of these patients changes over the days, weeks and months after the onset of the condition when they were in the acute stage. Pain and complaint are unremitting and often a more and more elaborate search for treatment becomes a major activity. In other respects, the patients show all aspects of a deepening depression. Movement is restricted, thought is slow, and attention to the outside is limited. Suicide may occur. There is loss of appetite, constipation, loss of libido, disturbance of menstrual periods, disturbance of sleep pattern and disturbance of family and social relations. As this pattern of sick behaviour settles and appears to fix, the original signs of disease may disappear or resolve to some minimal scar. Here we have again a mismatch between the amount of pain and the amount of injury. Needless to say, relatives and doctors begin to express their frustration at being unable to help by suspecting that 'there is nothing wrong'. Here we have a practical expression of the dualistic thinking of our society. A pain is a mental process associated with a body process and damaged tissue. If pain seems disproportionate to the apparent damage, the external observer becomes suspicious. 'Nothing wrong' in the obviously sick and suffering person implies that nothing is wrong with the body and therefore the disease is of the mind. The patients are then examined to determine whether there is some cause other than injury for their sick behaviour. In

Skinnerian terms, have they been rewarded for their sick behaviour? Are they gaining some secondary benefit by getting more love and attention than previously, by avoiding the tensions of ordinary life, by getting a pension or an insurance settlement? These uncharitable thoughts may begin to dominate people's thinking about these patients and lead to counter-conditioning and behaviour therapies or even to abandonment of the patients. Sometimes the patients respond but more often they steadfastly remain convinced that they are in pain and sick and need specific treatment. Antidepressant treatment is frequently very useful. Training in techniques for shifting of attention also helps. These patients in their search for treatment are frequently taking high doses of multiple drugs and often become narcotic addicts. Especially in rich societies, they seek and get multiple surgical operations, often repeats of previously unsuccessful surgery.

The chronic pain syndrome has been described as a specific state. I wish now to propose that this is the extreme of a common condition seen in injured people or animals. I suggest as a subject for investigation that all postoperative patients show some degree of this condition. Furthermore I suspect that one of the factors in the intensity and duration of the phase is the amount of tissue damage. The condition is often missed because the patients have been sick before the operation and the effects of the operation are confused with the resolution of the sickness. However, accidents and war injuries occur suddenly in people who were previously healthy, yet they too suffer a period of pain, lassitude and inactivity. Some diseases show the syndrome without pain. Infectious hepatitis is an example where activity, sleep, mood and behaviour patterns take many months to recover, even after liver function tests have apparently returned to normal. As proposed above, animals also show prolonged periods of relative inactivity, sleep, eating, grooming and social behaviour disturbances while recovering from localized injuries which do not themselves prevent the animals from leading an active life.

There are certain striking exceptions to the proposed generality of this chronic state, and they prove the rule. Where pain is intermittent, a different state develops. Angina pectoris is an example where each attack evokes a repetition of the acute phase, putting fear and anxiety into the patients. If attacks are frequent and severe, the patients very reasonably reach a chronic anxiety state. They are pale, sweating, jumpy, limiting activity because activity precipitates further attacks. Similarly, patients with triggered attacks of trigeminal neuralgia very reasonably feel a rising terror and adopt extremely alert and cautious protected ways of moving to prevent recurrence.

CONCLUSIONS

Pain is taken not as a simple sensory experience signalling the existence of damaged tissue. The presence and intensity of pain is too poorly related to the degree of damage to be considered such a messenger. Pain is a poor protector against injury since it occurs far too late in sudden injury or very slow damage to provide a useful preventive measure. Instead it is proposed that pain signals the existence of a body state where recovery and recuperation should be initiated. This places the word pain in the same class as words such as thirst and hunger which signal not only a body state but also the impending onset of a form of behaviour. The curative recovery mode of behaviour is undoubtedly associated with general changes of body chemistry and endocrine changes as well as with central nervous system changes. Hungry people change not only their mode of motor behaviour but also their body chemistry. Just as there are disorders of hunger such as obesity and anorexia, so there may be disorders of the pain–recovery system where invalid behaviour is excessively prolonged or abbreviated. Just as hunger is associated with the search for food and eating, so it is proposed that pain is associated with the search for treatment and optimal conditions for recovery.

References

1. MOUNTCASTLE, V. B. (1968) *Medical Physiology*, 12th edn., Mosby, St Louis
2. BEECHER, H. K. (1959) *Measurement of Subjective Responses*, Oxford University Press, New York
3. CARLEN, P. L., WALL, P. D., NADVORNA, H. & STEINBACH, T. (1978) Phantom limbs and related phenomena in recent traumatic amputations. *Neurology 28*, 211–217
4. STERNBACH, R. A. (1968) *Pain: Psychological and Psychiatric Aspects*, Academic Press, New York
5. STERNBACH, R. A. (1974) *Pain Patients: Traits and Treatment*, Academic Press, New York

The emotion of pain and its chemistry

C. D. MARSDEN

University Department of Neurology, Institute of Psychiatry, and King's College Hospital Medical School, London

Abstract Pain is not an electrical impulse derived from tissue injury but an emotional experience arising when a nervous input is interpreted in the light of experience and emotional context as being 'painful'. Pain may thus signify tissue damage, vivid sensory experience or inner turmoil. Pain may be distressing but it can also be pleasurable. Whether a given stimulus provokes pain and whether that emotional feeling causes distress varies from individual to individual and from moment to moment. The brain possesses chemically mediated mechanisms that can exert control over the experience of 'pain'. An understanding of such mechanisms suggests new approaches to the relief of distressing pain (and to the artificial production of pleasurable pain).

'Pain is a physical sensation which is always, always, always modified by the patient's psychological emotional reaction to it. It follows from this that pain is modified by mood, morale and meaning. It is the third point – meaning – which so often makes cancer pain so severe.

'Looked at another way, the same sensory input, from the same noxious stimulus, can be experienced as anything from an 'ache' to agony. We see this particularly in the young child who is in agony until mother comes along and caresses the part hurt in a fall or injury'.

Dr Robert Twycross

'There is a pleasure in poetic pains Which only poets know'.

William Cowper

The Task, part ii, The Timepiece

305

The English language sometimes lets us down, and 'pain' is a case in point. The word is used to describe the agony of terminal cancer invading bone, the beauty of music and poetry, the grief of loss, and the emotions of love. The only clear thread that links such varied experiences is that they all provoke identical bodily responses which we outwardly recognize and inwardly feel as intense physical turmoil. Indeed, it is quite possible that all such events cause similar changes in autonomic function—a dry mouth, fast heart beat, abdominal tightening, tremor and sweating—which we can consciously appreciate as the 'feelings' associated with physical pain. By that we mean the bodily 'feelings' that occur in response to the physical pain produced by tissue damage. If such bodily 'feelings' occur spontaneously, or in response to some other sensory or emotional disturbance, it is reasonable to recognize them as 'feelings' of pain, even though they are not provoked by the stimuli produced by tissue injury. Such 'feelings' of pain may cause distress (or pleasure), but they are not accompanied by the localized sensory discomfort associated with physical pain.

The experience of physical pain usually involves the interaction of many nervous functions:

> *(a)* Injury causing tissue damage, provoking nervous input to the brain;
> *(b)* Recognition of such an input into the brain;
> *(c)* Concurrent assessment of the situation in which such injury occurs, by analysis of visual, auditory and other sensory stimuli;
> *(d)* Association of such injury and its context with past experience stored in memory;
> *(e)* Analysis of the impact of the injury, its context, and memories in the light of current mood;
> *(f)* Appreciation of the secondary physical responses to the whole experience.

Thus, I *recognize* the *cut hands*, in the *context* of the car crash and I *remember* the pain of the bacon slicer, it is late at night and I am *alone and afraid*, I feel *sick and cold* with sweat—'I suffer pain'.

RECOGNITION OF TISSUE INJURY

Injury causes signals to be transmitted to the central nervous system. If the signals travel up to the brain, specifically to the cerebral cortex, they arouse sensations that are more or less restricted to the damaged part. However, whether such signals intrude upon the stream of thought, and the extent to which they do, depend on the person's state at the time. The classical example is the footballer who does not notice the gash on his leg until he feels the blood in his sock, or until the game is finished. In other words, there must be nervous mechanisms that prevent stimuli produced by tissue injury from intruding into consciousness under certain circumstances.

The 'gate control' theory of pain proposed by Melzack and Wall[1] provided such a mechanism. According to this theory, peripheral pain receptors relay impulses to the dorsal horn of the spinal cord via small (C and delta) fibres. Whether such impulses excite cord cells responding to injury (T or transmission cells) depends on how much concurrent impulse traffic there is in large sensory fibres. It is supposed that to rub away pain is to excite a massive input from larger fibres that gates or stops the impulses from small fibres that signify tissue damage. There are objections to the theory in its original form[2,3] but in principle it provides a simple spinal mechanism for controlling pain.

The paraplegic does not feel pain below the level of the spinal cord lesion, so impulses generated in transmission cells must extend to the brain to be perceived. Many other sites thus exist in brain-stem and thalamus for further gating of this input before it reaches the cerebral cortex to intrude into consciousness. Some such higher 'gates' may be stimulus-specific—for example, the impact of arresting sights or sounds which can distract one from the pain of toothache. On the other hand, removal of all distractions will intensify the perception of pain, as happens in the dark silence and solitude of night, when pain is always at its worst.

One of the most exciting recent discoveries in neuroscience has been the demonstration of a pharmacological system in the brain which, by acting as an inbuilt source of an opiate-like substance, appears to be able to control the sensation of pain.

ENKEPHALINS AND PAIN

In 1973 a group led by Dr S. Snyder at the Johns Hopkins School of Medicine, Baltimore, demonstrated the existence of specific recognition sites in the brain for morphine and its analogues.[4] By 1975 the endogenous morphine-like enkephalins had been isolated by Hughes and Kosterlitz at the Unit for Research on Addictive Drugs in Aberdeen, and identified by the same team in collaboration with Dr H. R. Morris of Imperial College, London.[5] Subsequent work has established the pharmacological potency of such enkephalins and related opiate peptides (the endorphins).

Opiate receptors in the brain were identified and localized by being labelled with [^{3}H]naloxone or other ^{3}H-labelled opiates.[6] Specificity was established by the extent to which (−)-isomers of opiates displaced the ligand in comparison to (+)-isomers, e.g. levorphanol versus dextrophan. Such stereospecific opiate binding was found in fractions enriched in synaptic membranes. The density of the opiate receptor sites varies considerably in different parts of the brain. The highest concentrations of such sites have been found in areas of the limbic system in rat, monkey and humans, in particular in the amygdala and in the medial thalamic and midbrain periaqueductal grey matter. These areas correspond to the non-specific slow-conducting somatosensory projection pathways concerned with pain perception, as against the rapidly conducting site-specific spinothalamic pathways. High concentrations of opiate receptors have also been found in sensory input areas of the spinal cord. (Other cerebral sites of dense opiate receptor concentration are the head of the caudate nucleus and the hypothalamus, but their relevance to pain mechanisms is less certain.)

A series of opiate-like active peptides have been found in the central nervous system, derived from the C-terminal fragment of lipotropin. Lipotropin is split into its N-terminal fragment (amino acids 1–38), β-MSH (41–58) and C-fragment (β-endorphin; 61–91) (MSH is melanotropin, a peptide hormone). The C-fragment has many pharmacological effects when injected into the cerebral ventricles, including long-lasting analgesia—which is reversed by the specific narcotic analgesic drug, naloxone. Indeed, the C-fragment has an analgesic potency about 100 times that of morphine. (The smaller C^1-fragment [61–87] has much less analgesic activity.)

Smaller fragments still are derived by cleavage of the C-fragment of lipotropin into the endorphins (γ-endorphin [61–77], α-endorphin [61–76]) and the pentapeptide endorphins (methionine-enkephalin [61–65] and leucine-enkephalin [leucine^{65}-61–65]). The large opiate peptides—C-fragment (β-endorphin) and α- and γ-endorphin—have been identified definitively only in the pituitary, but the pentapeptide enkephalins are found throughout the brain. In contrast to the long-lasting biological action of C-fragment, that of enkephalins is very brief, possibly because they are rapidly metabolized by aminopeptidases. This explanation seems likely because synthetic analogues (obtained for example by replacing glycine in position 2 with D-alanine) are highly potent and long-acting analgesics.[8]

The distribution of enkephalins closely follows that of the opiate receptors, and enkephalin has been identified by immunochemical means in nerve terminals in the brains of animals and man.[9] Enkephalins are contained in the synaptosomal fractions of brain homogenates, are released by K^+ from brain synaptosomes,[10] and generally inhibit single neurons when applied to them iontophoretically (an effect reversed by naloxone).[11]

All this evidence is compatible with the notion that the enkephalins are neurotransmitter (or neuromodulator) agents in pathways acting at sites concerned with the transmission of signals indicating tissue injury. Indeed electrical stimulation of the periventricular and periaqueductal grey matter of the human brain can substantially relieve chronic pain, an effect blocked by the specific opiate antagonist naloxone.[12]

THE FUNCTIONAL CONTROL OF THE ENKEPHALIN SYSTEM

Is there a neural 'pain-controlling' system in the brain that constantly regulates the pain threshold by releasing enkephalins so that inputs signalling tissue injury are gated? And, if so, what controls this system?

Proof of the hypothesis has been difficult. If such a pain system is acting normally, then administration of naloxone or other specific opiate antagonists might be expected to provoke pain. In fact, naloxone given to normal subjects does not have this effect, even in heroic doses. However, it does appear to lower the pain threshold in some circumstances[13] but not in others.[14] This evidence is, perhaps, best interpreted as indicating that the activity of the enkephalin mechanism is low in normal circumstances. If this is the case then naloxone should intensify any pain already present, when presumably the pain control mechanism would be active. To some extent this has been found to be true.[15] Furthermore, people with severe chronic pain have been reported to possess less endorphin-like material than controls.[16] So far, however, the evidence for a significant naloxone-sensitive opiate/enkephalin system which controls the pain threshold in human beings is scanty. No doubt further work will resolve the matter.

If a pain control mechanism exists, it is easy to envisage it as causing pathological pain states. Indeed, since naloxone can objectively restore the transmission of pain impulses in the condition of congenital insensitivity to pain,[16] this illness has been attributed to an over-production of enkephalins. On the other hand, failure of enkephalin synthesis or action might cause spontaneous pain; if the deficit was localized, such pain might affect only specific parts of the body.

So far we know little about the factors that control the enkephalin system, or about the parts of the brain involved. Obviously it would be attractive to assume that electroanaesthesia and acupuncture activate enkephalin release. Also it is fascinating to contemplate the consequences of the brain controlling its own enkephalin system, either subconsciously or consciously. Such a mechanism would allow us to determine our own pain threshold at will. Perhaps that is just how saints, monks and fanatics allow themselves to be burnt alive or undergo tortures inflicted by themselves or others.

That the mind may control the brain's enkephalin system, at least subconsciously, is suggested by the recent experiments of Levine, Gordon and Fields.[15] These workers suggest that the opiate antagonist, naloxone, reversed the analgesia produced by a placebo in postoperative dental patients. In other words, they conclude that the pain relief generated by the patient's belief in an inactive drug substitute is brought about by the release of enkephalin. This observation certainly hints at the possibility of a subconscious cerebral control of enkephalin pain-relief mechanisms.

THE CEREBRAL CORTEX AND PAIN

As a generalization, human consciousness is a function of the cerebral cortex. Appreciation of pain depends on activity in the cerebral cortex and it is probably at this level that the various factors determining the significance and severity of pain interact. Thus when signals indicating tissue injury arrive in the somatosensory cortical areas, they will be shaped and interpreted in the light of visual, auditory and other information, and modified by memory and emotional context stored elsewhere in the brain. The final output may be interpreted as consciousness of pain, but where such a synthesis occurs is not known.

The cerebral cortex of man is not sensitive to pain, a fact that allowed early neurosurgeons to use local anaesthetics when they operated on the brain. Penfield,[17] in the course of such operations for epilepsy, also established that electrical stimulation of the human cerebral cortex did not evoke pain. Indeed, spontaneous focal electrical discharges in epilepsy do not, as a rule, cause an aura of pain, wherever they arise in the cortex. It appears that electrical stimulation of a single cortical point cannot cause the feeling of pain, so perhaps there is no one area in which pain is identified. Rather it may be necessary for a number of brain sites to be activated concurrently before this feeling is evoked—a situation that cannot be mimicked by spontaneous or surgically delivered electrical stimulation of one area.

The role of enkephalins in controlling cortical function is not yet known. However, opiates are renowned for their effects on mood and behaviour, and at least part of their analgesic action is the result of an effect on the individual's psychic reaction to pain, rather than a change in the perception of the stimulus causing it. Opiates allow the patient to dissociate the pain from the rest of mental life, which can then proceed in a more normal fashion. The vivid symptoms of narcotic addiction and withdrawal also presumably indicate the impact of opiates on cerebral function generally. Endogenous enkephalin systems may exert similar effects on higher mental function, and their role in psychiatric disease is currently under scrutiny.

MOOD, AMINES AND PAIN

Pain can provoke misery, but depression makes pain worse. Studies of the biochemistry of mood stemmed from the impact of drug action. Soon after the anti-hypertensive drug, reserpine, was introduced, it was found to provoke in some individuals a severe depression indistinguishable from the spontaneously occurring illness. Subsequent biochemical studies established that reserpine causes a profound depletion of the brain monoamines—dopamine, noradrenaline and serotonin. There followed the discovery that isoniazid lifted mood in patients treated for tuberculosis, and this lead was exploited to develop monoamine oxidase inhibitors for the treatment of depression. The antidepressant action of monoamine oxidase inhibitors was held to be due to their ability to increase the levels of amines in the brain by preventing metabolic breakdown of the amines. Such evidence led to the concept that depression arose as a result of decreased monoamine function, and various 'amine hypotheses' were proposed to explain affective disorders. Some held depression to be due to decreased noradrenaline and/or dopamine function in the brain —the 'catecholamine hypothesis'.[18] Others favoured a deficiency of serotonin.[19] These proposals received added support from the discovery that newer antidepressants also affected brain amine function.

The tricyclic antidepressants were found to inhibit amine reuptake mechanisms, thus increasing the concentrations of amines in the synaptic cleft.[20] Lithium, discovered to exert prophylactic action against manic-depressive illness, was found to enhance the cerebral action of serotonin, while electroconvulsive therapy was shown to increase the brain's sensitivity to serotonin and dopamine effects.[21] Furthermore, a disturbance of tryptophan, the precursor of serotonin, was linked to depression.[19]

Thus, there is a considerable body of evidence linking disordered amine function to altered mood states, so suggesting that opiates affect brain amines.

OPIATES AND AMINES

In experimental animals opiates have been found to influence amine function, and amines have been shown to affect the analgesic actions of opiates. Morphine and other opiate analogues cause behavioural changes reminiscent of those produced by inhibition of catecholamine action[22] and after brain catecholamine turnover.[23] Recently, enkephalins have also been found to stimulate striatal dopamine synthesis.[24]

Depletion of cerebral monoamines by reserpine has been found to reduce the analgesic actions of morphine in mice.[25] This has been taken to indicate that opiate analgesia is mediated via amine mechanisms, but whether this is via adrenergic[26] or serotonergic systems[27] is a question for debate. Most studies suggest the latter, for increasing brain serotonin or blocking cerebral serotonin uptake enhances morphine analgesia.[28] Recent studies have also shown that analgesia provoked by electrical stimulation of the brain, which is supposed to be opiate-mediated, depends on brain amine function.[29]

Thus there is now good evidence to suggest:

(1) That brain amine mechanisms control pain threshold in part at least by manipulating opiate action;

(2) That brain amines affect mood; and

(3) That opiates affect brain amines.

It follows that mood influences pain appreciation and that opiates alter mood. Such facts provide a chemical basis for well-established clinical observations, and open new avenues for the pharmacological control of pain. They also indicate that the brain may control its own input by specific chemical mechanisms. Abnormalities of such mechanisms may, therefore, generate spontaneous or distorted impressions of sensory input, including those interpreted as pain. The emotion of pain could even be produced by the brain itself, without external input. Finally, the distribution of the enkephalin system beyond the classical pain pathways raises the possibility that this system is concerned, not only with pain control, but also with these motor, emotional and social expressions of 'being hurt'.

References

1. MELZACK, R. & WALL, P. D. (1965) Pain mechanisms: a new theory. *Science (Wash. D.C.) 150*, 971–979
2. NATHAN, P. W. (1976) The gate-control theory of pain. *Brain 99*, 123–158
3. WALL, P. D. (1978) The gate control theory of pain mechanisms (a re-examination and re-statement). *Brain 101*, 1–18
4. PERT, C. B. & SNYDER, S. H. (1973) Opiate receptor: demonstration in nervous tissue. *Science (Wash. D.C.) 179*, 1011–1014
5. HUGHES, J., SMITH, T. W., KOSTERLITZ, H. W., FOTHERGILL, L. A., MORGAN, B. A. & MORRIS, H. R. (1975) Identification of two related pentapeptides from the brain with potent opiate agonist activity. *Nature (Lond.) 258*, 577–579
6. SMYTH, D. G., AUSTEN, B. M., BRADBURY, A. F., GEISOW, M. J. & SNELL, C. R. (1978) Biogenesis and metabolism of opiate active peptides, in *Centrally Acting Peptides* (Hughes, J., ed.), pp. 231–239, Macmillan, London
7. SNYDER, S. H., PASTERNAK, G. W. & PERT, C. B. (1975) Opiate receptor mechanisms, in *Handbook of Psychopharmacology*, vol. 5: *Synaptic Modulators* (Iversen, L. L., et al., eds.), pp. 329–360, Plenum Press, New York
8. PERT, C. B., PERT, A., CHANG, J. K. & FONG, B. T. W. (1976) D-Ala²-Met-Enkephalin-amide: a potent, long-lasting synthetic pentapeptide analgesic. *Science (Wash. D.C.) 194*, 330–332

9. Cuello, A. C. (1978) Endogenous opioid peptides in neurons of the human brain. *Lancet 2*, 291–293

10. Hughes, J., Kosterlitz, H. W., McKnight, A. T., Sosa, R. P., Lord, J. A. H. & Waterfield, A. A. (1978) Pharmacological and biochemical aspects of the encephalins, in *Centrally Acting Peptides* (Hughes, J., ed.), pp. 179–193, Macmillan, London

11. Bradley, P. B., Gayton, R. J. & Lambert, L. A. (1978) Electrophysiological effects of opiates and opioid peptides, in *Centrally Acting Peptides* (Hughes, J., ed.), pp. 215–229, Macmillan, London

12. Hosobuchi, Y., Adams, J. E. & Linchitz, R. (1977) Pain relief by electrical stimulation of the central gray matter in humans and its reversal by naloxone. *Science (Wash. D.C.) 197*, 183–186

13. Buchsbaum, M. S., Davis, G. C. & Bunney, W. E. Jr. (1977) Naloxone alters pain perception and somatosensory evoked potentials in normal subjects. *Nature (Lond.) 270*, 620–622

14. El-Sobky, A., Dostrovsky, J. O. & Wall, P. D. (1976) Lack of effect of naloxone on pain perception in humans. *Nature (Lond.) 263*, 783–784

15. Levine, J. D., Gordon, N. C. & Fields, H. L. (1978) The mechanism of placebo analgesics. *Lancet 2*, 654–657

16. Yanagida, H. (1978) Congenital insensitivity and naloxone. *Lancet 2*, 520–521

17. Penfield, W. & Rasmussen, T. (1955) *The Cerebral Cortex of Man*, Macmillan, New York

18. Schildkraut, J. J. (1965) The catecholamine hypothesis of affective disorders: a review of supporting evidence. *Am. J. Psychiatry 122*, 509–522

19. Editorial (1976) Tryptophan and depression. *Br. Med. J. 1*, 242–243

20. Iversen, L. L. (1973) Monoamines in the mammalian central nervous system and the action of antidepressant drugs. *Biochem. Soc. Spec. Publ. 1*, 81–96

21. Grahame-Smith, D. G. (1946) Cerebral mechanisms of mood and behaviour. *Psycholog. Med. 6*, 523–528

22. Kuschinsky, K. & Hornykiewicz, O. (1972) Morphine catalepsy in the rat: relation to striatal dopamine metabolism. *Eur. J. Pharmacol. 19*, 119–122

23. Sugrue, M. F. (1974) The effects of acutely administered analgesics on the turnover of noradrenaline and dopamine in various regions of the rat brain. *Br. J. Pharmacol. 52*, 159–165

24. Biggio, G., Cada, M. & Corda, M. G. (1978) Stimulation of dopamine synthesis in caudate nucleus by intrastriatal encephalins and antagonism by naloxone. *Science (Wash. D.C.) 200*, 552–554

25. Schneider, J. A. (1954) Reserpine antagonism of morphine analgesia in mice. *Proc. Soc. Exp. Biol. Med. 87*, 614–615

26. Verdernikov, Y. U. P. & Aflikanov, I. I. (1969) On the role of a central adrenergic mechanism in morphine analgesic action. *J. Pharm. Pharmacol. 21*, 845–847

27. Genovese, E., Zonta, N. & Mantegazza, P. (1973) Decreased antinociceptive activity of morphine in rats pretreated intraventricularly with 5,6-dihydroxy-tryptamine, a long-lasting selective depletor of brain serotonin. *Psychopharmacologia 32*, 359–364

28. Messing, R. B. & Lytle, L. D. (1977) Serotonin-containing neurons: their possible role in pain and analgesia. *Pain 4*, 1–21

29. Sandberg, D. E. & Segal, M. (1978) Pharmacological analysis of analgesia and self-stimulation elicited by electrical stimulation of catecholamine nuclei in the rat brain. *Brain Res. 152*, 529–542

Pain and the senses [Commentary]

DANIEL WIKLER

Program in Medical Ethics and Department of Philosophy, University of Wisconsin, Madison

Abstract There has been considerable philosophical debate over whether pain is a form of perception. A point of controversy is what pain is perception of; the best answer is neither pain-causing stimuli nor pain sensation but injury or the threat thereof. This answers the argument that pain cannot be perception because its 'objects' are private and exist only when perceived. A more potent argument is that pain is too poorly correlated with injury to count as perception of it. This issue is to be settled, in part, by determining the *function* of pain. The standard view of pain's function has here been contested and the resolution of the controversy will affect our inclination to ascribe to pain the status of perceptual faculty.

The papers of Professors Wall and Marsden show that pain and mood are intimately related. Professor Marsden points out the interaction of the biochemical determinants of each while, on the psychological level, Professor Wall postulates the existence of a comprehensive drive mechanism following injury in which both pain and mood alterations have important roles. Some of the effects of pain on mood, and vice versa, have been evident to clinical and even lay observers; but in these two papers the connections are present within the context of systematic neurological and psychological theory.

These positive theses accompany a negative one: that, contrary to the usual view of the matter, to have a pain is not to perceive. Wall finds pain ill-suited for inclusion in the class of senses such as vision and smell, suggesting that it belongs instead to the class of bodily feelings attendant to the major drives, such as those for food, water and oxygen.

It happens that one can also find considerable scepticism within the philosophical literature concerning the status of pain as a mode of perception. The doubts philosophers have voiced are different from Professor Wall's, but I believe them to be related, as I hope to show here.

The philosophical objections to classifying pain as a sense are to a degree independent of doubts about the inevitability of pain following injury—and in this way they differ from the objections listed by Professors Marsden and Wall. Some of the philosophers' objections would be pressed even were there an exact correlation, in both occurrence and magnitude, between injury and pain. The objections fall into two groups, distinguished by choice of the sort of thing which pain, were it a mode of perception, would be perception *of*. (For a full discussion of the points which follow, see Refs. 1 (ch. 14), 2, 3 and 4.)

The first sort of claim[4,5] proceeds from a general view of the nature of perception as the obtaining of information about the objective environment through the actions of the nervous system. The reason that pain is not perception, on this view, is that it does not give much information about the environment; at least, not information of the right kind. Floors and walls can cause pain in a person when the person falls on them or bumps into them but this does not give the victim information about any of their abiding qualities. These external objects are 'painful' in those encounters, but they do not have the abiding quality of painfulness and there is thus no quality to be perceived by a putative sensory mode of pain. This point, however, does not itself show that pain is not a mode of perception, in my view. It shows only that if pain is perception, it is not perception of such things as floors and walls. It remains possible that pain may be perception of some other kinds of things, namely states, events or qualities within the body. Of course, this latter possibility would appear to be blocked by the contention, mentioned above, that perception must be perception of the 'external world'. But this can be answered by a claim that much of a person's body is external in a relevant sense: external to the mind, or to the central nervous system. Limbs and other body parts are thus just as much elements of the external environment as the rest of the furniture of the world. Besides, hearing does not cease to be perception when it is used to monitor one's own heart beat; nor taste when one investigates the state of one's own mouth.

Objections have been put forward, however, even to the thesis that pain is perception of internal states. It is suggested that pain has several qualities which the classical modes of perception do not have, and which they could not have, given our concept of perception. They are:

(1) That pains are essentially *private*. Only I can feel my pains. The trees I see and the onions I smell, however, can in principle be perceived by others. In a way this is a restatement of the idea that perception must be of the objective world; pain is seen rather as a feature of the observer.

(2) That pains exist only when perceived; for a pain to exist *is* for it to be perceived. The things I see and hear exist independently of whether I (or anyone else) takes notice of them.

(3) Our perception of pain is incorrigible, i.e. one's belief that one is in pain cannot be doubted. This claim must be qualified a bit—it holds only for pains of substantial intensity and requires that the subject be attentive and not confused about what pain is. One still might quibble with this proposition but I think some version of it is true. The classical senses, on the other hand, are held to be inherently fallible: we hallucinate, encounter illusions, and have after-images. This does not mean that mistakes are inevitable; it would be conceptually possible that a lucky individual would never err in his or her life. The claim is rather that unless there exists the conceptual possibility of error in the use of a faculty, that faculty is not a mode of perception. Again, the picture is of the mind obtaining data about the contents of the world, not about its own contents, with which it is supposed to be immediately acquainted.

There are a number of moves open to the philosopher who wishes to maintain that pain is a mode of perception. One can try to argue that some or all of these features are inessential for perception. Or, one might insist that pain does meet these requirements. For example, it might be contended that pain is in principle public, its evident privacy being a result of the merely contingent fact that no one's pain sensors penetrate the skin of others (Siamese twins are perhaps the exception which proves the rule). Still another approach is to argue that when we speak of pain perception, the perception in question is not of pain *per se*—we *have* pain, are *in* pain, but do not perceive pain—but of injury. Injury is a public phenomenon (in principle) which exists even when unperceived by the victim who has a pain, and about which one can make perceptual mistakes. The experience of pain in the phantom limb would thus constitute a pain hallucination, the occurrence of which would prove the conceptual possibility of perceptual error cited as a requirement of perception in the third objection listed above.

Thus some degree of error would be essential for pain to be perception of injury; or at least the possibility of such error is essential. The mere existence of painless injury and of pain without injury would not cast doubt on the thesis that pain is perception, but would support it.

The existence of too much error, on the other hand, would undercut that thesis. A very low correlation between a kind of sensation or other mental event and some feature of the external world would be insufficient to establish that sort of sensation as perception; it would hardly serve as a means for obtaining information. This leads me directly to Professor Wall's remarks. Professor Wall informs us that pain-free injury and pain without injury occur frequently; perhaps regularly, in certain contexts. His findings indicate a far looser correlation of pain and injury than most lay observers realize. We must thus choose between demoting pain from its status as a mode of perception and continuing to ascribe that status to pain while admitting that it is a sense of the most rudimentary and inefficient kind. The various senses do vary a great deal in their informativeness and accuracy. As Armstrong[4] has noted, the use of vision as a paradigm of perception in this respect is misleading because (in human beings, at least) it far surpasses the other senses in precision and informativeness. What is needed is an account of the standards of accuracy which are to be required. This task will, I believe, be of more interest to philosophers than to scientists.

Professor Wall's attack on the characterization of pain as perception of injury, however, goes deeper than this. He is not merely questioning whether pain is sufficiently accurate as an indicator of injury to count as perception of it. As I understand it, his argument is about the function of pain (thus he speaks of seeking to learn the 'common biological significance' of pain as it occurs in various species). That pain is only a rough indicator of injury is no surprise, on his argument; for that is not what pain is for. Rather, it is (or is an element in) a drive, one directed at ensuring recovery.

If I am correct in interpreting Professor Wall's view as an ascription of function, then it consists of more than a mere claim that pain is correlated with the behaviour he describes. Other senses similarly point to behaviour. Bad smells drive us away from their source. It is true that the sense of smell is not always tied to avoidance, but perhaps this is, theoretically speaking, a biological accident. One can imagine a person—or a species—so constituted as to be unable to smell any but the vilest odours, so that any use of this faculty would lead to at least the holding of the nose. This eventuality would not cause us to revoke the status of sensory mode from smell. Nor would we do so, I believe, even were the impetus to cut off smell so overwhelming as to dominate the creature's thought and behaviour.

The thesis that pain's function is tied up with a drive to permit recovery is destructive to the characterization of pain as perception just because this classification rests on an assumption that pain has a different function. The function in question is, of course, transmission of information on injury, to be used for learning to avoid injury-causing stimuli, and for cutting injury short (where possible), as well as for arranging treatment. If this is not the function of pain, then the pain sensation is merely a sign or indicator which can be used to infer the desirability of these steps being taken but it does not exist for that purpose. By way of analogy: one can sometimes infer from the fact that one is shivering that one's body is cold, but shivering is not perception of cold; its function, so I have been told, is to stimulate the body to warm itself.

The designation of a different function for pain thus suggests that a search for standards of reliability for sensory modes is out of place and will not address the question of whether pain is a form of perception. Thus I believe I appreciate the significance of Professor Wall's project. I find myself left with some questions about it, however, which I would like to state briefly. Since I am neither biological theorist nor observer, I put these forward primarily as requests for elaboration.

The first is merely the personal observation that many injuries—perhaps most minor ones—do not feature the three stages Professor Wall outlined. And many occurrences of pain do not occur as parts of such sequences. This is true especially of relatively minor pains; but—or so I am told—it is at least sometimes true of excruciating pains, such as the passage of a kidney stone. Perhaps Wall's is a theory of injury (and its sequelae) as much as, or rather than, a theory of pain.

Second, it still seems that pain at least sometimes serves the purposes usually ascribed to it, such as teaching us to avoid future contact with hot stoves, which involve its serving as an information conduit. Professor Wall points out that hunger and other drives can also serve these ends, but if so this might only show that they too serve also as modes of perception (though this classification is dubious for other reasons).

My third and principal query concerns the exact role played by pain in the sequence of events following injury. The desirability (selective advantage) for any organism of at least part of this sequence is self-evident. But what is the desirability of pain's being an element in it? The attack on the injuror, the flight from the source of injury, and the organization of efforts to secure treatment can all occur in the absence of pain; indeed, in Professor Wall's Stage I this is what standardly occurs. The typical appearance of pain is only in the acute phase, his Stage II. The aggressiveness and agitation of creatures in this phase are characterized by Professor Wall as an irrational continuation of the first stage; if pain is responsible for this behaviour it serves no apparent purpose. What, then, is the function of pain? Professor Wall has shown that it 'announces' or 'signals' the onset of the third-stage depressed activity. For pain to have a function here, however, it would have to not only mark the transition to the much-needed Stage III but actually *cause* it. My question, then, is whether pain does cause the third stage to appear. If it does not cause it, it seems to be but an unfortunate, and dysfunctional, by-product of the reaction to injury. I might add that the existence of pain is unfortunate even if pain does have a causal role. As Professor Wall points out, hepatitis produces Stage III inactivity without the intervention of pain; and one could, perhaps, say the same of exhaustion after running a race. Pain, in comparison, would be a costly means to the end of recuperation.

It is conceivable that upon thorough acquaintance with the stages of reaction to injury, we would alter our concept of pain. The move I have in mind would be a definition of pain as whatever state it is that leads from Stage I to Stage III. If this were the case then my question about the function of pain receives an automatic answer. And this would be to assimilate pain to the other drives Professor Wall mentions. For hunger is, I take it, that state which disposes the organism to search for food. It is thus entirely proper to characterize a person as hungry even in the absence of any subjective sensations of hunger; if I deny that I feel hungry and then proceed to wolf down a large meal my hunger is retrospectively established. Perhaps some reservation is in order concerning this linguistic change, however, since pain seems to differ from hunger in this respect: if you do not feel it (and are not unduly distracted), you are not in pain (for an opposing view, see Palmer[7]).

If pain is not productive of the adaptive behaviour of Stages I and III, and if, as Professor Wall states, it is not of much use for avoiding injury either, then it is difficult to see why we do endure pain. This will, of course, be more bad news for theists. Though they are burdened with explaining how a benevolent God could permit injuries and other calamities to occur in the first place, the received view of pain which Professor Wall criticizes gave them the comfort of believing that the capacity for pain helps to keep the incidence and extent of injury under control. But an absence of an important causal role for pain would also have implications for Professor Wall's attack on the thesis that pain is perception of injury, as I reconstruct it. Though there is a sequence of states following injury of which pain is an element, it would not establish this role as the function of pain; and it was the identification of an alternative function for pain which suggested that the attempt to fix standards of accuracy should be abandoned so that classification of pain as a *bona fide* —if imprecise and limited—mode of perception could be justified. It remains possible, of course, that pain has *both* functions: that it be at once perception and drive.

I have but one point to make about Professor Marsden's paper, and it is a decidedly minor one. Considerable attention has been paid of late to the ethics of prescribing placebos. This practice is thought to involve several evils, but prime among them is the misrepresentation of the placebo by the physician as a potent analgesic. The experiment of Levine and colleagues[8] which Professor Marsden referred to suggests that the placebo relieves pain by stimulating the release of enkephalin, the endogenous opiate-like agent. If this is correct, future physicians can faithfully tell patients that the wonder drug they prescribe stimulates the production of biochemical agents which constitute the body's natural mechanism for pain control. Indeed, if scientists were to search for the perfect analgesic, perhaps a pill stimulating enkephalin release would be the result. The placebo-prescribing physician is thus giving patients now what pharmacologists may not be able to produce without years of scientific labour.

Of course, what the physician cannot tell the patient is that the pill works only because the patient does not believe that the reason that the pill works is that the patient believes that it does not work because of the patient's belief that it does work. But perhaps this slight mental reservation will have fewer untoward consequences than the more straightforward deception involved in current practice.

ACKNOWLEDGEMENTS

The author wishes to thank the Joseph P. Kennedy, Jr. Foundation for financial support and Fred Dretske, Dennis Stampe, and Abraham Wikler for helpful discussion and suggestions.

References

1. ARMSTRONG, D. M. (1968) *A Materialist Theory of the Mind*, Ch. 14, Routledge & Kegan Paul, London
2. PITCHER, G. (1970 Pain perception. *Philos. Rev. 79*, 368–393
3. CORNMAN, J. W. (1977) Might a tooth ache but there be no toothache? *Austr. J. Philos. 55*, 27–40
4. ARMSTRONG, D. M. (1972) *Bodily Sensations*, Routledge & Kegan Paul, London
5. GRICE, H. P. (1964) Some remarks about the senses, in *Analytical Philosophy (Series 1)* (Butler, R. J., ed.), Barnes & Noble, New York
6. McKENZIE, J. C. (1968) The externalization of pains. *Analysis 28*, 189–193
7. PALMER, D. (1975) Unfelt pains. *Am. Philos. Q. 12*, 289–298
8. LEVINE, J. D., GORDON, N. C. & FIELDS, H. L. (1978) The mechanism of placebo analgesics. *Lancet 2*, 654–657

Discussion: Pain and mood

Wall: I liked Dr Wikler's summary very much. There are just three points I want to correct. I spent perhaps too long talking about the poor relationship between injury and pain. In the paper as printed I emphasize that there is a very exact relationship between pain and actual behaviour. I relate pain not to injury but to the recovery process.

Second, I did not state that pain causes something. I said that pain is an awareness of a need state in which the body is moving towards a certain type of adaptive behaviour. That is very different from saying that pain causes that adaptive behaviour.

On the third point, I want to emphasize the common nature in man and animals of the chronic recovery phase. The deer show a period of restricted movement, disturbed eating, sleeping and social behaviour. On the one hand, one can say that this animal is demonstrating an adaptive process which is best suited to allow recovery from the wound. On the other hand one may say that the animal appears depressed. I suggest that an identical pattern is seen in humans during the late stages of the recovery process. There are some psychiatrists who believe that depression in a human who is not injured may have similar aspects except for pain. The depressed and grieving widow is reacting to the slings and arrows of outrageous fortune. The depressed recovering injured patient is reacting to real slings and arrows and has pain in addition. If the injury is real, the recovery state is associated with pain. If the injury is to the sense of well-being, the recovery process is identical except that there is no pain.

Wikler: My question remains, what is pain for? If we can get into the state without pain and if pain isn't what we thought it was, why did pain evolve?

Searle: I was brought up to believe that from an evolutionary point of view the function of pain is to make me want to get injured less. Indeed the paradigm case is the patient who can't feel any pain and is busy biting her tongue off, which I take it decreases her 'genetic fitness', as they say. You seem to be challenging that received view and it wasn't absolutely clear that you intended to.

Wall: I don't think pain necessarily does anything. It is correlated with learning to avoid future injury and with the state of treatment and recovery.

Fried: Wikler has again made what I consider to be a mistake about the way evolutionary explanations work. He somehow suggested that unless there is a necessary or sufficient connection between the phenomenon and what it is for, you haven't demonstrated that the phenomenon has that evolutionary function. That simply is not so. The argument that pain is *for* a number of things, in the only sense in which things are *for* anything in an evolutionary way, is not refuted by the observation that sometimes pain does not serve a function and that that function is sometimes served without pain.

An interesting way to look at pain and to show the way it does correlate with functions is this. Lawyers speak of pains and penalties and in a real sense pain is a sanction. If we regard pain as a penalty or fine imposed upon the organism, that explains why it is correlated, and why in an evolutionary way it would be correlated, with things in the way that Patrick Wall put it. For instance it explains why the pain need not invariably follow the stimulus. The pain has to be something which the animal will associate with the injury but it needn't follow it immediately. If it becomes a sanction then of course it can perform its evolutionary adaptive function of teaching the animal to avoid the painful stimulus, though not necessarily by immediately following the stimulus.

Itches and nausea also bring this out very well. An itch is a less acute form of pain. Is an itch a form of perception, or is nausea a form of perception? One wouldn't be inclined really to put that question, yet itches and nausea strike me as being very similar to pain. What is much more important, they serve the same function in adaptive and survival terms, and they show the same kind of looseness of fit to that function which Dr Wikler's insistence on necessary connections refuses to allow. Nausea is presumably connected with the vomiting of harmful substances but there are some harmful substances that we don't vomit and we die from them and there are other substances which we vomit which are not harmful. That doesn't mean that nausea doesn't have this adaptive function.

Wikler: If pain were a sanction, I presume it would have to have a causal role. If it had no causal power, it would not be an effective sanction. I take it that you believe pain's causal role and function to be that of steering organisms away from injurious stimuli. That seems to contradict, rather than support, Professor Wall's account. The question which I put to Professor Wall is what the causal role of pain actually is, if it is not the one you mention.

I agree with your statements about functions in biology. A faculty needn't invariably take a certain role for the role to be its function; nor must its action be necessary, since there may be fall-back systems in the body. Still, to determine the function of an organ or a faculty, one first finds out what it does, what role it plays in the organism's overall functioning. There is still considerable philosophical controversy over what *else* might be involved in making function statements.[1,2]

Bennett: Couldn't you put it in terms of whether it has a causal role and keep the word 'necessary' out?

Putnam: When you used the word *necessary*, Dr Wikler, the question was, would an organism have to develop a pain mechanism to serve these functions? The whole point of François Jacob's remark that *evolution is a tinker* is that evolution doesn't produce mechanisms which an organism has to have to do X. It finds one way of doing X.

Wikler: The question is, does it do X? Does it have a role at all?

Cooper: The question of what pain is for is a relevant question. Eighty per cent of the people sitting here will one day ask that as the most relevant question of their entire existence, as it obviously was in the mind of the man with prostatic cancer pictured by Professor Marsden. Perhaps one purpose of pain is to give the impulse to a freebooting doctor to find the cause of that pain or try to relieve it.

Blakemore: Surely the kind of pain induced by looking at other people in a state of injury is specifically the function of a social animal. I would predict that non-social animals don't have the sort of induced pain that we have when we look at a sick man. It is a way of identifying the state of another individual, of appreciating his feelings and therefore predicting what will be his reactions and needs.

Trevarthen: I am unhappy with the theory that pain is a sanction because babies rarely have the behavioural capacity to profit from experience of that kind. They are initially capable of projecting a general state of pain very powerfully. Quite soon they can indicate what part is hurting. I suggest that in humans pain is fundamentally associated with a need to 'tell' someone else that the pain exists. That makes it very difficult to ascribe pain to animals who are carrying out movements of self-care and recovery that are identical with the ones that humans do if they don't make any appeal. However, many animals such as dolphins and elephants make specific appeals for physical assistance from other animals. They indicate what kind of help they need and they don't need to do it linguistically. We use pain to tell doctors, surgeons and social workers what is wrong with us.

Armstrong: I have no objection to regarding itch as perception. (Nausea is harder!) Dan Wikler said that pain may be both perception and a drive. I think that is right. It is a perception, and in the cases that Professor Wall was pointing to, we simply don't have that perception. In massive injuries you don't get those perceptions. Pain helps you not to cut your fingers on razor blades and so on. What I suggest is that it is a perception that characteristically causes a drive. The perception and the drive can be dissociated. In some conditions which produce intractable pain, if a leucotomy is performed the patients report that they still have the pain, but that it doesn't worry them, there is no more drive. I take it that some causal pathway has been cut there, with the result that the patients don't have drive but simply have the perception.

Wall: That is another example of an *ad hoc* hypothesis for explaining the first stage of injury without pain. I spoke of massive injury because it is so surprising, both to the victim and the observer, but of course this applies even more to trivial injuries. It applies in the experimental laboratory where small stimuli are neglected or reacted to, depending on all sorts of contingencies. People are always introducing technical tricks to allow the maintenance of stimulus–response locked characteristics. The fact is that minor manipulations allow you to achieve any relationship you please between injury and pain.

Dunstan: I have been reflecting on the way in which we complicate our problems by the words we use. Earlier we did it with 'dualism'. The whole discussion was overshadowed by that dreadful defection of Platonism and Neoplatonism from Aristotle in the use of *psyche, anima,* 'the soul', Our western sentiments are thoroughly and incorrigibly dualistic: 'John Brown's body lies amouldering in the grave, but his soul goes marching on'—a sentiment that half the world would associate with Christianity, but which is in fact alien to it. This shadow hovered over our discussion when we used 'dualism' for a totally different purpose in the body–mind discussion, and it clouded it. Today we do the same, with different words.

In England we have used 'pain' for the experience of being hurt only since the later Middle Ages. That highly legalistic and moralistic epoch took the word 'pain' out of *poena,* the Latin for penalty or punishment; this was the earlier meaning of 'pain'—Charles Fried has alluded to it. Before we thus confused suffering with the notion of inflicted 'pain' we used the word 'hurt'; we took it from the Old French and so from Germanic roots, and we gave it a peculiarly English development to mean an injury or wound. We also used, in those early times, the word 'smart', another from the German, whose first meaning was a sharp physical pain. It is very interesting to me that we now use the words 'hurt' or 'smart' for sensations of lesser intensity, and 'pain' for those of greater intensity. Mediaeval poets and mystics (like Richard Rolle of Hampole) used 'smart' for the sufferings of the crucified Christ, with no intention whatever of making light of that suffering. Similarly we have altered the meaning of 'injury'. An injury, from the Latin *injuria,* is primarily a wrong—*volenti non fit injuria,* we can say, in a context divorced from physical harm. Now we use it for precisely that, and nothing of the old sense remains, except the notion that the body ought not to be so harmed, even by accident.

Then a crude theology, or cosmology, intrudes into the question of cause and effect. When trouble strikes, the ancestral cry is 'Why should it happen to me?'—as though an omnipotent but unpredictable deity had inflicted it as a pain, a punishment for sins unknown. This compound of legalism, moralism and a primitive cosmology masquerading under the name of religion complicates and clouds our understanding of pain as a physiological phenomenon and response.

Crow: On a biological and anatomical basis it seems to me that pain is like gustation or olfaction, which are other modalities which seem to have a direct relationship to a drive. These seem to have an *a priori* biological significance that vision and hearing do not have. There is an anatomical differentiation: vision, hearing and somatic touch have somatotopic representations in the cortex whereas, as far as I know, gustation, olfaction and pain have no such representation. There seems to be a dichotomy of sensory modalities. One group (gustation, olfaction and pain) has a direct relationship with drives and the other does not (vision, hearing and somatic touch).[3]

In embryological terms there is a sense in which the modalities in the first group (gustation and olfaction, in particular, and perhaps pain also) are related to visceral afferent pathways, whereas those in the second group are more closely related to somatic afferent structures. When one considers the phenomena of learning and conditioning, the stimuli which can act as primary reinforcers or unconditioned stimuli are all in the first group whereas conditioned stimuli and discriminative stimuli are generally those which utilize visual, auditory and somatic sensory pathways, i.e. those modalities which have a spatially organized representation in the cerebral cortex. Thus it seems that, in the course of learning, significance is imparted to neutral stimuli arriving in the cerebral cortex by way of the specific visual, auditory and somatic sensory pathways by the association of these stimuli with 'drive-related' stimuli in the gustatory, olfactory and nociceptive pathways.

Young: Although pain and gustation do not have those representations they do have the overall representation that we have heard about from Marsden. For example the locus coeruleus projects to every part of the cortex. Indeed this must be so because we can learn, and we need to learn, about correlations of events with taste, smell, and pain. The information gets to the cortex somehow but there is no specific area for them. The gustation signals are everywhere and the pain signals are everywhere.

Ploog: I think that sensation is something which basically does not have to be learnt. If you put a sugar solution in the mouth of a newborn baby it will show you by its facial expression that it senses sweetness.[4]

Young: I didn't mean that we had to learn sweetness or pain but that the information on sweetness and pain had to be associated with other things.

Ploog: I quite agree, but it is perhaps somewhat different for the emotions. A certain set of emotions seems to exist for all humans, but we cannot learn those emotions; there is no copy to learn from; there is no firm association between certain emotions and certain objects as there is with sensations and objects.

In regard to pain it is peculiar that in German these things are mixed up. We have the word *Schmerzgefühl* for the emotion of pain and the word *Schmerzempfindung* for the sensation of pain.

This brings me to what Colin Blakemore said. It seems that what I really sense is context-dependent and nearly always related to a social situation. And the more it is related to a social situation, the more it is related to emotion. That is, there are not two categories but a continuum. Professor Wall's discourse on emotion and sensation in regard to pain shows us that this pain sensation has a very specific place in our evaluation of stimuli that we experience.

Young: It is also correlated with learning.

Blakemore: I want to question the criteria that we seem to be adopting for believing that there is a dichotomy between things like pain or hunger and other 'real' sensations. There are three grounds that are being raised for this. One is a lack of understanding of the stimulus. That is a relatively trivial reason: just because we don't understand the physical stimuli involved in pain, we can't see a constant relationship between stimulus and sensation. But that is not a good reason for abandoning the idea that there *is* such a simple sensory relationship. We don't understand much about the olfactory stimulus, yet no one will challenge the idea that smelling is a basic sensation.

Secondly, Pat Wall raised the question of the reliability of pain as an indicator of stimulation. Although there is clearly a difference in degree I don't think there is a difference in kind between, say, vision and pain in this respect. We all know of cases where we have *seen* things that did not exist, and we sometimes fail to see things that do exist, or even see things that change their form from moment to moment.

Finally, the idea that hearing and seeing are ends in themselves whereas things like pain and hunger lead only to expressions of drive is surely a matter of the information content and the choice of action presented by each particular sensation. The availability of action presented by a pain is very limited. Therefore the direction of action is much more concentrated than the plans of action that can be elicited by a particular visual sensation. Seeing a visual scene presents almost an infinite variety of possible actions. Perception isn't an end in itself even for vision, but is a large set of plans of action.

Crown: When the physiologists, neurologists, sociologists, surgeons and lawyers have finished with pain, psychiatrists often end up with the problem. Organic medicine assumes that if people say they have pain, they have pain. Psychiatrists are put in the paradoxical position of telling patients that they haven't 'really' got pain because other relevant specialists have 'shown' that they can't possibly have it.

Another difficulty is what therapy to give to people who think they have pain but who haven't 'really' got it. Psychoanalysts might try to get their patients to see what else the pain symbolizes. Behaviourists, such as Fordyce,[5] have developed forms of behaviour modification for modifying pain behaviour. Fordyce attempts to modify the environmental rewards patients get from having pain, e.g. extra attention, until they learn not to have pain or at least not to show pain behaviour.

Marsden: There is a category of psychiatric patients who complain of pain but do not exhibit the suffering of pain. There are also large numbers of patients who complain of pain and exhibit the suffering of pain but whose doctors cannot explain why they have pain, so they too may end up in psychiatric hands. Those are two separate categories.

Blakemore: Do patients in the second category respond to morphine?

Marsden: No.

Brazier: Nobody has mentioned the problem of memory in discussing whether pain is a sensation or a perception. Neuroscientists will tell you that pain fibres do not reach the association cortex. We can reconstruct our other sensations or perceptions such as seeing or hearing but I have no way of reconstructing the sensation of pain. That last remark is about myself because we can only judge pain in other people by their behaviour.

Crow: But you can't construct olfactory and gustatory sensations either, can you?

Brazier: I wouldn't absolutely agree with you. I think I can taste caviare. A different neuronal circuit is involved in smell and taste.

Putnam: David Armstrong said that pain may be a perception which normally triggers a drive. This sounded very plausible to me but I didn't see how it was compatible with what he said in his paper, and I didn't understand what he said there. If pain is a perception of an injury then it is not a proprioception of a mental state. I take it, David, that you think there can be unconscious perception, that the truck drivers in your example may not be conscious, but are nevertheless perceiving? So there is a distinction in your view between conscious pain and unconscious pain, and we have a conscious pain when we have a proprioception of the unconscious pain. At this point I lose my grip totally. First I would ask the Popperian question, what would falsify that? One way of interpreting your view would be to identify it with Dennett's[6] view that a conscious sensation is something like an *input to the speech centre*. You might say that we have a conscious pain when there is not only whatever takes place when we have what you want to call unconscious pain, but also a *judgement* that that has taken place, an input to the speech centre. But then I think you will get into trouble with the phenomenon of automatic speech.

Armstrong: I think that you have confused proprioception with introspection. Proprioception is perception of one's own bodily states. Introspection is perception of one's own mental states. They are quite different from each other. I think that pain is proprioceptive perception (but one which characteristically causes a drive) and that one may or may not introspect that perception. If you introspect it you are aware of it, you are conscious of it; if you don't introspect it, which happens in some odd cases, you have unconscious pain.

Bunge: Instead of asking what is the purpose of pain, we should ask, as others have already done: what, if any, is the biological value or evolutionary advantage of pain? Feeling pain is not a purposive action, though it may trigger such actions. If we don't ask this we will be taken for vitalists.

Professor Marsden claimed to be a dualist and a phenomenalist but I haven't seen any evidence in his paper that he regards the mental as being immaterial or as not being in the brain. Everything he said is compatible with the materialist view that mental events are brain events.

Thirdly, what is wrong with regarding pain as a drive, provided one regards it not as causing or as being caused by the drive but as being a physiological imbalance, which in turn may of course trigger behaviour of some kind?

Wall: There are many different ways of measuring pain. They all amount to helping the subject to verbalize.

Bunge: So they are not objective measures?

Wall: No.

Bunge: Couldn't you measure, let's say, the firing frequency of nerve fibres to assess the intensity of pain?

Wall: No. You can measure nerve impulses to assess the intensity of injury but not of pain.

Bunge: Do you mean it is possible in principle to measure pain but that no one has succeeded in doing this yet?

Bennett: Have I understood that the answer is that something can be measured but it won't be pain?

Marsden: We can measure nerve impulses which are going to the brain, which may or may not be interpreted as pain.

Plum: Does painless trauma ever occur in settings where vigorous activity is not involved?

Wall: I spoke of the dramatic circumstances of no pain in the presence of massive injury. Irrespective of the amount of activity, if attention is focused on some more impelling event than the injury, pain may be absent. A sewing-machine operator may have needles pass through the finger without noticing any pain, if attention is intensively directed at some other part of the task. A much more common event which presents a serious clinical problem is that even when pain occurs, its intensity is poorly related to the amount of tissue damage.

Creutzfeldt: The discussion is leading us again to the problem of mixing up phenomenological levels, which I won't talk about now. As neurophysiologists, however, we should realize that what might be called pain pathways are different from other sensory pathways. The activity elicited by fibres that are supposed to transmit pain is transmitted to the nervous system in a very different way from, say, the activity of auditory nerve fibres. There is no localized cortical representation of pain. On the other hand, if one produces a painful stimulus in the muscle, for example, the activity of the whole spinal cord, including motor neurons, is upset. So it looks as if the activity of 'pain fibres' produces a very dramatic and very generalized effect on nervous activity, unlike activation of the specific senses which we were discussing earlier. We are dealing with different neurophysiological mechanisms as well as with different types of sensations.

Regarding the distinction between protection and recovery I think these are not mutually exclusive but rather complementary, and they are certainly both true.

Blakemore: In thinking about pain as a social response a very pertinent case to consider is childbirth. Pain is partly a response to the expectation of whether the situation should be painful. In some societies childbirth is not considered to be worthy of pain and pain is not reported under those circumstances.

Wall: That is really anecdotal.

Searle: I don't believe it, so far.

Blakemore: Then what about the situation in which cervical dilatation during delivery produces intense pain, whereas episiotomy a few seconds later produces no painful reaction at all? What do you say to that?

Wall: That is an example of the contingent effect of the circumstances. What you or what somebody else is doing has a strong effect on the amount of pain evoked by equal amounts of injury.

Towers: The pain fibres which enter the spinal cord end on nerve cells almost immediately. There is a decussation almost immediately at the spinal cord level, whereas sensations which are dealing with much more localized and sensitive things such as fine touch tend to go a long way up the central nervous system and synapse very high up before decussating. This implies to me that the pain fibre is likely to have a much wider distribution than other modalities, because the second-order neuron is much longer. The trigeminal nerve is the most sensitive of all the somatic nerves of the body and has the largest representation in the cerebral cortex because the whole face area has such large cerebral representation. The trigeminal nerve enters at the level of the pons; the trigeminal nucleus descends all the way to the substantia gelatinosa in the spinal cord. The first-order neurons conveying fine touch end at a high level and are then distributed by point to point localization up to the thalamus and then to the cerebral cortex. The pain fibres are represented by the descending tract of the trigeminal nerve and they synapse way down in the spinal cord. Therefore when they go back up again in the second-order neuron presumably they have a wider distribution. It is very interesting that enkephalins are found in the substantia gelatinosa at a high level of the spinal cord. This has always seemed to me something like the difference between the sympathetic and the parasympathetic innervation of organs in the body, where the sympathetic tends to have its second-order neurons a long way from the organ innervated. The sympathetic thus innervates over a very wide area, whereas the parasympathetic system has its second-order neurons starting very close to the organ innervated and tends to be very localized.

Wall: One of my theses here is that we should consider the sensation of pain as being in a different class from the sensation of touch. In tissue there are nerve endings which detect injury and give a very accurate account of its location, nature and extent. These are injury detection fibres and should not be called pain fibres. If we see an action potential from them we can make a very definite statement about what has happened at the periphery. But we cannot make a prognostic statement about what will happen. We heard from Colin Blakemore a proper defence of the classical proposal that a spectrum of events occur, some of which are neutral in terms of what one does about them and others which have an imperative order associated with them. We have also just heard about the transmission pathways and various links going upwards to the cortex. I would add that there are very strong feedback pathways, so that the input is under control, partly from the brain and partly from other events in the periphery. The classical view is that a very highly organized afferent pathway provokes first something called 'sensory pain'. First there is a stimulus which provokes a pure sensation, then the sensation is dressed up with memories, feelings, etc. and becomes a perception, and then the perception is used to trigger a drive. Thus, the route from stimulus to reaction passes through a set of blocks for which I would maintain there is absolutely no evidence. You are not aware consciously of the input. The input must exist for you to have pain but you are not aware of it until it has triggered an internal body state. That state is what you are aware of and what you call pain. That summary refers to many of the things we have been talking about. I am challenging the concept that a stimulus leads to sensation as an independent event examinable by the consciousness, and leads after that to something called perception, which is again examinable and which may or may not lead to action. I am proposing that there are non-examinable events which trigger examinable events. In the case of pain, we are speaking of the awareness of the consequence.

Cooper: Fred Plum suggested that there may be pharmacological factors which we do not yet know. Professor Marsden, is your example of people who innately never feel pain a model which suggests that pain, before we add anxiety and learning, is in fact a perception which depends on precisely the pharmacological factors that you outlined so beautifully?

Marsden: I agree entirely with Professor Wall's concept. I would add that people who are taking opiates for pain tell you that they perceive the pain still but they are not distressed by it. They experience a perception which they describe by the word pain, but they can dissociate themselves from it and from the unpleasant consequences.

Wikler: It seems to me that though both physiologists and philosophers are concerned over whether pain is perception, the sources of concern are different. The scientific issue is pain's location in the causal sequence of events proceeding from injury; specifically, whether adaptive injury-related behaviour is mediated by awareness of pain. The philosopher's interest is in a conceptual question: how a faculty's function, causal role and degree of reliability are to be understood as determining whether it is a perceptual faculty. The criteria derived from the philosopher's efforts, combined with factual results of the scientists, would yield a judgement on whether a patient in pain is perceiving.

References

1. WRIGHT, L. (1976) *Teleological Explanation*, University of California Press, Berkeley and Los Angeles
2. CUMMINS, R. (1975) Functional analysis. *J. Philos. 72*, 741–765
3. CROW, T. J. (1973) Catecholamine-containing neurons and electrical self-stimulation: a theoretical interpretation and some psychiatric implications. *Psychol. Med. 3*, 66–73
4. STEINER, J. E. (1974) Innate, discriminative human facial expressions to taste and smell stimulation. *Ann. N. Y. Acad. Sci. 237*, 229–233
5. FORDYCE, W. E. (1976) *Behavioural Methods in Chronic Pain and Illness*, Mosby, St Louis, Mo.
6. DENNETT, D. (1978) *Brainstorms*, Bradford Books, Montgomery, Vermont

Schizophrenia: the nature of the psychological disturbance and its possible neurochemical basis

T. J. CROW

Division of Psychiatry, Clinical Research Centre, Northwick Park Hospital, Harrow, Middlesex

Abstract The diagnosis of schizophrenia is established principally by the presence of certain psychological symptoms which although subjective can be reliably assessed by standardized interviewing procedures. The most characteristic symptoms (Schneider's first-rank symptoms) fall into three groups: (a) auditory hallucinations of particular types, (b) 'ego-boundary disturbances', including intrusions into the stream of consciousness attributed to external agencies, and (c) delusional perception. Symptoms closely resembling those seen in schizophrenia can be induced in non-schizophrenic individuals by amphetamine-like drugs, and both these symptoms and those of schizophrenia are ameliorated by neuroleptic drugs (the major tranquillizers). Amphetamines facilitate and neuroleptic drugs diminish neural transmission mediated by the chemical substance dopamine. In recent post-mortem studies on patients who had suffered from schizophrenia, it was found that dopamine release was not increased. However, in some cases there was evidence of increased sensitivity of the dopamine receptor.

THE CONCEPT OF SCHIZOPHRENIA

Schizophrenia is the term introduced by E. Bleuler to denote those disturbances of psychological function which Kraepelin had previously grouped together under the heading of dementia praecox. Kraepelin attempted a great simplification of the previously chaotic psychiatric nosology by giving a single label to a number of diverse but overlapping symptom-clusters which he considered to have a similar course and outcome. In developing Kraepelin's disease concept Bleuler thought he could discern a pattern of fundamental symptoms from which the more variable 'secondary' symptoms could be seen to be derived. Although the disease concept of schizophrenia has been widely accepted, it is increasingly recognized[1] that neither Kraepelin nor Bleuler

335

achieved their objectives of delineating a group of psychiatric illnesses of similar outcome or underlying psychological dysfunction, and of distinguishing them with precision from other psychiatric syndromes. Yet because these illnesses are common, with a lifetime prevalence perhaps as high as 1% in many populations,[2] and include the most severe, progressive and debilitating psychiatric diseases, the question of the definition of schizophrenia continues to be of considerable practical importance.

This question may also be of more general scientific and philosophical interest. Firstly the aetiology, or primary causation, of these illnesses is still obscure. Many psychiatrists, probably a large majority, believe that some specific alteration of brain function is involved. They hope that in due course this abnormality will be revealed and it may then be possible to diagnose schizophrenia on the basis of a laboratory test. However, until that time the diagnosis remains one which is based upon a description by the patient of his or her own subjective symptoms. This is the second point of general interest. The patient describes particular subjective experiences which are qualitatively different from normal experience, are not shared by the examiner, but are recognized by the examiner as belonging to a class of experience regularly reported by other patients with similar life problems. It is on this foundation that the disease concept, and inference of specific abnormality, rests. The third point is that, with increasingly sophisticated methods for eliciting psychological symptoms (i.e. the development of standardized interview techniques), it appears that those symptoms which are the most reliable discriminators of the illnesses that psychiatrists call schizophrenic are abnormalities of mechanisms for establishing beliefs about the nature of the external world, for distinguishing internal subjective from external perceived experience, and for establishing the identity and limits of the self.

THE DIAGNOSIS OF SCHIZOPHRENIA

In principle schizophrenia (or the group of schizophrenias) is readily distinguished from two other major classes of serious psychiatric disturbance, the 'organic' disorders and the affective psychoses. In the organic disorders (i.e. the confusional states and dementias) there is often an identifiable physical cause of the mental disturbance. These illnesses are associated with what psychiatrists refer to as disturbances of consciousness. By this they mean principally that there is loss of orientation with respect to time or place. Orientation in this sense depends on the ability to receive and assimilate sensory information, and it appears that the disturbance of orientation in the organic psychoses is part of a more general impairment of the neural mechanisms for acquiring new information, i.e. of learning. It is generally held, and was emphasized by Bleuler in particular, that consciousness in this sense is not impaired in schizophrenia. There is doubt whether this is true of some chronic schizophrenic patients[3,4] but it appears generally to be the case in acute schizophrenia.

Affective disorders are defined as those in which the primary disturbance is one of mood. Disturbances of perception, e.g. hallucinations, or of thought content, e.g. delusions, if they occur are seen as secondary consequences of the disturbance of mood, e.g. of depression or elation. Mood disturbance occurs frequently in schizophrenic illnesses but the other psychotic phenomena which are likely to be present cannot be seen as arising from the mood change. This criterion provides a rule of thumb for distinguishing the affective from the schizophrenic psychoses: but it is not a reliable one since what can and cannot be seen as secondary to mood change will vary considerably, depending on the assessor.

Kraepelin's own criterion for distinguishing the affective from the schizophrenic psychoses (in his terminology dementia praecox) was outcome. From an affective illness complete recovery can be expected, while schizophrenic patients seldom return to their premorbid personalities, and there may well be progressive deterioration. Kraepelin himself recognized that this was no more than a generalization, and recent work[5,6] has established that even with the most stringent diagnostic criteria the outcome of illnesses described as schizophrenic is highly variable. Moreover, a diagnosis which is established only on the basis of outcome has lost one of its principal functions: to predict the course of the illness over time.

Thus it is apparent that to define a disease either by the exclusion of other diseases or retrospectively in terms of its outcome is unsatisfactory. It is highly desirable that it be defined by the presence of features or symptoms which are specific to that disease. It was to this problem that Bleuler addressed himself in formulating his 'primary' (or 'fundamental') symptoms which were regarded as characteristic of schizophrenia and present to some degree during all stages of the illness. These symptoms included a disturbance of the associations between ideas, specific changes in affective responses, and ambivalence, or the presence at the same time of positive and negative attitudes to a person, action or idea. Unfortunately neither Bleuler nor subsequent workers have been able to devise operational definitions which can be applied reliably to the individual case. Therefore, Bleuler's hypothesis that these symptoms are always present remains untested and may be untestable.

FIRST-RANK SYMPTOMS

A more direct and practical approach was proposed by K. Schneider, who suggested that there are certain symptoms ('symptoms of the first rank') whose presence defines an illness as schizophrenic. These symptoms need not be present, and in particular need not be present at all times, for an illness to be schizophrenic, but if they are present, Schneider suggests, we can agree that the disturbance is in the category which we wish to label as schizophrenia. Schneider adds the exclusion clause that organic illness (i.e. known structural disease of the brain) must be absent, but in practice this is seldom an issue.

Schneider's first-rank symptoms are:

(1) Hearing one's thoughts spoken aloud within one's head;
(2) Hearing voices arguing;
(3) Hearing voices that comment on what one is doing at the time;
(4) Experiences of bodily influence;
(5) Thought withdrawal, thought insertion, and other forms of thought interference;
(6) Thought diffusion;
(7) Delusional perception; and
(8) Everything in the spheres of feeling, drive and volition which the patients experience as imposed or influenced by others.[7,8]

Schneider regarded these symptoms not as a description of the central disturbance, as Bleuler had intended of his fundamental symptoms, but as a pragmatic approach to diagnosis. Schneider's symptoms, unlike Bleuler's, can be reliably assessed by independent observers. This has been demonstrated in work with the Present State Examination (the PSE), a standardized interview developed by Wing and his colleagues,[9] which has been quite extensively tested in cross-national studies of the reliability of psychiatric diagnosis.[10] The PSE includes items relating to each of Schneider's first-rank symptoms and specifies both what the feature to be elicited should consist of and how it should be searched for.

For example, *thought insertion* is described in the glossary thus: 'the essence of the symptom is that the subject experiences thoughts *which are not his own* intruding into his mind. The symptom is not that he has been caused to have unusual thoughts (for example, if he thinks the Devil is making him think evil thoughts) but that the thoughts *themselves* are not his. In the most typical case, the alien thoughts are said to have been inserted into the mind from outside, by means of radar or telepathy or some other means . . .'.

The symptom is to be sought for, at the appropriate point in the structured interview, by the question: 'Are thoughts put into your head which you know are not your own?', with the follow-up questions 'how do you know they are not your own?' and 'where do they come from?' if the examiner feels the response to the first question suggests the symptom may be present.

The first of Schneider's symptoms (sometimes referred to as *thought echo*) is elicited by the question: 'Do you ever hear your own thoughts repeated or echoed?', with 'what is it like?', 'how do you explain it?, and 'where does it come from?' as possible follow-up questions.

Delusions of control, a category which includes the last of Schneider's symptoms, is described as: '... the subject experiences his will as replaced by that of some other force or agency... The basic experience may be elaborated in various ways—the subject believes that someone else's words are coming out using his voice, or that what he writes is not his own, or that he is the victim of possession—a zombie or a robot controlled by someone else's will, even his bodily movements being willed by some other power'.

Delusional perception is a type of delusion which is exceptional in that it arises directly from a perception. For this reason the examiner is able to discern that it is not secondary to some other pathological process.[11] Such delusions are sometimes referred to as primary delusions, the patient suddenly becoming convinced that a particular event has special meaning.

Two examples illustrate this phenomenon:

A young Irishman was at breakfast with two fellow-lodgers. He felt a sense of unease, that something frightening was going to happen. One of the lodgers pushed the salt cellar towards him (he appreciated at the time that this was an ordinary salt cellar and his friend's intention was innocent). Almost before the salt cellar reached him he knew he must return home, 'to greet the Pope, who is visiting Ireland to see his family and reward them ... because our Lord is going to be born again to one of the women ... And because of this they (all the women) are all born different with their private parts back to front'.[12]

An Englishman was standing in a bar in a small town in New York State when his American brother-in-law picked up a long straight biscuit from the counter and said, 'Have one of these. They are salty'. Immediately the patient realized that his brother-in-law was accusing him of being a homosexual and was organizing a gang to spy on him.[13]

The essence of the symptom is that the delusion arises *de novo*, and that the patient invests a particular event or perception with a significance which cannot be understood either in terms of the event itself or the patient's previous life history.

THE MEANING OF FIRST-RANK SYMPTOMS

Although at first sight they appear quite heterogeneous Schneider's symptoms fall into three categories:

(1) Special forms of auditory hallucinations (symptoms 1 to 3 above).

(2) Varieties of what has been referred to as 'ego-boundary disturbance' —this group includes apparent loss of subjective control over thought processes, actions and emotions, and the attribution of subjectively experienced mental phenomena to an external agency (symptoms 4, 5, 6 and 8 above), and

(3) Delusional perception (symptom 7 above).

In spite of Schneider's denial that he was attempting to describe the disease process, it seems plausible that if these symptoms discriminate a schizophrenic illness, or a particular type of schizophrenic illness, they do in some way reflect on the underlying disturbance. An explanation either in psychological or neurological terms of how these symptoms originate would surely greatly illuminate the pathophysiology of schizophrenia.

Auditory hallucinations presumably arise when internally generated stimuli acquire the attributes of stimuli from the external world. The origin of two of Schneider's symptoms, hearing one's thoughts spoken aloud and hearing voices comment on what one is doing, can be relatively easily traced. Frith[14] has pointed out that much processing of sensory and other information normally takes place below the level of consciousness. If the schizophrenic became aware of part of this normally subconscious process, these symptoms could be understood. What is not entirely clear, however, is why such sensory processing should be experienced as external stimulation. Is there something about the mechanism of consciousness which determines that any intruding activity shall be treated as information from the external world?

The ego-boundary disturbances are not unrelated in form to the auditory hallucinations. Again patients appear to have lost control of their sequences of thought or actions, and mental contents which they do not recognize as their own appear in their conscious awareness.

Delusional perception by contrast seems unrelated to either of these two groups of symptoms. In this case it appears that a mechanism which normally operates either to attach significance to sensory stimuli which in reality have turned out to have particular meaning for the individual, or to terminate a problem-solving sequence of thoughts by recording and labelling the correct solution, is operating autonomously without regard to the facts of the external situation or to the correctness of the solution.

Any neurophysiological explanation of the subjective phenomena of schizo-phrenia should take into account that:

(1) The normal individual has no difficulty in distinguishing those mental events which arise from stimuli in the external world from those which arise internally, while the schizophrenic treats much that arises internally as relating to the external world. It seems likely that the schizophrenic is abnormally aware of internally-arising stimuli, and may be conscious of classes of information-processing activity of which the normal individual has no awareness.

(2) Normal individuals have a control over their sequences of thought and action which is a coherent and continuous process, and is experienced by them as relating only to themselves. For schizophrenic patients this process is disrupted by events unrelated to this sequence of willed thoughts and actions, and they experience the interruption as arising not from their own irrelevant mental activity but from outside themselves.

(3) Some mental mechanism for evaluating the significance of events or stimuli in the external world and for registering the successful conclusion of a sequence of problem-solving mental activity must operate in the normal individual, and apparently operates inappropriately in schizophrenia.

A POSSIBLE NEUROCHEMICAL BASIS OF SCHIZOPHRENIA

For over twenty years it has been recognized that the symptoms of schizophrenia can be significantly alleviated by administration of certain drugs (termed neuroleptics) of which chlorpromazine is the prototype. More recently it has been found that schizophrenic symptoms can also be exacerbated, and can be mimicked in normal subjects, by administration of amphetamine and related compounds. Individuals who self-administer the amphetamines[15,16] and volunteers who have received increasing doses of amphetamine in an experimental situation[17,18] are reported to experience many of Schneider's first-rank symptoms, including the development of primary delusions.

These pharmacological observations may throw light on the neurochemical basis of schizophrenia. Amphetamine exerts at least some of its central actions by facilitating the release of the neurotransmitter dopamine from certain localized neural pathways within the brain. Thus the psychological effects of the amphetamines, and by analogy the changes in schizophrenia, may be due to excessive activity of central dopaminergic pathways. Neuroleptic drugs also have actions on dopaminergic mechanisms but diminish rather than facilitate transmission. There is good evidence that the antischizophrenic effects of these drugs are related to their actions on central dopaminergic transmission.[19] There is also evidence from post-mortem studies that although the activity of dopamine neurons probably is not increased, there may be an abnormal increase in the response to dopamine, i.e. in the dopamine receptor.[20]

For these reasons the normal functions of dopamine neurons are of particular interest. Although these systems have been associated with control of motor function, there is evidence that they may also be involved in motivational[21] and attentional[22,23] processes. Activation of dopamine neurons is apparently rewarding to the organism[24] and it has therefore been suggested that these systems may function as a mechanism for energizing and directing the organism's motor responses towards potentially rewarding environmental stimuli.[25] It seems plausible that such a system may in some way be related to schizophrenia, but the manner in which a change in the functioning of this system (e.g. an abnormal increase in transmission) might give rise to the complex subjective changes experienced by the schizophrenic patient remains obscure.

References

1. WHO International Pilot Study of Schizophrenia (1975) *Schizophrenia: a Multinational Study (Public Health Papers No. 63)*, World Health Organization, Geneva
2. LIN, T.-Y. & STANDLEY, C. C. (1962) *The Scope of Epidemiology in Psychiatry (Public Health Papers No. 16)*, World Health Organization, Geneva
3. CROW, T. J. & MITCHELL, W. S. (1975) Subjective age in chronic schizophrenia: evidence for a sub-group of patients with defective learning capacity? *Br. J. Psychiatry 126*, 360–363
4. JOHNSTONE, E. C., CROW, T. J., FRITH, C. D., STEVENS, M., KREEL, L. & HUSBAND, J. (1978a) The dementia of dementia praecox. *Acta Psychiatr. Scand. 57*, 305–324
5. STRAUSS, J. S. & CARPENTER, W. T. (1974) Characteristic symptoms and outcome in schizophrenia. *Arch. Gen. Psychiatry 30*, 429–434
6. KENDELL, R. E., BROCKINGTON, I. F. & LEFF, J. P. (1979) Prognostic implications of six alternative definitions of schizophrenia. *Arch. Gen. Psychiatry*, in press
7. SCHNEIDER, K. (1939) *Psychischer Befund und Psychiatrische Diagnose*; (later editions renamed *Klinische Psychopathologie*); English translation: *Clinical Psychopathology* (1959) from 5th edn., Grune & Stratton, New York
8. SCHNEIDER, K. (1957) Primare und sekundare symptome bei der Schizophrenie. *Fortschr. Neurol.-Psychiatr. Grenzgeb. 25*, 487–490 (translated in *Themes and Variations in European Psychiatry* (Hirsch, S. R. & Shepherd, M., eds.), John Wright, Bristol, 1974)
9. WING, J. K., COOPER, J. E. & SARTORIUS, N. (1974) *The Measurement and Classification of Psychiatric Symptoms*, Cambridge University Press, London
10. WING, J. K. & NIXON, J. (1975) Discriminating symptoms in schizophrenia. *Arch. Gen. Psychiatry 32*, 853–859
11. SCHNEIDER, K. (1949) Zum Begriff des Wahns. *Fortschr. Neurol.-Psychiatr. Grenzgeb. 17*, 26–31 (translated in *Themes and Variations in European Psychiatry* (Hirsch, S. R. & Shepherd, M., eds.), John Wright, Bristol, 1974)

12. MELLOR, C. S. (1970) First rank symptoms of schizophrenia. *Br. J. Psychiatry 117*, 15–23
13. HAMILTON, M. (1974) *Fish's Clinical Psychopathology*, John Wright, Bristol
14. FRITH, C. D. (1979) Consciousness, information processing and schizophrenia. *Br. J. Psychiatry 134*, 225–235
15. CONNELL, P. H. (1958) *Amphetamine Psychosis (Maudsley Monogr. No. 5)*, Oxford University Press, London
16. ELLINWOOD, E. H. (1967) Amphetamine psychosis: I. Description of the individuals and process. *J. Nerv. Ment. Dis. 144*, 274–283
17. GRIFFITH, J. D., CAVANAUGH, J., HELD, J. & OATES, J. A. (1972) Dextroamphetamine: evaluation of psychotomimetic properties in man. *Arch. Gen. Psychiatry 26*, 97–100
18. ANGRIST, B., SATHANANTHAN, G., WILK, S. & GERSHON, S. (1974) Amphetamine psychosis: behavioural and biochemical aspects. *J. Psychiatr. Res. 11*, 13–23
19. JOHNSTONE, E. C., CROW, T. J., FRITH, C. D., CARNEY, M. W. P. & PRICE, J. S. (1978*b*) The mechanism of the antipsychotic effect in the treatment of acute schizophrenia. *Lancet 1*, 848–851
20. OWEN, F., CROSS, A. J., CROW, T. J., LONGDEN, A., POULTER, M. & RILEY, C. J. (1978) Increased dopamine receptor sensitivity in schizophrenia. *Lancet 2*, 223–226
21. UNGERSTEDT, U. (1971) Adipsia and aphagia after 6-hydroxydopamine induced degeneration of the nigro-striatal dopamine system. *Acta Physiol. Scand. 82, Suppl. 367*, 95–122
22. MARSHALL, J. F., RICHARDSON, J. S. & TEITELBAUM, P. (1974) Nigrostriatal bundle damage and the lateral hypothalamic syndrome. *J. Comp. Physiol. Psychol. 87*, 808–830
23. UNGERSTEDT, U. (1974) Brain dopamine neurones and behaviour, in *The Neurosciences: Third Study Program* (Schmitt, F. O. & Worden, F. G., eds.), MIT Press, Cambridge, Mass.
24. CROW, T. J. (1972) Catecholamine-containing neurones and electrical self-stimulation, Part I. A review of some data. *Psychol. Med 2*, 414–421
25. CROW, T. J. (1977) The neuroanatomy of intracranial self-stimulation: a general catecholamine hypothesis. *Neurosci. Res. Program Bull. 15*, 195–205

Communication and abnormal behaviour

SIDNEY CROWN

The London Hospital (Whitechapel), London

Abstract In this paper the similarities between normal and abnormal behaviour are emphasized and selected aspects of communication, normal and aberrant, between persons are explored. Communication in a social system may be verbal or non-verbal: one person's actions cause a response in another person. This response may be cognitive, behavioural or physiological. Communication may be approached through the individual, the social situation or social interaction. Psychoanalysis approaches the individual in terms of the coded communications of psychoneurotic symptoms or psychotic behaviour; the humanist–existential approach is concerned more with emotional expression. Both approaches emphasize the development of individual identity. The interaction between persons and their social background is stressed. Relevant are sociological concepts such as illness behaviour, stigma, labelling, institutionalization and compliance. Two approaches to social interactions are considered: the games-playing metaphor, e.g. back pain as a psychosocial manipulation—the 'pain game'; and the 'spiral of reciprocal perspectives' which emphasizes the interactional complexities of social perceptions. Communicatory aspects of psychological treatments are noted: learning a particular metaphor such as 'resolution' of the problem (psychotherapy), learning more 'rewarding' behaviour (learning theory) or learning authenticity or self-actualization (humanist–existential).

COMMUNICATION IN SOCIAL SITUATIONS

Communication within a social situation means that signals from one person lead to a response in another or others. This response may take three forms: a change in attitude; a change in behaviour; or a change in physiological responsivity. By change in attitude is meant change in cognition, emotion or will. Behaviour includes both motor and verbal behaviour. Changes in attitude and behaviour may or may not be reflected in the third parameter, physiology, particularly autonomic responsivity. In ordinary life this would be clear when, in response to a provocative remark, one may be aware of

345

an attitudinal change, or a slight change in behaviour or a physiological change such as increased heart rate, none of which may be noticed by the other person. Conversely in a stressful situation one may be quite certain that one is not reacting in any noticeable way only to be challenged by the other person who suggests that 'something is wrong'.

The major channels of communication in social situations are verbal (what we say), and non-verbal, the latter including para-linguistic communication (how we say things) and gesture, expression, bodily attitude, gait, gaze and eye contact.[1] Verbal and non-verbal communication are important in all forms of communication, normal and abnormal. The same basic principles apply to normal social intercourse as to communication in the psychoneuroses and the psychoses.

Communication and its relation to behaviour may be considered from the viewpoint of the individual, the social situation and social interaction.

COMMUNICATION AND THE INDIVIDUAL

Two approaches will be considered: psychoanalysis and humanist-existentialism.

Psychoanalysis

Freud differentiated primary process thinking from secondary process thinking. Secondary process thinking is rational thinking. Primary process thinking is related to emotion and is governed by three mechanisms: condensation, whereby complicated ideas and feelings are expressed in a single image; displacement, whereby emotion and thought belonging to one source are displaced to another; and symbol formation, a coding system whereby one image stands for another. Freud suggested a link between the thinking process characteristic of normal persons, as in rational thinking, day-dreams, night-dreams, fantasy, and the creative process; and the thinking of persons characterized as neurotic or psychotic.

Psychoneurotic symptoms represent a compromise. A person who combines aggressive personal ambition with religious feeling may remain psychologically stable by becoming a philanthropist; another person with a similar problem may become psychoneurotic, developing anxious, phobic or obsessional symptoms which express the conflict in symbolic form. Neurotic symptoms are disguised communications both to the person with those symptoms and to others. Freud and his followers with a special interest in the field[2] realized that much of the unusual or even grossly aberrant verbal and non-verbal behaviour of psychotics consisted of communications coded according to the principles of condensation, displacement and symbol formation. Thus the withdrawn, grotesque and unbelievably fatiguing posture of a catatonic schizophrenic may express the conflict between fear and hatred of the world together with self-punishment for having such intense feelings.

The second relevant area of psychoanalytic theory is the study of anxiety and methods of coping with anxiety—defence mechanisms. It is postulated that the ego (or self) experiences anxieties coming from outside stresses, from within, especially from the major drives, sexuality and aggressiveness, or from the conscience (superego). Defensive manoeuvres are adopted to cope with these anxieties, the constellation of these defences being characteristic of the individual. There are also characteristic defensive constellations of psycho-neuroses such as hysteria or obsessive–compulsive neurosis. Psychotherapist and patient need to unravel these convoluted modes of existence and to replace constricted by freer expression.

Within the psychoses the mechanism of projection is characteristic of paranoid illnesses. Thus unwanted facets of a person's personality are projected outwards so that they are experienced as coming from another source. The projections may be experienced either in the content of hallucinations or delusional ideas. This mechanism may be used, after the initial impact of a psychotic break with reality, to re-establish primitive contact and communication with others.

Humanist–existentialism

The theoretical analysis of abnormal behaviour has rested heavily on concepts drawn from psychoanalysis and theories of learning. In the last twenty years or so a psychology characterized by the term humanist–existential, loosely based on European existential philosophy combined with the current social-political climate of individual freedom, fulfilment and authenticity, has become influential. This is appropriately called the 'third force' in psychological theory. The uniqueness of people is stressed in relation to battles with the shaping forces of convention, whether in the family or in broader society or culture. Premature crystallization of individual personality or relationships by an outsider such as a psychotherapist must be avoided by stratagems such as 'going on looking' rather than diagnosing, labelling and hence dismissing. The humanist–existential approach is preoccupied with how people grow and develop, or grow and do not develop; how they interact and establish authentic communication with each other, or how they fail to grow or establish destructive or false communications and relationships.

Identity

A major concept in both psychoanalysis and humanist–existentialism is identity.[3] Through facing the 'crises' of normal development our sense of ourselves and our place in the world becomes sharper. In early life we establish (or fail to establish) 'basic trust' in significant other people; we learn to separate geographically, and to individuate psychologically, from them; and we learn to establish our early autonomy. Later gender (sexual) identity as a boy or girl is established and the early vicissitudes of complex relationships and psychological conflict are experienced with love and jealousy between the child and the parents of the same and opposite sex. In adolescence identity becomes more firmly established in the average child although there may be delays, backward movement under stress—'identity crises'—which may even present in adulthood or middle and old age. Laing[4] has noted how identity or the 'true self' as he prefers to call it may not develop and a false self or multiple false selves—false self systems—may establish an unstable equilibrium.

Intrapsychic immaturity or identity confusion may present to the outside observer as odd, unaccountable, 'abnormal' behaviour. Thus a crisis in a working-class family in the East End of London reveals at its centre a young man, immaculately dressed in a dark suit as befits his position in a bank, his appearance made incongruous by old, battered, inappropriately coloured suede shoes. A severe hysteric living in a mental hospital for many years and incapable of functioning outside comes towards a visitor with hand outstretched in elegant posture as if offering hospitality to a friend in a grand house. These persons communicate facets of their malformed or fractured identities to the world and their abnormal behaviour may be labelled eccentric, neurotic or psychotic according to the perception, psychological sophistication or training of the onlooker.

COMMUNICATION AND THE SOCIAL SITUATION

Deviance

If the communicatory aspects of normal and abnormal behaviour can be related to individual psychology, it also relates to the social context or social situation within which the behaviour takes place. Sociology has helped to sharpen our perspectives. The basic viewpoint is that of ethnomethodology.[5] This postulates a relationship between what is perceived and the personal background and experience of the perceiver. A young woman at lunch pushes aside potentially fattening foods and follows this with black coffee. This behaviour may communicate attraction and sexual provocation to a male fellow guest; anorexia nervosa and probable sexual frigidity to a psychiatrist. Effeminate behaviour may be sufficiently abnormal to appear deviant[6] and labelled[7] as such in a conventional group; ignored in a bohemian group. A similar conventional group, if a potentially deviant individual is known to be unusually talented, may 'normalize' their perception of the individual and refuse to assign a deviancy label. Illness behaviour[8] in a favourite person has to be extreme indeed before such a person is stigmatized[9] and not granted full social recognition. On the other hand a physically handicapped person may be stigmatized by those who feel threatened by the disability. Thus a dynamic relation exists between observer and observed, leading to flexibility in defining the boundaries of deviance.

Sociology has provided a striking terminology for describing abnormal aspects of social behaviour as it is related to, determined by and observed within the social situation. As Jones[10] has suggested, however, in an eloquent paper, these concepts can combine conviction on the one hand with conceptual vagueness on the other. Their definition and measurement are indeed difficult.

Institutionalization and compliance

Conventional forces within institutions lead inmates to 'normalize' their behaviour, to adjust, but at considerable personal cost. Goffman[11] shows how in a 'total institution', such as a psychiatric hospital or prison, attitudes and behaviour may be modified so as to reduce the inmates' adjustment to the world outside: in a word to make them 'institutionalized'. Group pressures —of peers, of relatives, of special interest groups or change agents such as psychiatrists—may reward conformity and punish deviance. From the viewpoint of individual psychology this area of theory has been conceptualized as 'compliance'.[12] Thus, for example, in a surgical ward a 'good patient' is one who accepts the diagnosis without question, does not 'bother' the medical or nursing staff and may even agree to invasive, undignified or painful 'special' investigations or to having a physically and emotionally valued part of the body removed after relatively little questioning as to how and why the decision was arrived at.

This behaviour has complicated communicatory facets. Prisoners who conform and earn maximum remission of their sentences may see themselves as shrewd, playing the system; to the authorities they are 'old lags'. Patients in psychiatric wards may conform to the therapeutic community approach because they soon realize that in this way they show how well they are 'settling down' and 'relating'—as recorded in the weekly 'business round' before weekend leave or discharge is granted. Conversely other patients whose usual behaviour is to spend the time alone on their beds reading or listening to classical music may receive reports which are less favourable. At the other extreme, a normal person who mimicks psychotic behaviour may be diagnosed as insane.[13]

Thus normal behaviour in the psychotic, psychotic behaviour in the normal, manipulative behaviour in the hysteric, compliant behaviour within a total institution, the normalization of deviant behaviour in a person who is socially highly regarded—all demonstrate the communicatory aspects of behaviour and show how these are in part dependent upon the social context in which they occur and the dynamic interaction between the actor or actors and their social context.

COMMUNICATION IN SOCIAL INTERACTIONS

While it is artificial to divide aspects of communication into self, situation and interaction, it helps to delineate this complex field. Two aspects of social interaction will be considered: games-playing and the relation of perception to communication.

Games-playing

Games and myths as metaphors of abnormal behaviour are appealing. Early in the field, and ironically perhaps far more influential now than when he published his major book *The Myth of Mental Illness*, Szasz[14] attacks the concept of 'illness' as applied to psychiatric disorder. He feels it is like confusing a fault in the TV set with a bad programme. The argument is most convincingly developed in relation to hysteria, the phenomena of which Szasz regards as communicatory. Thus hysterical blindness might signify defence against or rejection of a relationship problem. The variability of hysterical symptoms is supportive of a communication hypothesis. Thus a man whose right arm is apparently paralysed and who maintains the symptom when doctors are in evidence may currently be the darts champion of the ward. A psychosomatic example using the games model is pain: people play the 'pain game' and, for example, people with rheumatoid arthritis may tyrannize their families by the 'use' of their painful disability.

Although relevant to a smaller segment of psychotic behaviour, paranoid patients, as Laing[15] suggests in his brilliant existential analysis of the phenomenology and interactional aspects of paranoia, always have some basis to their delusional beliefs. Witness the number of psychiatrists who have been formulating a 'paranoid' diagnosis in their minds during a diagnostic interview only to have their thoughts interrupted by the patient accusing them of hostility. Seligman's concept[16] that depression is a behavioural pattern of learnt helplessness also seems related to a games-playing model.

The games analysis of abnormal behaviour helps in the understanding of a significant segment of people's communicatory behaviour: in normal social interaction; in the disability of physical and psychosomatic disease; in understanding psychoneurotic reactions; and in comprehending some aspects of psychotic behaviour.

Communication and perception

The general laws of perception are basic to experimental psychology; individual differences in perception are basic to the psychology of personality. Here we are concerned with interpersonal perception in a social context and its relation to abnormal behaviour. Laing, Phillipson and Lee[17] remark on the extraordinarily complex ways in which human beings perceive one another and, following this, react to one another: a 'spiral of reciprocal perspectives'. Husband sees wife and wife observes husband and they both observe the other observing them and they both observe themselves observing the other observing them, and so on. To take an example from a poem by Laing[18] about how one of a couple becomes addicted to alcohol:

She has started to drink
   as a way to cope
   that makes her less able to cope

the more she drinks
the more frightened she is of becoming a drunkard
the more drunk
the less frightened of being drunk

the more frightened of being drunk when not drunk
   the more not frightened drunk
   the more frightened not drunk

the more she destroys herself
the more frightened of being destroyed by him

the more frightened of destroying him
the more she destroys herself

Within a family there may be authentic relationships leading both to individual and joint fulfilment within accepted constraints for all members. When perception and communication go awry, however, they contribute to the development of deviant behaviour. Thus the families of male homosexuals seem characterized by a constellation of a dominant, close-binding intimate mother and a weak, despised and negated father.[19]

All groups—friends, occupational, in marriage, in the family, politico-social, therapy, encounter, self-help—can lead to aberrant perceptions between self and other. Paradoxically, apparently not dissimilar forces can lead to constructive human groupings and to sublime creations as in music, art and literature.

COMMUNICATION AND PSYCHIATRIC TREATMENT

Psychiatric treatment is intimately bound up with the personality, social background, training and philosophy of both psychiatrist and patient as well as with the socio-political matrix within which these person-altering treatments are based. These forces relate also to the system of referral to care, whether formal, as through links in the medical establishment (general practitioner, hospital, etc.) or informal—through friends, acquaintances, others who have had breakdowns, etc. The only clarity existing in this area is in the minds of those who unequivocally embrace the medical model: to such persons the modification of the symptoms of, say, a schizophrenic illness by phenothiazine medication constitutes a 'cure' at least as much as insulin medication provides a 'cure' for diabetes.

Other models of treatment of abnormal behaviour lead to basic queries as to the meaning of 'cure'. The psychotherapies aim to achieve new understanding and insight, leading to personality alterations. The learning therapies aim to alter aberrant behaviour, insight being irrelevant. What is interesting, however, is that with behavioural modification, as with a person who is socially phobic, the personal–social environment may alter so greatly that social feedback may secondarily lead to increases in insight and understanding of self. A similar argument applies to developments in behavioural modifications relating to schizophrenia. If schizophrenics are trained by being rewarded for 'normal' as opposed to psychotic behaviour, for example for holding their heads up rather than bowing down, their lives are altered largely because of other people's changed reaction to them. Is this a 'true' change, is it acting or is it education? The 'new' therapies[20] based on the humanist–existential framework add a further dimension: emotional release and catharsis. If you hate your mother let the pillow represent her and hit it if that is how you feel.

How should the changes that follow the psychotherapies be regarded? As new roles and action patterns or as fundamental, underlying personality change? Or is there no difference? Sociological writers persistently refer to the 'actor' when dealing with psychological phenomena in individuals. On the other hand the concept of identity assumes that we develop a basic core, a 'true' self. If a physiological dimension is included as well as behaviour and attitude, an interesting additional dilemma appears: thus homosexual behaviour and attitude may be modified by treatment but homosexual preference as measured by penile erection may remain. Which of these measures is of 'true' sexual orientation?[21]

I have no answers to these questions but there is a need to pose them. Do persons communicate with true selves? Or with false selves? With egos? With action patterns? With expressed attitudes? With occult physiology? The understanding of communication is one facet to the understanding of normal and abnormal behaviour.

References

1. ARGYLE, M. (1967) *The Psychology of Interpersonal Behaviour*, Penguin Books, Harmondsworth, Middlesex
2. FREEMAN, T. (1971) Psychoanalysis and the treatment of the psychoses. *Br. J. Psychiatry* *119*, 47–52
3. ERIKSON, E. H. (1965) *Childhood & Society*, Penguin Books, Harmondsworth, Middlesex
4. LAING, R. D. (1965) *The Divided Self*, Pelican Books, Harmondsworth, Middlesex
5. TURNER, R. (ed.) (1974) *Ethnomethodology.* Penguin Education, Harmondsworth, Middlesex
6. BECKER, H. S. (ed.) (1964) *The Other Side. Perspectives on Deviance*, Free Press, New York
7. ROMAN, P. M. (1971) Labelling theory and community psychiatry. *Psychiatry (Wash. D.C.) 34*, 378–390
8. MECHANIC, D. (1972) Social psychologic factors affecting the presentation of bodily complaints. *N. Engl. J. Med. 286*, 1132–1139
9. GOFFMAN, E. (1964) *Stigma*, Pelican Books, Harmondsworth, Middlesex
10. JONES, K. (1978) Society looks at the psychiatrist. *Br. J. Psychiatry 132*, 321–332
11. GOFFMAN, E. (1970) *Asylums*, Penguin Books, Harmondsworth, Middlesex
12. BLACKWELL, B. (1976) Treatment adherence. *Br. J. Psychiatry 129*, 513–531
13. ROSENHAN, D. L. (1973) On being sane in insane places. *Science (Wash. D.C.) 179*, 250–258
14. SZASZ, T. S. (1972) *The Myth of Mental Illness*, Paladin (Granada), St Albans, Hertfordshire.
15. LAING, R. D. (1971) *Self & Others*, Penguin Books, Harmondsworth, Middlesex
16. EASTMAN, C. (1976) Behavioural formulations of depression. *Psychol. Rev. 83*, 277–291
17. LAING, R. D., PHILLIPSON, H. & LEE, A. R. (1966) *Interpersonal Perception*, Tavistock Publications, London
18. LAING, R. D. (1972) *Knots*, Penguin Books, Harmondsworth, Middlesex
19. BIEBER, I. (1962) *Homosexuality. A Psychoanalytic Study*, Basic Books, New York
20. LISS, J. (1974) *Free to Feel*, Wildwood House, London
21. MCCONAGHY, N. (1976) Is a homosexual orientation irreversible? *Br. J. Psychiatry 129*, 556–563

Commentary on papers by Tim Crow and Sidney Crown

HILARY PUTNAM

Department of Philosophy, Harvard University

The papers by Drs Crow and Crown pose any philosopher who reads them with the problem of explicating the dichotomy between *physical* and *functional* as it applies to mental disorders. Dr Crow explicitly argues against the view that schizophrenia is a functional disorder and for the view that it is a purely physical disease. He speculates that it is related to excessive dopamine sensitivity on the part of certain neural structures. Dr Crown discusses the psychoneuroses, and his discussion ranges over the large number of therapies on the market today, both from the patients' point of view and from the practitioners'; and he asks what concepts we should use in thinking about them. The point of view is explicitly 'functional': the 'talking cures' do work, in Dr Crown's view, or at least they work for some types of patient.

While there is no inconsistency between these views (since no one would class schizophrenia among the psychoneuroses), they clearly reflect a difference in approach and expectation with respect to strategies of diagnosis as well as cure. The nature of the difference indicates some of the factors that are involved in the physical/functional dichotomy itself. Someone who regards a psychological disorder as 'physical' apparently expects the cause to be genetic or, if not genetic, to be explained by physical properties of the environment which do not, in themselves, have much emotional or 'psychological' significance, e.g. the presence or absence of certain chemicals in the diet. Correspondingly, the therapy indicated would tend to be chemical or physical intervention of some kind. Someone who regards a disorder as 'functional' apparently expects the cause to be environmental, and not just environmental but emotional (i.e. to have to do with emotional relationships with people in the environment, be it the childhood or post-childhood or present environment) or else (if the therapist is 'behaviour modification'-oriented) to lie in the learning of dysfunctional habits (and, thus, to be susceptible of both diagnosis and cure by methods derived from learning theory). I say 'apparently' in both cases because the notions 'physical' and 'functional' themselves are far from clear, and many theorists would regard physical and functional explanations as in some way compatible and complementary. Be that as it may, there is some tension between the viewpoints, and the remarks I have just made may indicate where a degree of incompatibility lies between them. There is a difference between viewing a disorder as purely genetic, at one extreme, and viewing it as due to unresolved emotional problems and/or dysfunctional habits at the other.

If we think of the brain as a computer, and of experience as supplying the 'inputs', then we may say that a 'physical' theory of a nervous disorder sees the patient as a *damaged* computer, one whose 'hardware' needs to be repaired, while a 'functional' theory sees the patient as a *misprogrammed* computer, one whose 'software' needs to be altered by reprogramming.

This way of putting it can be misleading, however, because of the interplay between 'hardware' and 'software' both in people and computers. One simple example is dreaming. Dreaming obviously has a physical basis; the brain is 'wired' for dreaming, one could hope to learn more about the specific neural processes involved, etc. Yet, even if we found out exactly where in the brain dreams take place, this would not, in and of itself, tell us why some dreams are stories. Some dreams have quite complicated plots, have characters, and have dialogue. Moreover the 'composer' of the dream is an unconscious mechanism, on any theory, not just on Freudian theory. Thus some account of the program that enables this 'composer' mechanism in the brain to produce stories complete with plots, characters, and dialogue is necessary and not *just* an account of the localization or biochemistry of the mechanism.*

A similar example occurs in Dr Crow's paper. The phenomenon he calls 'delusional perception' involves the production of quite complex stories by patients, stories full of 'primary process' material, to use psychoanalytic jargon (e.g. the female relatives with their genitalia reversed, the second coming of Jesus). Although the cause of the disorder as a whole may be something as simple as 'dopamine sensitivity', this does not explain the functionally described symptoms of the disorder; it does not explain the 'plot, characters, and dialogue' of these stories (which quite resemble dreams except for the important detail that the patient believes these 'delusional perceptions', whereas people do not normally believe their dreams).

Dr Crow's own conjecture is that the schizophrenic may be 'monitoring unconscious processes'—i.e. such stories are being produced all the time in all our brains and it is only the inability of the schizophrenic to repress, or in

---

*See Putnam[1] for a fuller discussion of problems of reduction in psychology.

some way remain unconscious, of these stories that requires explanation in terms of chemical malfunctioning in the brain. This conjecture is plausible and something like it is a commonplace in the published studies of schizophrenia, but it is a typical functional explanation (i.e. it is in terms analogous to the following: 'the story stored in such-and-such an address got transferred to the wrong address'), even though it appears in the context of a 'hardware' diagnosis.

Nothing I have said is meant to be critical of Dr Crow's very carefully researched and argued paper. What I *am* arguing against is the widespread tendency to think that 'hardware' explanations totally dispose of the need for 'software' explanations—a common reductionist error in the biological sciences (Ref. 2, p. 135). Localizing the dream process in the brain or confirming that schizophrenia is a genetic disorder would not in any way show that talk of the unconscious in connection with dreams and schizophrenia was wrong or silly (although it might show that 'talking cures' cannot work in the case of schizophrenia. But even this is not certain*).

Before I discuss Dr Crown's paper, it may help if I indicate what my own background beliefs are about psychotherapy. Of course, I cannot even attempt to defend these in so short a space; I shall simply set them out as a set of assumptions, if you will, for the aid of the reader.

First of all, I am not impressed by the 'validation studies' which purport to show that all psychotherapies work equally well (or badly). In part these studies *may* show that most psychotherapists aren't very good, whatever their theoretical persuasion. Indeed, there are studies which show considerable differences in the 'success' ratios of individual therapists within every 'school' of psychotherapy, and which show that these differences correlate with the ability of the therapist to show affect, to empathize, to confront, etc. But even these latter studies assume the crudest possible notion of 'cure': you are well, in effect, if a committee of experts says you are well (and you agree). Such a notion of cure cannot distinguish between successful neurosis (and there are successful neurotics, at least for a time) and grown-up people. Especially in a time when many therapies aim at promoting successful selfishness, the refusal to distinguish between different types of 'success' amounts itself to a systemic narcissistic bias in the studies themselves.

My own view is that statistical information, while always welcome and interesting, is no more decisive in psychotherapy than it is in history. My

---

*Even where there is a 'hardware' disorder, it could be that a degree of compensation for it can be achieved by therapy. The occasional success of massive psychological treatment with autistic children is a case in point.

choice of this comparison is not accidental; psychotherapy is a historical discipline, at least in its analytic versions, in that it attempts to reconstruct the life history of an individual, and to separate what truly happened from selfish fantasy. The problems—that one is dealing with unique unrepeatable events, that there is little in the way of 'scientific theory' to rely on, that individual wisdom and sensitivity are important—are similar in the two cases.

Since I don't believe that 'all methods are equally good', it follows, of course, that I regard the problem of finding out which methods are better and why as a genuine problem.

Secondly, while recognizing that psychoanalysis has often become a closed circle of ideas, and that it is as futile to try to understand all individual lives by forcing them into the mould prescribed by Freud as it is to try to understand all of social history by forcing it into the mould prescribed by Marx, I think that Freud was correct in insisting on the great importance of the emotional events that take place in early childhood. More than this, I think that the postulating of the unconscious as the source of emotional problems was correct, and that unconscious processes are to some extent knowable. But, as the comparison with history already suggests, 'knowledge' in this area is likely to be controversial; and there is no answer to the perennial charge (in both areas) that one is 'reading in', except to try to look at the data impartially and wisely in the individual case.

Coming now to Crown's paper: what disturbs me is Crown's radical eclecticism. Crown seems to think that every therapy works (he mentions in his paper touchy-fccly-'humanist' therapies, analytic therapies, behaviour modification, etc.). But saying that every therapy works poses the 'drawing the line' problem: what counts as a therapy? Do some (or all) of the following *also* count as therapies: (1) Joining the Roman Catholic church? (2) Joining Jehovah's Witnesses? (3) Joining the People's Temple? (In private discussion Crown answered that *all* of these work 'for some people'.)

Coming to theoretical issues: Crown suggests that we can understand what goes on in the different therapies by employing the notion of *communication*. But the metaphor of communication goes with the correlative metaphor of *interpretation*. What theory does Crown suggest we rely on in interpreting these 'communications'? Or does he suggest that we be as eclectic in theory as in therapy? (Following our discussion, I would add another, related, question: if 'every therapy works for some people', then what theory do we use to tell which people to send to which therapists? Or to judge who is helped? Or, like Jeremy Bentham, do we say you are better off if you think you're better off? Of course, this last is a theory too.)

Crown also raises a question about which is one's 'core self': the stimulus-bound response (penile erection in the case of a former homosexual) or the conscious choice? It seems to me that the very notion of a 'core self' (like a needle lost in a haystack) is unhelpful here. Aristotle, many centuries ago, suggested that we *construct* our true selves, we don't *find* them (he speaks* of identifying oneself with one's excellences as these develop and of the close connection this process has with both self-respect and friendship). My preference for the Aristotelian view of the self as a sort of life-project is connected with my own preference for therapies that try to increase the insight of patients so as to make their behaviour less stimulus-bound and more subject to their autonomous control over therapies that seek to 'condition' them to behave in very specific ways.

This last remark suggests that Crown and I would perhaps agree in viewing the choice of a therapy (and a concept of 'cure') as in part a *moral* choice. And the 'eclecticism' that I criticized in Crown may spring from a value that I actually share with Crown: the value of *autonomy*. It is, I suspect, because he respects the autonomy of the patient that he wishes to let the patient define what 'better' is. He has a healthy suspicion of 'forcing people to be free'. Where I disagree is in thinking that the responsibility for choice cannot be evaded on the therapist's side either: 'let the patient decide' is a cop-out. But it may be that I have misunderstood Crown completely.

References

1. PUTNAM, H. (1973) Philosophy and our mental life. Published as chapter 14 of Putnam, H. *Mind, Language and Reality*, pp. 291–303, Cambridge University Press, 1978
2. PUTNAM, H. (1971) Reductionism and the nature of psychology. *Cognition 2* (1), pp. 131–146

---

*Here I am assuming a certain reading of Aristotle's *Nicomachean Ethics*, and particularly of the opening chapters of books VIII and IX.

Discussion: Psychosis and abnormal behaviour

Crown: It is we who are trying to classify what is therapy, not the people who come for help. Everyone gets help from different things, including spiritualism, transcendental meditation and so on. Although we have a certain idea of conventional therapies such as psychotherapy or behaviour therapy, I think one of our aims should be to get people into the psychotherapy that is correct for them. Much of the weight of current research in psychotherapy is to try and decide which therapy, given by which person for which condition, is likely to be effective under which social situation. Each of those variables is highly complicated and the whole is a difficult multifactorial problem. I agree with Putnam that the emphasis should be on producing self-determination rather than other-determination.

Crow: Eclecticism is all very well but unless you measure something everything is possible. For example, it may be true that you can influence psychotic symptoms by rewards, reinforcement and so on. You might infer from that that psychotherapy was sometimes of value. But the studies of psychotherapy with psychotic patients suggest rather that psychotherapy delays recovery.[1] Everything may indeed be of value sometimes but you have to specify the circumstances and you must measure something.

Khin Zaw: It may well be true that everything will help somebody, but there is still the problem of what helping someone consists in. You may say that your model of psychiatric intervention is not governed by some ideal state of flourishing, but if you are not aiming at that, what are you aiming at? If you are allowing judgement of whether they are sick or not to rest entirely with the individuals concerned, you have a situation in which absolutely anything goes. I doubt in fact if any psychiatrist really does believe the judgement rests with individuals. What sort of expertise could the psychiatrist claim if it did?

Crown: One must differentiate between the patients I work with and the sort that Crow talked about. The usual psychotherapy patient has a personality disorder, or a psychosexual or psychosocial problem. Whilst such persons may need psychotherapy this must also include encouragement to fulfil their lives in their own way. When it comes to more aberrant behaviour, for example self-destructive behaviour, the psychotherapist, like the psychiatrist, may be forced to decide what to do. I would not be 'eclectic' about that.

361

Khin Zaw: In talking about self-destruction aren't you appealing somewhere along the line to a biological model? You don't count self-destruction as a possible acceptable choice, whereas some therapists would say that if a person wants to destroy themselves that is up to them.

Searle: This is the dissatisfaction that one feels with Szasz and people like that who think that somehow we are politically oppressing these poor patients. There is an example of an eight-year-old girl who was trying to tear her eyeballs out. It seems to me to be oppressive on the other side to allow her such complete self-expression. I gather you don't go all the way with Szasz, Dr Crown?

Crown: No, certainly not. Suicidal behaviour is common and is therefore a good example. If people say they want to commit suicide I discuss it with them, just as if they were saying they wanted to do something harmful but less dramatic—for example, drive too fast. If they don't then resolve the suicide wish, I attempt honestly to face up to the new position. I usually try to get them to come into hospital for a time and then see how they feel. One does of course equivocate but, at least in principle, if a man wants to kill himself I would not think it unreasonable if that is what he really wishes to do.

Searle: So you draw the line at the eyeball but not at the suicide?

Crown: Murder and suicide are of course difficult examples. Medical students always challenge, saying 'what would you do if'? It is difficult because you can of course decide to behave like any other doctor—that is be directive, possibly punitive, and get patients into hospital. I don't approve of that in principle and I try to avoid it.

Fried: If that is how you act in practice but you don't approve it in principle, shouldn't you reflect on your principles a little more?

Crown: One is not often pushed so far. Fortunately these situations are rare.

Fried: We are pushing you to that now.

Crown: I think I can usually resolve these situations in a way that is true to my principles of encouraging individual freedom of choice.

Trevarthen: In families, children are not allowed total self-expression, in part because the children do not want that. You are talking about the problem of communication, of getting the person to reveal themselves to you. You can help by not telling them to keep quiet or to be someone else. But you still have the problem in some form or another of getting people to come forward, to ask other people to have relationships with them and tell them or make them do something for which they know they need help.

Crown: You have to get patients to establish their own boundaries, not your boundaries.

Trevarthen: This is part of the problem of getting to know what they want you to do or make them do.

Young: They may be partly your boundaries, as in the family.

Crown: Yes, you can't help it altogether.

Ploog: I am glad to see that Kurt Schneider's first-rank symptoms, which he conceived in our institute in Munich, have now made their way into the textbooks and that they are of diagnostic value. As a clinical psychiatrist I want to draw your attention to the fact that when schizophrenic patients talk about their delusional experiences, it seems that they have experienced them as an absolute reality that is unquestionably the truth. This is important if one reflects on the problem of brain and mind. In Dr Crow's presentation I think we all felt the big jump from the experiences of these people to the biochemistry in their brains. The discoveries of the last twenty years surpass everything that has taken place in medicine. Millions of people get relief by the neuropharmacological mechanisms to which he referred. The specific experiences that schizophrenic patients undergo and which are relieved by neurotropic drugs occur all over the world, independent of cultural influences. These experiences must have very specific brain mechanisms at very specific sites of the brain. Then the question comes in, where in the brain is that specific experience manufactured? How is it manufactured? There are many possibilities. At present it is supposed that certain drugs change the balance of transmitters in the brain, with the result that the patients recover from their deviant experiences.

I want to suggest how one could look at these brain mechanisms in a slightly different way to the way biochemists look at them. In our discussions here we have always come back from different angles to the problem of dualism and monism and other 'isms'. Most of the allusions to these mechanisms were as if we were talking about the interaction of physical events. We never took into account that while we can talk about communication between individuals we can also talk about communication in the internal system of the brain. The thesis from communication research that information is information, not matter or energy, didn't come into the picture. In a system such as the brain that means that we do not always have to think of causal effects in terms of physical events. Using information theory, one could try to find, from birth to adulthood, what kind of informational basis the concept of self-awareness might have in terms of brain mechanisms. For instance one's own thoughts that are experienced as if coming from outside might be due to feedback mechanisms in certain areas of the brain being out of order. Similarly, non-verbal or verbal social communication, based on certain brain mechanisms, might be upset and experienced as if externally governed, etc.

Bunge: Two of Schneider's symptoms of schizophrenia are thought withdrawal and thought insertion. In both cases patients have the impression that thoughts enter the head or leave it. This is precisely what dualists have been telling us all along—that disembodied thoughts can exist. I invite those of you who still believe that to make an appointment with Dr Crow!

Secondly, I do not believe in the computer model of the mind, or even of the brain, because you cannot clear a brain, short of killing it. Professor Young has emphasized that you cannot really make the distinction between software and hardware in a living brain. The analogy between software and the mind on the one hand and hardware and the brain on the other is also philosophically displeasing, at least to me. It is a modern version of psychoneural dualism, which is methodologically misleading. If we want to understand mice we study living mice, not clockwork mice. And if we want to understand the brain and its functions, in particular its physical functions, we ought to be studying the brain and the way it functions.

Something we must remember is that there is no information flow without energy. The fact that information theory is not interested in energy exchanges does not mean that there can be information without energy. This is the mistake that D. M. MacKay[2] makes. MacKay uses the information–theoretic model in order to support dualism.

As for psychoanalysis, I cannot take it seriously as a science. It ignores the central nervous system, it is practically immune to refutation, it does no experiments, it is a cult, and as a therapy it is inefficient.

Fried: I disagree with the idea that Hilary Putnam is leading us down a blind alley with his computer analogies. There are many fruitful examples in science of the construction of models which help us to understand things. Those models are not made of the same substances as the things modelled. So I don't understand why, particularly as you are a materialist, you would exclude computer models in this sense.

Young: The point is that all our computer models are one-line systems whereas the brain is a multi-channel system. I shall mention that later on.

Searle: Have Hilary Putnam and I been at the same meeting? He was struck by how much of this seemed to support cognitive psychology and artificial intelligence while I have been sitting here for three days absolutely delighted by the fact that we have had almost nothing about computer models, artificial intelligence and cognitive psychology. It seems to me that neuroscientists really don't need very much of that sort of talk.

Wall: There have been suggestions that pain is for communication, but what would happen if you were a totally hidden observer on a desert island with Crow's patient? My gut feeling is that this man would be expressing his madness in a somewhat different way. If another man developed appendicitis, he would not address the land crabs and say 'please send for an ambulance, I need surgery', but his general behaviour and his own reports of his feelings would probably be somewhat similar whether he was on a desert island or in London. A real example of people on a desert island for a very brief time is provided by parachutists. Israeli paratroopers call out 'mother'. I don't believe that they are mad. They are saying 'I wish someone was here to hold me'. They are not communicating—they are sending a message with no one to receive it. We can therefore dissect off the question of communication and all its complexities from another reality going on within the person.

Trevarthen: I agree. Earlier we were up against the problem of not being able to explain why pain evolved, and you were definitely not answering that question properly. What I was suggesting was that many aspects of human pain, though they might be regarded in isolation, did not evolve in isolation.

Plum: I don't think either Dr Putnam or Dr Crown discussed the fundamental differences between the psychotic illnesses. The diagnosis of schizophrenia runs remarkably true to type and could seldom be confused with other psychoses when first-rank symptoms are present. The genetic studies of identical twins with schizophrenia indicate that they have an identical frequency of clinical expression despite their upbringing in entirely different environments.

Putnam: I didn't suggest that the psychotic illnesses were functional disorders.

Plum: If one excludes the psychotics, where does diagnosis rest? The trouble with schizophrenia is that it doesn't have a verifying laboratory test such as high blood sugar. Therefore people argue heatedly about its cause and sometimes even its expression, although typical examples of the disorder run predictably true to form. My guess is that we will find that as an inherited disease schizophrenia bears no more specific relationship to the environment than does diabetes or perhaps acute intermittent porphyria.

Trevarthen: What does that sentence mean? Why should an inherited disease have absolutely nothing to do with the environment?

Plum: I mean within the framework of identifying a specific influence.

Trevarthen: You mean immediately; it has nothing to do with the present circumstances?

Plum· One cannot identify anywhere, within any environment which has been examined up to the present time, consistent root causes even for the precipitation of the schizophrenic state.

Trevarthen: That surprises me.

Plum: There is no consistency.

Bunge: It is environment invariant.

Armstrong: If it is environment invariant, and if it is also a disease of intro-spection, that suggests that Trevarthen is wrong when he thinks that intro-spection is very closely tied in with socialization.

Young: By invariant don't you merely mean 'manifest in many environments'? You don't mean that the environment is unimportant but that no specific environment is associated with the disease.

Plum: What I meant to say was that one is unable to identify consistent or predictable factors in the environment associated with the precipitation of the disease.

Crown: Genetic research shows that about 40 % of schizophrenia is genetically determined. Objective studies in events research suggest that the exacerbations of this illness are often environmentally determined, for example a too close or too distant family is harmful.

We are talking almost as if schizophrenia is a single disease whereas it is a whole spectrum of diseases. One end of the spectrum is likely to be environ-mentally determined and the other end almost totally genetically determined. I do not believe that the social environment or aberrant communications 'produce' schizophrenia or hysteria. I believe they modify them.

So far as psychotherapy for schizophrenia is concerned, I don't think Crow and I really differ. I certainly don't think that insight psychotherapy has been demonstrated as useful in schizophrenia. I think behaviour modification techniques are likely to be helpful, for example in suppressing some of the 'psychotic' behaviour of schizophrenia.

Putnam: Mario Bunge said that the mind cannot be cleared, but not all computers can be cleared. Some of them have some programs hard-wired in; some are single-purpose computers whose entire program is hard-wired in. The important thing about a computer is that it has a finite set of rules which collectively define an algorithm. The line between a computer and a non-computer need not be sharply defined. One observes something carrying out an algorithm. For any device, natural or artificial, that is computing, for example, the decimal expansion of π, it would be far more useful to ask what *rule* is followed than merely to have the hardware description. Hubel and Wiesel's work on neurology is fascinating but at certain points there are tricks which could very easily be simulated with a computer. What they have provided is an elegant algorithm. Part of that algorithm is in the eye, for detecting the orientation of a line in terms of excitatory and inhibitory cells. People working on artificial intelligence are trying to figure out how a left-eye picture and a right-eye picture could be coordinated. Once you know that one piece in the left-eye picture is the same as one piece in the right-eye picture, then you are home. How to solve that problem is very relevant to work on vision and to work on motion perception.

Young: I absolutely agree that computers are useful in many senses. I was only concerned to point out some of the senses in which they are not useful.

Putnam: It might be better to say that the brain is a whole lot of computers, with maybe some things which are not computers.

One fascinating suggestion that comes out of the computer model is that most of the programs that we have been able to write for doing anything difficult involve the manipulation of representations, the manipulation of something very much like a language, so that the problem to be solved can be cut into a set of categories. This is why I was especially interested in Elizabeth Warrington's paper (pp. 153–166), which showed some of the physical reality of categories.

Crow: Earlier you posed a question about the biological function of consciousness and I want to answer this by using some of Elizabeth Warrington's findings in a way that she may not like. The solution I want to offer is that consciousness is really the same as what she calls short-term memory. Although she has several types of short-term memory it seems to me that they have much in common. This fits in with Dr Creutzfeldt's point that the cortex looks like a mechanism that operates on different inputs in a similar way. My suggestion[3] is that short-term memory (identified with consciousness) is a mechanism which is a read-in and read-out from long-term memory. One could suggest that long-term memory traces are only modified if they pass through the short-term memory mechanism. As Griffith[4] put it, consciousness could be defined as the rate of change of long-term memory. The question then is why there has to be a short-term mechanism. Professor Young[5] has put the point very clearly that there has to be a short-term trace mechanism which holds inputs from the external environment (and also from long-term memory). These inputs then have to be acted on by something which selects out whatever is biologically significant. The things which do the selecting are stimuli in drive-related modalities (see p. 327) such as gustation, olfaction and pain. The crucial point is that the stimuli (generally visual and auditory) which are acquiring significance arrive first. Some neural trace of these stimuli must be maintained until what J. Z. Young has called the 'results of action signal' (the drive-related stimulus signalling the biological value of subsequent events) arrives. Short-term memory (and consciousness), according to this viewpoint, is the mechanism necessary to maintain the neural trace. Thus consciousness in this sense is a mechanism for selecting neural traces which have survival value, and it thus has a biological function.

References

1. MAY, P. R. A. (1968) *Treatment of Schizophrenia*, Science House, New York
2. MACKAY, D. M. (1978) Selves and brains. *Neuroscience 3*, 599–606
3. CROW, T. J. (1968) Cortical synapses and reinforcement: a hypothesis. *Nature (Lond.) 219*, 736–737
4. GRIFFITH, J. S. (1967) *The Neural Basis of Conscious Decision*, Bedford College, London
5. YOUNG, J. Z. (1974) *A Model of the Brain*, Oxford University Press, Oxford

Triunism: a transmaterial brain–mind theory

JOSÉ M. R. DELGADO

Centro Ramon y Cajal and Autonomous Medical School, Madrid

Abstract Triunism postulates that the mind is a unity with the following three structural elements so essential that the absence of any one will prevent its existence:

(1) Brain cells and pathways possessing material and transmaterial properties.

(2) A flow of environmental information, coded and transduced at the sensory receptors and forming part of the working brain through modifications of its anatomy and physiology.

(3) Detectable manifestations derived from (1) and (2) which are expressed inward as perceptions and outward as behaviour.

The outside world enters through the senses and becomes a material and functional part of the maturing brain. Without a brain, the mind cannot exist. Without sensory inputs, the mind will not be structured and cannot appear. Without manifestations of inner perceptions and outward motor expression, the mind cannot be recognized by the individual or the environment.

Transmaterial entities require the existence of supporting matter and may be represented by patterns of material organization or by temporal or functional relations between parts of the material substratum. They may transcend the existence of specific materials, changing carriers while preserving their non-material identity, but do not possess intrinsic properties of matter such as mass and energy. Transmaterial aspects of reality, including material substratum, patterning, and relative, temporal, and functional characteristics may be subjects of experimental research.

BIOLOGICAL ELEMENTS OF THE MIND

In their approach to the mind, modern neurobiology and philosophy differ in methodology although they share the common objective of trying to understand the structural, functional and transcendental aspects of mental activity. Neurobiologists design and conduct experiments to investigate the anatomy and physiology of living organisms, whereas the role of philosophy

369

is to interpret man's discoveries in the light of other systems of knowledge. The two approaches serve as a mutual challenge and reinforcement, and their spokesmen often listen to and learn from each other.

In the past, a practical dualism pervaded science and philosophy because consciousness and other mental manifestations were beyond experimental reach and were therefore considered subjects of philosophical speculation which could be ignored by scientific investigators. Recent developments, however, have modified these positions, demonstrating that physical manipulation of the brain by electrical stimulation, electrolytic lesions, section of pathways, psychosurgery or intracerebral injections may produce changes in mental activities. The Brain–Mind problem has been continuously emerging in experiments performed in cats and monkeys as well as in surgical interventions in the human brain. Scientists have been obliged to consider the philosophical and humanistic implications of their research. Philosophers have ventured by necessity into the field of neurological sciences.

A classical dichotomy has also existed between science and values. Science deals with objective facts and cannot formulate value standards or enter into the domain of subjective value. In the context of current brain–mind theory, however, '. . . this traditional separation of science and values and the related limitations it has implied for science as a discipline are no longer valid'. 'Science deals with values as well as facts'.[1]

The mind is an ill-defined concept, usually described as active processes and not as a passive object. Most definitions express what the mind does, but not what it is or when or how it is formed. The main mental functions are the reception, interpretation, storage and retrieval of both inner and outer stimuli through processes of consciousness, thinking, remembering, feeling, willing and other phenomena.

In contrast with the difficulties of defining the mind, the brain is a well-identified object, and the centre of intensive experimental research. It has a physical existence and most of its internal structure persists and may be investigated even if this organ is dead and preserved in formalin. After brain injury, a large part of the cortex and thalamus may be destroyed and the remaining structures may continue to regulate respiration, blood pressure, temperature and other vegetative functions, while mental activities such as consciousness, intelligence and speech have been lost forever. Therefore the brain may perform some functions in the absence of a recognizable mind, whereas the reverse is not true, for without a functioning brain there can be no mental activities.

The brain, which is the site of mental activities, is never in direct contact with environmental reality because all information from the surroundings must be electrically and chemically coded in order to enter the nervous system. Thus the brain deals not with material reality but with its symbolic representation which is transduced at the sensory receptors, originating neuronal codes through which information is circulated, evaluated, stored and retrieved, subsequently triggering the organism's behavioural responses.

From the biological point of view, the prerequisites for the existence of the mind include:

(1) A functioning body to provide nutrients, oxygen and other elements necessary for cellular metabolism;

(2) Sensory receptors to provide portals of entry of information;

(3) A functioning brain to provide suitable mechanisms for the input, throughput and output of messages;

(4) Organs of expression for the manifestation of cerebral activities.

One biological approach to investigation of the mind is to study the flow and modifications of information codes as they circulate from the environment to the brain and from the brain back to the environment, recognizing the consequences of this flow and their role in the emergence of consciousness, feelings and intelligence. An issue to be considered is whether, without this flow, the mind can exist. For example, visual inputs are essential for the patterning of neuronal responses in the occipital cortex. The visual structures of the brain of a blind person differ from those in normal people. The lack of understanding of written language in illiterate people represents a lack in their optic system. Coding and decoding mechanisms have not been acquired and this fact must have anatomical and functional neuronal consequences.

Another approach is to study the brain substance itself—its anatomical and physiological characteristics—in order to understand the properties, mechanisms and possible participation of cerebral areas in specific mental activities. For example, Area 4 of the motor cortex plays an essential role in mobility and not in consciousness; the amygdala is important for the organization of aggressive behaviour and not for the understanding of speech; and the frontal lobes are activated during planning of future behaviour although they are dispensable for visual recognition.[2]

In experimental studies investigators can concentrate their efforts on specific aspects of cerebral mechanisms, but in interpreting the results they should avoid the misleading localization of mental qualities in specific anatomical structures, or the identification of non-specific carriers with specific messages. The paper and ink of a book are non-specific material carriers of messages. The same information may be given visually, acoustically or even by touch.

If the paper of this page burns, the carrier and therefore its message are certainly destroyed. Materials are necessary but should be differentiated from written concepts and also from reactions evoked in the readers. Information is related to the pattern of words and the agreed meaning of symbols. The same letters are used to form different words. The same object has a variety of names according to the language used. Identification of reality is coded by cultural agreement, and if we do not know the code we cannot understand the meaning. Some codes are highly complex, and the same spoken word may have a wide range of meanings in relation with its context, intonation, accompanying gestures and type of audience. The word *red* may have thermal, luminous, emotional, psychological, political and other meanings.

In spite of the complexity involved in coding, sending, receiving and interpreting messages, all the intervening elements may be investigated, including carriers, cultures and codes. Information exists in the material carrier without being an intrinsic property of the matter, and its deciphering requires the existence of an observer with suitable decoding mechanisms and experience. To discuss whether these temporal and experiential relations are material or immaterial is perhaps less important—at least from a biological point of view—than to investigate existing elements, functional mechanisms and related consequences.

In a similar way the brain cells (neurons and glia), which are essential as material carriers of information, should not be identified with the messages originating in the environment, with the mechanisms for extracting meaning from those messages, or with the sensations and reactions that the messages evoke. Neural material carriers are not passive elements comparable to paper and ink but reactive components which may be modified in their composition and structure by the patterns of electrical and chemical events which carry the information. The problem is therefore complex. The study of unitary activity has not been able to explain emotions, memory or thoughts, but we know that some neurons are related to conscious perceptions, while others are not.[3] Electrical stimulation applied directly to the primary sensory cortex or thalamus may produce a conscious sensory experience in the awake human subject, while a similar stimulation applied to the frontal lobes or to the pulvinar fails to reach consciousness.

Apparently there is a neuronal time factor in conscious perceptions which differs in sensory receptors and in the brain. A single shock delivered to the skin is clearly perceived and evokes a primary potential with a surface positive wave in the somatosensory cortex. A similar single pulse applied to the thalamus (VPL nucleus) may produce a larger evoked cortical potential without any reported sensation. For conscious sensations to be elicited from the thalamus or cortex stimulations must be applied for about half a second. Conscious perception of skin stimulation may be blocked by cortical excitation, providing an opportunity for timing and the electrical events required for conscious sensations to be investigated. Further research about interacting neuronal fields, and *Gestalt* and holistic conceptions of brain functions, should provide needed information and ideas that will increase our understanding of some neurological mechanisms of mental activities.

The differentiation between basic neurological mechanisms, triggered non-specifically by sensory inputs, and the symbolic meaning of coded messages was vividly demonstrated by the late British neurologist and Nobel Laureate, Lord Adrian, known as the scientist who photographed thought and made nerves audible. In one of his experiments, Adrian placed electrodes in the cat's ear and connected them to a system of electronic amplification. Then, as he talked to the animal, his words could be heard—with some distortion— through a loudspeaker. The explanation was simple: the cat's auditory system was transducing the human voice into electrical patterns which were picked up, instrumentally amplified, and reconverted into sound. Obviously the animal had not suddenly learnt to talk: the experiment demonstrated only that the cat's ear could be used as a biological microphone. Voice communication with an animal produces electrical phenomena which are transmitted by auditory pathways through the brain. Animals are unable to understand human language. Some may obey elementary commands but cannot grasp the grammatical and symbolic complexity of a conversation because they lack the cerebral organization for the acquisition and use of language. Only the human species has this ability. The basic neurological mechanisms that transform sound into electrophysiological codes are similar in both animals and humans, but the more sophisticated neuronal anatomy and physiology which permit understanding and production of articulated speech are an exclusive human privilege. The anatomical substrate may be some specific modes of intercellular activity and a distinctive pattern of transcortical fibre connections.[4]

Chimpanzees have been taught to use symbols, plastic cards, and even computers to make requests, form new phrases, and communicate with people.[5,6] This ability may be considered the phylogenetic beginning of the use of language by primates, but it is still very elementary, and the symbols and instruments used are the creations of man, not of chimpanzees.

The use of language is a sophisticated means of communication and one of the most important manifestations of the mind, permitting symbolic thought and transmission of culture and placing human beings far above other animals in this capacity. Possession of a complex brain, however, does not automatically provide humans with language, which is an acquired skill like playing the piano or driving a car. Each individual must learn to code and decode symbols. Neurological structures must be developed through training. Symbols used in English are useless in Chinese.

In early childhood, the cerebral hemispheres are not yet specialized for language, and the left-to-right polarization resulting in dominance is easily blocked by different types of disorders.[7] Anatomical and functional development of the brain depends not only on genetically determined and time-dependent sequences of maturation but also on individual experience. As shown by several investigators, the binding capacity of synaptosome fractions, the local amount of cholinesterase, the amount of RNA, the number of excentric nucleoli, and other morphological, physiological and chemical characteristics of the neurons are decisively influenced by the quality and quantity of received sensory stimulation.[8,9,10]

Sensory inputs are essential for the development of material and functional elements of the brain, and these in turn are essential for the development of mental qualities. Information is materialized as memory traces. In this way, a continuous feedback is established between the anatomical and physiological properties of the brain and the functional manifestations of the mind. The sounds of words are heard by the individual who talks, constituting an indispensable feedback for the functional structuring of the brain.

Clinical study of aphasias reveals that these language deficits may be related to (1) production, when the patient understands but cannot talk; (2) cognition, when understanding is very difficult although production of words is possible; and (3) amnesia, when words are difficult to find but understanding and talking are fairly normal. These and other types of aphasias correspond to different types of brain damage, an indication that language is an extremely complex activity with different functional aspects represented anatomically and physiologically in different parts of the brain. For research and diagnosis, as well as for therapy, it would be a gross error to pool together all human beings with speech difficulties.

In summary, possession of language by the individual depends on three groups of elements: (1) genetic determinants responsible for the growth and maturation of the brain; (2) sensory inputs which influence the anatomical and physiological development of specific brain structures; and (3) acquisition through learning of symbols, decodification mechanisms and motor skills. Each of these three elements is essential; in the absence of any one of them, the use of language will be disturbed or even completely blocked.

In this neurophysiological discussion, language has been selected as a typical mental activity related to many others, including intelligence, memory, emotions and understanding. A specific mental function is considered in order to avoid the problem inherent in many debates, in which the mind is regarded as a unit when in reality it is complex and heterogeneous in its qualities, biological mechanisms and functional consequences. We should expect disagreement among those who theoretically refer to the same subject—the mind—although one of them is considering free will, another consciousness and still another aggressive behaviour. The intervening related neurochemical and neurophysiological mechanisms, brain structures and manifestations are different in each case.

OWNERSHIP OF THE MIND

Personal ownership of our body is usually taken for granted. We feel our skin, use our senses and command our muscles. In a similar way, we assume proprietorship of our ideas, emotions and experiences. Personal identity is based on the possession throughout life of a determined set of physical and mental characteristics. These ideas should, however, be discussed in the light of recent biological findings.

The concept of possession of the air in our lungs may be valid for a brief period of time because the gas within our chest is not shared with anyone else and is separated momentarily from the environment. Most of the air we breathe flows in and out of our lungs. A percentage of oxygen penetrates the blood, to be combined with the haemoglobin and transported to the capillaries of muscles, liver and various organs where oxidative processes occur. Some of this oxygen is transformed into carbon dioxide and transported through the veins back to the lungs, from where it is expelled to the environment. The possession of air, therefore, is of rather limited duration.

The water we drink passes to the stomach and intestines, is absorbed, transported by the circulation, retained in small amounts, and mostly eliminated by the lungs, kidneys and perspiration. We 'own' much of our body water for only a short period.

Property rights are also debatable for the content of the intestines, for clipped nails and hair, or for our own blood, which is in a continuous process of renovation. Modern biology shows that most of the material substratum of the body is constantly being transformed. The bones of a child change in structure, strength, shape and chemical composition according to the amount and direction of mechanical forces. Musculature is modified in relation to its use and disuse. The human central nervous system consumes ten times more oxygen than most other tissues, due to its very active metabolism which includes a rapid rate of protein synthesis. Neurons do not regenerate like other less differentiated cells, but their submicroscopic content and structure are in a process of continuous change and renovation, involving the release and uptake of different chemicals. The traditional concept of neuronal stability should consequently be re-evaluated.

Learning in rats is known to be related to an increase of protein S 100 in the nerve cells of the hippocampus.[11] Apparently, short-term information is stored near the synapses at which signals arrive and are read out, while lasting memory traces involve RNA-dependent mechanisms of the nucleus. Neuronal membranes involved in these processes are morphologically, biochemically and functionally different mosaics. Structural changes in the synaptic membranes occur under the influence of different types of transmitters. Synaptic regions are modified through the influence of pre- and post-synaptic areas; altered uptake, availability and release of several transmitters; variations in the number, size and sensitivity of the receptor sites; structural changes in the synaptic cleft; and modifications in the diffusion rate and extent of the neural transmitters.[12] The presence and characteristics of glycolipids and glycoproteins of neuronal surfaces may play an essential role in specific interneuronal recognition.

The dynamic complexity of neuronal activities is under the continuous influence of genetic determinants, inducer gradients, reactive tendencies, metabolic and humoral factors, electrophysiological phenomena, received inputs and many other elements which shape the composition, structure and functions of the neuronal units and responses of neuronal pools. Most of these processes depend on genetically established mechanisms, on automatic reactivity and on the flow of information reaching the brain from the environment. Pacemaking of the respiratory centre, electrical coding of sensory inputs, and complex neuronal activity do not depend on personal preferences; moreover, many of their mechanisms are similar in cats and in humans. We do not personally 'own' these mechanisms, which are given to all mammals. We do not 'own' the material and functional elements of the brain or the information flowing in and out of the brain.

Ownership of these materials, mechanisms and information is a matter of interpretation. Air and water, like sensory inputs, are elements which originate outside the organism and penetrate it for a limited time. Each organism could be considered either as the centre of these transactions and the proprietor of elements circulating within it, or as a miniscule short-lived unit involved in these transactions. A similar problem is whether to accept the earth as the centre of the universe, which has relative validity from the human point of view, or as a tiny particle lost in the immensity of the galaxies, which is more accurate from a cosmic position. The privilege of human intelligence is to understand both concepts within their frames of reference and to accept each as supplementing the other.

Perhaps a more important question than ownership is the study of the origin, properties, timing and evolution of the different elements which form each human being. What is preserved and what is altered from birth to death? Fingerprints are a permanent individual characteristic; personal experiences stored in memory are unique although usually modified by time; skills may be learnt, modified and forgotten; taste may be educated and changed; ethics may be influenced by social factors; beauty may fade. Is a person the same at 50 years of age as at 15, or when he or she was born? On which characteristics shall we base personal identity?

Many of these factors can be investigated with the aid of neurobiological technology. If personal identity is determined by elements which can be known and manipulated, should we let natural chance be the decisive power in structuring each individual brain, or should we use our intelligence in order to encourage the development of neuronal and behavioural qualities selected with a human purpose?

BUILDING BLOCKS OF MENTAL ACTIVITY

If we compare the brains of bees, frogs, monkeys and human beings, the most surprising observation is the similarity of their neuronal structures, chemical mechanisms and physiological activities. Much of our information about the release of neurotransmitters, spike potentials and dendritic activation seen in the rat is valid for the human brain, and in fact neurophysiological and psychopharmacological investigations are usually performed in rats and cats. How, then, does the human brain differ from that of lower species? The human brain does *not* have special, larger or more sophisticated nerve cells which could account for its higher mental capacities. As Ramon y Cajal suggested 70 years ago, these higher capacities seem to result from the greater amount of small neurons, neuronal branching and synaptic multiplicity.[13]

How can we explain the appearance of human qualities in the brain of apes as they became transformed into hominids? How many 'human' mental functions were present—or lacking, or undeveloped—in the pithecanthrope or in Neanderthal man? Anthropological research has provided data about the weight and shape of the evolving brain in chronological parallel with achievements such as the invention of tools, the ability to make fires, the use of signs and alphabets, and other indications of increasing intelligence. Progressive humanization of the primate brain was a slow process, taking hundreds of thousands of years, and we can only speculate about the biological bases. Fortunately we may approach this problem experimentally in existing primate species. For example, we know that contemporary monkeys and apes possess rudimentary manifestations of consciousness, intelligence, symbolic communication, use of tools, recognition of their own image and other mental attributes, while they lack articulated language, culture, scientific and artistic creativity, and other human qualities. The most careful and time-consuming education of baby chimpanzees, reared in human households, has been able to teach them only a limited repertoire of symbols, a smattering of grammatical associations, and a few skills and tricks, but nothing comparable to the growth of human children who quickly forge ahead of the chimpanzees, revealing their cerebral superiority in many ways. If the same environment and the most painstaking teaching efforts produce such different results in training the minds of chimpanzees and human babies, an explanation should be sought in the biological differences between their brains.

In the reverse situation, some cases have been described of feral children who developed in the wilderness among animals, without contact with other humans. These 'human' children, when recovered and returned to civilization, behaved with animalistic reactions, and in spite of subsequent efforts to train them to act like other people, they were practically unable to understand or learn to speak any language. Their brains lacked the functional coordinates needed to produce most of the behaviour considered 'human', because these children had not been exposed during early development to appropriate cultural and social sensory inputs.

The process of humanization is a daily experience for every baby. Starting from birth, mental functions develop over the years. Biological and mental correlations may be investigated by examining victims of genetic defects, traumatic accidents and nutritive insufficiencies, and also members of different cultural environments. It is very difficult to determine when and how the mind is formed, and many theories have been proposed, ranging from acceptance of a pre-existing mind given to the body at a specific moment (perhaps at birth), to the concept of mindless newborn babies (not yet human?) who slowly acquire the materials, functions and structural elements necessary for the formation of a mind.

Ancient beliefs about the existence in the germinal cell of a compressed 'homunculus' with microscopic eyes, arms, legs and an unveiled but preformed mind have been disproven by experimental embryology. Chromosomes do not contain a heart, brain or any other organ. They carry only a set of architectonic plans able to direct the organization of the building elements formed by proteins, fats, carbohydrates and other components supplied from the outside via the maternal placenta. These materials will be shaped into new sets of instructions and into multiplying cells that start the formation of organs and functional systems.

It should be emphasized that an architect's plans are only instructions, not real buildings. The most beautiful project is only a promise which without bricks, cement, steel and other materials will remain a collection of papers. A germinal cell and even the embryo are only possibilities, not realities, of human beings. Plans are unfulfilled for millions of sexual cells and countless miscarried embryos.

In spite of these facts, many respected authors believe that the fertilized ovum contains the primordia of 'what we later call mind'.[14] 'The appearance of recognizable mind in the soma would then be not a reaction *de novo* but a development of mind from unrecognizable into recognizable'.[15]

The controversy between heredity and environment (nature and nurture) as determinants of mental functions and personality is classical in the literature. The importance of the prenatal period for future behaviour crystallized in the concept of ontogenetic zero,[16] and is accepted by most child psychologists.[17] An even more controversial issue is the starting moment of human existence, as well as the human mind. Could it be at the time of fecundation? When the ovum is implanted in the uterus? As soon as there is a rudiment of heart and brain? When there is viability at six or seven months of fetal life? At the moment of birth? Or perhaps the human being starts later, at the onset of detectable mental functions in the baby?

At present, the debate of nature versus nurture and its dichotomy of percentages (50%–50%?) is losing interest. Research and evaluation of data are directed towards analysis of the specific roles of the many intervening elements and the study of their mutual relations. It is not very useful to discuss what is more important in a house—the plans of the architect, the bricks, cement, decoration or activities of the owner. Each element is essential; many substitutions are possible, and what may be discussed are the consequences of each choice with respect to the integrated functioning of the whole house. In a similar way, we should investigate the mechanisms and consequences related to the selection of events leading to the acquisition of human cerebral functions.

The set of chromosomes, and therefore the genetic characteristics of each individual, derive from paternal and maternal sexual cells linked together by pure chance, without the intervention of human intelligence and without consideration for parental desires. They are given automatically to the embryo without its consent and without concern for that individual's future success or failure. Under the guidance of genetic organizers, using the available materials provided by the maternal placenta, and with suitable or unsatisfactory adjustments to possible alimentary deprivations, the new being will be structured according to pre-established rules and mechanisms, developing to term in the uterus, and finally being born and detached from the umbilical cord.

Partners may be chosen for their physical aspect, cultural background and personal qualities, but there is no way of selecting and encouraging a specific spermatozoa to win the swimming competition inside the Fallopian tubes and, alone, to reach the target of the waiting ovum. We are ignorant of the wonderful possibilities and tragic handicaps hidden in the genetic codes carried by innumerable parent cells.

In summary, plans for the structural and functional beginning of individual life are established by chance, without intelligent choice of the parents and obviously without intervention of the new being who is in a state of creation and lacks cerebral mechanisms for knowing or choosing.

The question whether, in the newborn human brain, there is a coexisting mind is difficult to answer because it depends on our concept of mind. The possibility of conscious experience in the fetus was a classical philosophical and psychological problem (see, for example, Locke[18] and Peterson and Rainey[19]). Modern studies indicate, however, that for the fetus immersed in the night of amniotic fluid—without visual, auditory, olfactory, or gustatory sensations—the possibility of awareness is extremely limited.

To clarify discussion, instead of referring to the vagaries of an undefined mind, it is preferable to focus attention on the appearance of specific qualities such as: upright posture, purposeful motor activity, comprehension of sensory inputs, language, substitutive or symbolic behaviour and intelligent choice. Some of these functions, for example motor skills, are present in animals but far below the mature human level. It is well known that human beings are born with very immature brains and that babies are unable to survive by themselves, requiring care and feeding. At birth, a baby cannot have upright posture or purposeful motor activity because of the absence of a myelinated pyramidal tract, the lack of branching dendrites in the basal ganglia, the development of only a small fraction of future synaptic connections in the cerebellum, and the absence of ideokinetic formulas in the brain.

The problem is not that motor skills are dormant somewhere in the brain, waiting only to be unveiled. The newborn brain does not have the anatomical support, functional mechanisms or experiential background for skilful mobility. Each of these three elements is essential for motor skills to appear. The crucial fact is that anatomical and functional development of the brain proceed by genetic determination but *under the guidance of sensory experience*. Learning leaves material traces in the neuronal flesh, influencing synaptic anatomy, enzymic activity, functional selectivity of pathways and chemical composition of the neurons.

Initial learning will modify brain structures and transmitting systems, making possible further and more complex learning. At birth, the brain is so immature that its learning capacity is very limited. Skills are not unveiled: *their mechanisms must be constructed* inside the brain. The cerebral areas which organize hand movements may have the potential to learn the ideokinetic formulas necessary for playing musical instruments, but these abilities do not exist in the naive brain, nor will they be acquired without training. Motor coordination and skilful performance *do not emerge* from the brain but must be *absorbed* through the experience provided by sensory inputs entering the central nervous system and by trial and error learning. The received information which imprints neurons and creates feedbacks and correlations will later be *expressed* by the functioning brain.

In a similar way, the speech areas are undeveloped at birth and it is impossible for a newborn infant to learn to talk in a few days. Languages are not dormant somewhere in the brain. A baby must undergo many months of training before it learns, very slowly at first, to parrot some words and then to comprehend their meanings and start constructing phrases. Early sensory experience will be decisive for the physiological organization of speech areas.

This is precisely one of the important differences between animals and human beings. The instinctive repertoire of lambs and calves permits them to start walking as soon as they are born, and this advantage represents a neuronal rigidity which prevents a greater influence of the environment. In the human species, each individual must learn a multiplicity of non-instinctive behavioural responses, thus enriching the personal brain by the cultural acquisition of millennia of human existence. Genes do provide the initial neuronal mechanisms of learning but not the information to be learnt, which necessarily originates in the environment and must be introduced into the brain through sensory inputs.

Molecules carrying information have two fundamental characteristics: (1) the message; and (2) a specific address. Peptides, steroids, prostaglandins and other substances acting as messengers may be compared to orders sent in closed envelopes with well-marked destinations. The material substratum is within each organism, but the coded messages originate outside and are received as sensory inputs. These messages will trigger the established mechanisms into action.

Codes are recognizable patterns of a material substratum, where the material element is accessory and does not carry information *per se*. For example, we may write 'I love you' on a piece of paper, on a tree, or in the sand, without changing its meaning. Experimental neurophysiology may provide data with which we can understand the correlations between information (including values) and matter, and between brain and mind.

At birth the baby does not recognize the face of its mother, does not talk, does not understand sensory inputs, and is certainly unable to behave intelligently. We must conclude that at that moment the most fundamental mental properties do not yet exist.

It should be made clear that action potentials and the released neurohumors act as material carriers of coded information in a comparable manner to paper, tree bark, or sand. The meaning of a message will be lost to scientific recording instruments because the meaning is related to frames of reference stored with past personal experience. Memory traces are made by modifications of the neurochemical and synaptic structure of neuronal pools in specific cerebral areas. In this way, the non-material aspect of information (its symbolic meaning) is materialized, and shapes the anatomy and chemistry of neuronal structures. The reverse is also true: because of the material bases of memory storage in the brain, electrical and neurochemical carriers may be elicited by sensory inputs, triggering the non-material manifestations of language and behaviour. Of course the evaluation of messages as 'non-material' is a question of interpretation; the important aspect is the possibility of investigating the molecular and neuronal phenomena necessary for the reception, elaboration and expression of information. In any case, the process of interconversion between codes and neuronal substance may provide decisive clues for the understanding of relations between brain and mind. At least we may approach both subjects experimentally and study the properties of their relations and intertransformations.

The mind does not appear suddenly or synchronously in all its manifestations but evolves as a multifactorial entity with its many elements at different stages of existence and refinement. Most of these elements are acquired slowly, step by step. Harlow and Harlow[20] demonstrated that both monkeys and children must learn how to learn. Comprehension of reality, correlation of information, retention and recollection, power of abstraction, must all be learnt. Solving one problem facilitates the finding of solutions for other problems.

On the basis of these observations, the following statements are proposed which can be used as working hypotheses for further research:

(1) At birth, the human brain is so immature that it does not have the anatomical, chemical or functional mechanisms for mental activities such as language, understanding of sensory inputs, intelligent analysis of

information, knowledge and identification of the environment, decision-making, awareness of the future, planning of behaviour and other functions.

(2) For these reasons at birth the human mind does not and cannot exist.

(3) Mechanisms for and existence of many mental functions require as building blocks information provided by the environment which will modify physically and chemically the shape and functions of specific areas of the brain.

(4) The appearance of mental activities requires the conjunction of the following factors: (a) the existence of a brain; (b) its progressive maturation under the direction of genetic preprogramming, using the materials ingested as nourishment; (c) reception of sensory inputs; (d) physical and chemical imprinting of neurons determined by the circulating codes of messages; (e) codes of information necessary for forming a memory storage (personal experience) which will be the individual frame of reference for decoding and interpreting the further reception of stimuli; and (f) patterns of motility (ideokinetic formulas) for automating responses and permitting the concentration of awareness and intelligence on a few selected topics, leaving most of the processing of information and motor and emotional reactions to subconscious mechanisms.

Parents—and society—have only two alternatives: they may either close their eyes and let natural chance affect the development of children, or they may use their intelligence to influence natural development by genetic counselling, perinatal care and infant education. In this case goals for individuals must be chosen. Most human societies approve of intervening to guide the physical and mental growth of babies, without realizing that these actions, however well meaning, signify a very powerful brain control which the affected individual cannot evade.

MONISM, DUALISM AND TRIUNISM

In relation to the classical brain–mind problem, solutions proposed in the past fall into two categories:

(1) *Dualism* accepts the existence of two entities which, according to different doctrines, (a) are *independent* of each other; (b) have a *parallel* existence with close relations, in which (c) the brain *influences* the mind (epiphenomenalism); (d) the mind *controls* the brain (mentalism); and (e) mind and brain *interact* with each other (interactionism).

(2) *Monism* postulates the existence of a single entity. In the extreme doctrines, (a) everything is *mental;* or (b) everything is *material*. More conservative theorists propose that (c) the brain and mind are only multiple aspects of the same entity (neutral monism); (d) the mind is corporeal (reductive materialism); or (e) mental states form a subset of brain states, emerging from the brain although they do not exist within brain cells, synaptosomes, dendrites or other neuronal elements (*emergentist* materialism[21]).

The postulates of this programmatic hypothesis have been formulated by Bunge[21] as follows:

'(i)   All mental states, events and processes are states of, or events and processes in, the central nervous systems of vertebrates;
(ii) these states, events and processes are emergent relative to those of the cellular components of the CNS;
(iii) the so-called psychophysical relations are interactions between different subsystems of the CNS, or between them and other components of the organism'.

Emergent materialism is perhaps the most flexible and biologically oriented hypothesis and it has been a driving force in physiological psychology and in investigation of mental phenomena through normal scientific procedures.

The hypothesis proposed in the present article is termed '*triunism*' and postulates that the mind is a unity with three structural elements so essential that the absence of any one will prevent its existence. These elements are:

(1)   Brain cells and pathways possessing material and transmaterial properties as explained later.
(2)   A flow of transmaterial, environmental information, coded and transduced at the sensory receptors and forming an active part of the working brain through a modification of its anatomy and physiology.
(3)   Detectable manifestations derived from (1) and (2) which are expressed inward as perceptions and outward as behaviour.

Triunism also postulates a dynamic, evolutive interrelation among the structural elements of the mind with the parameter 'time' always going forward. We cannot stop the mind; we cannot study it in isolation from the transactions of messages. The mind is always changing and evolving. Exploration of the question 'who am I?'—even if it could be answered satisfactorily—would have only a brief, temporal validity. As the 'I' is continually reacting to the environment, it cannot be known or identified in absolute terms. We could only identify the statistical probability of determined sets of responses.

In contradiction with monistic conceptions, the mind is not an emergent property of the brain which will automatically appear after suitable periods of maturation and growth. The appearance of the mind is slow and its many functions develop at different speeds and times, directed by the conjunction of genetic tendencies, materials received from the outside, and the decisive role of referential systems provided by sensory inputs. There is pluralism in the origin of the structural elements of the mind, some of which reside in the material brain, others in the material environment, and still others in the non-material codes provided by material carriers.

In summary: the mind appears and develops when extracerebral elements (symbols, temporal relations between incoming information and codes of behaviour) conveyed by material carriers penetrate the brain, shaping the physical structure of neurons. This explanation provides the neurophysiological mechanism for mental humanization within our material body, for acceptance of a 'spiritual' element inside the brain, and for interaction between material and non-material events. There is no need for an individually-structured mind to enter the body to provide consciousness, identity and personality. The necessary elements enter as tiny fractions of a huge dynamic puzzle, and many bits are needed to construct each mental function. Triunism provides a working plan for investigating the constituent elements of the mind and should clarify some aspects of dualistic and monistic doctrines.

The term 'triune brain' has been used by MacLean,[22] who postulates that the human cerebrum has the remnants of structures which have evolved from reptiles and extinct mammals. Conflicts could derive from different activities of these three amalgamated brains: the reptilian, palaeomammalian and neo-mammalian. The triunism proposed in this paper is unrelated to the phylo-genetic structuring of the brain and refers to the triunity in the origin, structure and functions of the elements which integrate the mind.

Support for the postulates of triunism is provided by a reinterpretation of the research of Sperry and others (see a good summary by Sperry[23]) who have demonstrated that, after surgical separation of the cerebral hemispheres in cats, monkeys and human patients, each half of the brain is able to sense, perceive, learn and remember independently of the other, being cut off from and inaccessible to recall through the opposite hemisphere. Monkeys have been trained to perform contradictory tasks learnt through lateralized inputs reaching only one hemisphere. Thus a monkey using only the left eye, controlled by the right half of the brain, may be taught that a circle represents reward and a square means punishment, while when only the right eye is used the animal may learn the reverse values. The animal's reactions suggest that conscious experience may be different and independent in each of the disconnected hemispheres.

Splitting the brain also divides consciousness and awareness. After cerebral commissurotomy performed to control intractable epilepsy in patients, their surgically separated hemispheres are independently conscious. By using manual signs, a patient can indicate that the 'minor' and 'non-vocal' right side perceives and comprehends the same stimulus input for which the 'speaking' left hemisphere disclaims any awareness. At the same time, the minor hemisphere displays a lack of ability to respond to stimulus input restricted to the vocal hemisphere. It has been asked whether patients with surgically disconnected cerebral hemispheres have two consciousnesses; whether they are one or two persons; who is who; who is the original individual; and even whether they should have two votes!

These split-brain studies demonstrate that consciousness, awareness, learning, recall and other mental activities may be split when each hemisphere is shaped independently by the three structural elements of the mind postulated in triunism. As indicated by Sperry[23], consciousness has been considered a passive phenomenon in cerebral operations, whereas actually it depends on higher brain activities, and therefore inner consciousness and subjective experience are accessible as subjects of experimental research. Behavioural sciences are becoming more interested in mentalistic, subjectivistic and humanistic phenomena.

Some qualifications should be added to Sperry's[1] statement that '... mind moves matter in the brain just as an organism moves its component organs and cells or a molecule governs the molecular course of its own electrons'. Most authors referring to the brain disregard the origin of its constituent elements. An organism already contains its organs, but the essential elements of the mind are initially extracerebral sets of information, and only after their reception, coding and circulation will they form an integral part of the brain by influencing the structure of the material carriers, without necessarily changing their amount of mass or energy.

For similar reasons I should question Sperry's statement that '... human values are inherently properties of brain activity'. Human values are not genetically determined, but must be individually acquired through the information learnt after being transduced at the sensory receptors. Therefore personal values have an extracerebral source which depends on the cultural environment and are *not* inherent properties of neuronal functions. They are related to structural modifications of the brain acquired by personal experience.

MATERIAL CARRIERS AND TRANSMATERIAL INFORMATION

It could be argued that the concept of triunism is not very original because its three elements include (a) the brain, as in other theories; (b) the flow of information, which in reality is the environment; and (c) manifestations of perceptions and motility which are part of mental functions. Also, the term 'triunism' may sound theological, although as presented it is free from metaphysical overtones.

Triunism's possible merit is to emphasize the biological bases of the mind, analysing the origin and role of the necessary building blocks. With this approach, we may investigate (a) the onset and evolution of each mental function during the process of humanization of the newborn brain; (b) the disappearance of mental fragments due to cerebral disturbances; and (c) the progressive loss of mental activities during old age.

During the lifetime of every person, the mind appears, grows, changes and fades away. In these processes, each mental fragment may be in a different stage of development. We may question how many mental functions (and how much of each) must be present to establish the mind. Is the mind 'smaller' than normal in a blind, deaf and dumb person; in sensorially and culturally deprived children; in lobotomized patients; or in microcephalic individuals? These questions are misleading because it is difficult to consider the whole mind, and preferable to discuss the specific aspects which integrate it. Obviously a blind man is deprived of visual aspects of mental activity and has a physiological deficit in the occipital cortex, superior colliculus and other vision-related structures, but he may have compensations due to refinement of other mental functions such as tactual and auditory perception.

Triunism stresses the essentiality of the three proposed elements of the mind which are considered so interrelated that their separation would be artificial. There is general agreement that, unlike the brain, the mind cannot be located, touched, weighed or preserved in formalin. The mind cannot be seen: only the consequences of its activities are observable as 'mental functions' which are heterogeneous qualities including consciousness, perception, intelligence, memory, emotion, and many other ill-defined entities. These functions may be correlated with cerebral anatomy and physiology by the detailed study of determined structures.

In the brain–mind controversy, the brain is usually believed to possess a variety of structures and functions that, in dualism, can be correlated with mental activities. Triunism maintains that these concepts may be considered in the mature brain but not at birth, because the newborn brain does not have and cannot develop by itself the appropriate functions necessary for the appearance of the mind. *The outside world enters through the senses and becomes a material and functional part of the maturing brain.* The central nervous system, considered independently of its essential extracerebral constituents, cannot function properly.

Without a brain, the mind cannot exist. Without sensory inputs, the mind will not be structured and cannot appear. Without manifestations of inner perceptions and outward motor expression, the mind cannot be recognized by the individual or the environment.

In agreement with monism, the mind has a material and functional unity, but in triunism it is structured by elements originating from three different sources. Without these elements, mental functions cannot exist and, in reality, the mind is only the result of their dynamic interrelations.

The concept of blood pressure provides a simpler example. Pumping of the heart, velocity and viscosity of the blood, peripheral resistance determined by arterial and capillary tonicity and other factors are in continuous, dynamic equilibrium providing pressure to the circulating liquid. In the absence of heart, blood or arteries, blood pressure cannot exist. We may preserve the heart in formalin, but not the blood pressure. Many hormonal, chemical and physical actions may influence the level of the blood pressure. There is a relation between the heart and blood pressure (as between the brain and mind) but it would be incorrect to evaluate blood pressure as an independent entity when, in reality, it is a manifestation of heart activity with the intervention of many other factors.

The distinction between *material* and *non-material* is essential for an understanding of the mind. Matter has been described as an aggregate of elemental particles (electrons, protons and mesons) possessing the inherent property of inertia, capable of being located in space and time, and able to interact by the impact of gravitational forces. Matter may be destroyed, releasing energy. In the last analysis, the whole world—the universe—consists of massy material objects and empty spaces. Chemistry is reducible to physics through the quantum mechanical theory of the chemical bond, and biology is based on complex physical and chemical organization of matter, with special laws and new emergent properties.

The existence and properties of material particles may be demonstrated experimentally provided that the investigator possesses the intellectual tool of knowledge, and uses suitable frames of symbolic reference and instrumentation. For anyone without adequate scientific education, a conversation about protons and mesons would be meaningless. Although a painting is necessarily structured by elements of gravitational matter, this fact will not help our understanding of the artistic and symbolic meaning of a masterpiece. In its struggle to eliminate the vestiges of metaphysical divine designs, supernatural forces and Brentano's intentionality, materialism also tries to reject the existence of the immaterial without realizing the essentiality of a non-material concept in the study of natural phenomena.

The term 'immaterial' has considerable emotional and cultural loading related to souls, spirits and a dualistic conception of reality. For this reason, it may be preferable to distinguish three orders of entities, namely (1) *material*, as defined earlier; (2) relatively non-material but materially dependent, which I propose to call *transmaterial*, as explained below; and (3) *immaterial*, which as accepted by many authors includes elements without material support and not necessarily related to matter, although interaction with material phenomena would be possible. For example, the soul is conceived of as an immaterial entity endowed with supernatural destiny, which enters and leaves the body, persisting after biological death. Immaterial entities are beyond the realm of experimental research and may be discussed only as philosophical or theological concepts.

Transmaterial entities require the existence of supporting matter and may be represented by patterns of material organization or by temporal or functional relations between parts of the material substratum. They may transcend the existence of specific materials, changing carriers while preserving their non-material identity, but they do not possess intrinsic properties of matter such as mass and energy. Transmaterial aspects of reality, including the material substratum, patterning, and relative, temporal and functional characteristics may be subjects of experimental research.

Transmaterial entities such as symbols, information and meaning, are not emergent properties of matter because they are not related to intrinsic atomic organization, nor can they appear as the result of natural material characteristics, being related to physiological functions requiring temporal and spatial associations of experiences of individual brains. A mould gives shape to matter, transmitting information without exchanging substance or energy. A material carrier may influence the organization of another material carrier without mixing any of its intrinsic material properties. Transmaterial entities are *carried by but not necessarily related to* material carriers.

The concept of transmaterial may be useful in the understanding of cerebral processing of information because it allows the separate study of mechanisms involved in the flow of sensory inputs, the transduction of messages through different systems, and the decoding necessary for comprehension of meaning, for individual perception and for reactive responses.

Pattern detection by specific neurons of the cerebral cortex seems to be determined by early individual experience. Experiments in kittens have shown that, during a critical period of 3 to 14 weeks after birth, daily exposure for one hour to an environment with vertical stripes resulted in a specificity of response of most cortical neurons for the stimulus pattern received. Information-extracting neurons have been described as able to respond to universal features, such as temporal and spatial transients, or to species-specific features, for example bug detectors in the frog, rotation movements in the fly, and colour-sensitive cells in the monkey (see summary by Blakemore[24]).

In the auditory system there are also feature-sensitive neurons that abstract information from complex auditory environments. There are cortical neurons capable of differentiating noises, clicks, tones and species-specific calls. Some cortical neurons may 'respond' to questions such as 'Is the stimulus on?' 'Has it just commenced?' 'Is the frequency changing?' 'If so, in which direction and at what rate?' 'Where is the stimulus located in space?' 'Is it moving?' and so on; (see summary by Evans[25]).

The complex circuitry necessary for some of these functions does not seem to be preprogrammed by genetic determinants and apparently it depends on environmental information impinging on the developing sensory cortex. In this way, the received information shapes the functional characteristics of the neuronal systems.

The mechanisms for recognition of meaning are poorly understood and some models have been proposed. According to Pribram,[26] inputs are distributed in sensory systems into an 'alphabet' of spatial frequency-sensitive elements at the striate cortex. This alphabet is temporarily assembled for the purpose of a specific recognition. 'A parallel processing mechanism initiated in the inferotemporal cortex addresses (categorizes) the elements of the alphabet via motor structures (e.g. the putamen) much as a program tape organizes a program by addressing elements in the memory of a computer'.[26]

Information received, stored or expressed by pattern-detection neurons and by a 'recognition program-tape model' depend on codes which flow through brain cells and neuronal circuits. To illustrate this fact, let us consider the second element of triunism—the flow of sensory information from the environment to the individual brain. We may postulate that this process requires both *material carriers* and *transmaterial, coded symbols*. As already discussed, matter is a non-specific element in sensory reception, while the coded symbols are specific messages whose exact meaning may be conveyed by different material carriers such as light, sound and shapes. For example, the concept 'red' may be expressed in different languages, written with a variety of implements and materials, or conveyed in Morse code. The meaning by itself is independent of the eventual material carrier.

Several processes of transduction and different types of physical and chemical material carriers are involved in the transmission of a message from an environmental source to its conscious perception by the brain, and each carrier is at the service of the same meaning. The message has no gravitational fields or inertia; it cannot be smashed to release energy, nor has it any of the accepted properties of matter. The meaning of a message has no intrinsic existence because, in the absence of decoding mechanisms and perceptive minds, symbols have no significance although their material carriers may persist.

In the special orientation of electrical charges on a tape, there is no sound or music until it is detected at proper speed, amplified, transformed into waves and heard by someone. Melodies must be recreated by the transduction of electrical codes into acoustic patterns.

Codes, symbols and meanings are not intrinsic—or emergent—properties of matter but intellectual agreements of human minds, based on invented systems of reference, learnt individually through personal experience, and transcending personal existence. The alphabet was invented long ago and will be used for centuries to come.

Initially the brain and the sources of messages have independent existences. The role of the brain with respect to incoming messages is their reception, circulation, decodification, correlation, storage and reaction with sensory perceptions, emotional feelings and behavioural responses. Language, knowledge and symbols have been created by the mental activities of many brains through many centuries of accumulated culture, and are not the gift of unreachable metaphysical powers. To consider messages a property of matter may handicap their experimental study independent of material carriers.

The reverse phenomenon, of cerebral materialization of symbols, takes place during verbal expression. In this case, the material substratum in the neurons activates the codification and transduction of symbolic representations, producing at the end the vibration of vocal cords and production of sound waves carrying transmaterial messages. All these processes are unconscious and automatic.

Symbols may be shared by human beings and animals. Cats and monkeys can learn that a red light means punishment and a green light represents reward. Development of personality is primarily the experiential accumulation of symbols and frames of reference for decoding sensory information. Neurological processes are influenced by the transmaterial symbols of sensory perception, directing the material structure of neurons. In these neurological processes there is interaction between transmaterial symbolism and material structuring of memory traces. The usefulness of the concept of transmaterial is that we must deal with it as a research tool when we explore the meaning of matter.

Saying that symbolic understanding is an emergent property of matter may be basically true but it is not very helpful, whereas establishing the difference between material carriers and transmaterial codes allows the independent examination of intervening elements.

Acceptance of the transmaterial—like the concept of the non-material vacuum—does not signify an attempt to reintroduce metaphysical doctrines. With clarification and redefinition of the concept, we can hope to have better intellectual and experimental tools for the understanding of reality.

Centring attention on mental activity and its three elements, as in triunism, is only one possible way of interpreting reality. The advantage is its usefulness for experimentation, ideological conception and discussion. The mind does not require an integral definition. If we accept the mind as a group of functions structured by elements which can be identified and investigated, we may use human intelligence first to structure the newborn brain and later to direct and modify mental capacities according to techniques derived from psychophysiology. Perhaps the aphorism 'know thyself' should be supplemented by 'use your intelligence to construct a better self'.

Because newborn babies lack the experience to interpret sensory inputs, the responsibility for structuring their minds is not personal but social. The brain functions as a reactive recipient of information and patterns of response, most of which have evolved over centuries of human existence. These elements from the past shape each individual's brain and return through behavioural acts to the environment, modifying other brains and minds.

The products of mental activities transcend individual existence and each life contributes to the passage of information from the past to the future. Personal mortality takes on new significance if individuals consider themselves as torch bearers of culture to be transmitted to other generations. Personal material carriers of flesh, bones and brain have a limited duration of usually less than a hundred years, while symbols, ideas and creativity may be individual contributions to the long-lasting existence of mankind.

ACKNOWLEDGEMENTS

The experimental part of this paper was supported by funds from the Spanish Seguridad Social and the March Foundation.

The helpful criticisms of Professor Mario Bunge and discussions with Dr Federico Di Trocchio, as well as the editorial help of Caroline S. Delgado, are warmly acknowledged.

References

1. SPERRY, R. W. (1975) Bridging science and values: a unifying view of mind and brain, in *The Centrality of Science and Absolute Values*, vol. 1 *(Proc. 4th Int. Conf. ICUS)*, pp. 247–259, International Cultural Foundation, Tarrytown, N.Y.
2. DELGADO, J. M. R. (1969) *Physical Control of the Mind: Toward a Psychocivilized Society (World Perspectives Series*, vol. 41*)*, Harper & Row, New York
3. DOTY, R. W. (Chrmn.) (1977) Consciousness from neurons: where, how, why, and so what? *BIS* [Brain Information Service] *Conf. Rep. 45*, 24–39
4. GESCHWIND, N. (1965) Disconnexion syndromes in animals and man. Part I, Part II. *Brain 88*, 237–294; 585–644
5. GARDNER, R. A. & GARDNER, B. T. (1969) Teaching sign language to a chimpanzee. *Science (Wash. D.C.) 165*, 664–670
6. PREMACK, D. (1971) Language in a chimpanzee? *Science (Wash. D.C.) 172*, 808–822
7. LENNEBERG, E. H. (1970) Brain correlates of language, in *The Neurosciences: Second Study Program* (Schmitt, F. O., ed.), pp. 361–371, Rockefeller University Press, New York
8. BENNETT, E. L., KRECH, D. & ROSENZWEIG, M. R. (1964) Reliability and regional specificity of cerebral effects of an environmental complexity and training. *J. Comp. Physiol. Psychol. 57*, 440–441
9. DEFEUDIS, F. V. & DEFEUDIS, P. A. (1977) *Elements of the Behavioral Code*, Academic Press, New York
10. HYDEN, H. (1967) RNA in brain cells, in *The Neurosciences: A Study Program* (Quarton, G. C. *et al.*, eds.), pp. 248–266, Rockefeller University Press, New York
11. HYDEN, H. & LANGE, P. W. (1970) Protein changes in nerve cells related to learning and conditioning, in *The Neurosciences: Second Study Program* (Schmitt, F. O., ed.), pp. 278–288, Rockefeller University Press, New York
12. VON BAUMGARTEN, R. J. (1970) Plasticity in the nervous system at the unitary level, in *The Neurosciences: Second Study Program* (Schmitt, F. O., ed.), pp. 261–271, Rockefeller University Press, New York
13. CAJAL, S. RAMON Y (1909, 1911) *Histologie du Système Nerveux de l'Homme et des Vertébrés*, vols. I & II, Malorie, Paris
14. RAINER, J. D. (1962) The concept of mind in the framework of genetics, in *Theories of the Mind* (Scher, J. M., ed.), pp. 65–79, Free Press of Glencoe, New York
15. SHERRINGTON, C. S. (1941) *Man on His Nature*, Cambridge University Press, Cambridge
16. GESELL, A. L. (1928) *Infancy and Human Growth*, Macmillan, New York
17. CARMICHAEL, L. (1960) The onset and early development of behavior, in *Manual of Child Psychology*, 2nd edn. (Carmichael, L., ed.), pp. 60–185, John Wiley, New York
18. LOCKE, J. (1690) *Essay Concerning Human Understanding* (Harvard University Press, Cambridge, Mass., 1931)
19. PETERSON, F. & RAINEY, L. H. (1910) The beginnings of mind in the newborn. *Bull. Lying-in-Hosp. N.Y. 7*, 99–122
20. HARLOW, H. F. & HARLOW, M. K. (1949) Learning to think. *Sci. Am. 181* (8), 36–39
21. BUNGE, M. (1977) Emergence and the mind. *Neuroscience 2*, 501–509
22. MACLEAN, P. D. (1978) A mind of three minds: educating the triune brain, in *Seventy-Seventh Yearbook of the National Society for the Study of Education*, pp. 308–342, University of Chicago Press, Chicago
23. SPERRY, R. W. (1974) Lateral specialization in the surgically separated hemispheres, in *The Neurosciences: Third Study Program* (Schmitt, F. O. & Worden, F. G., eds.), pp. 5–20, MIT Press, Cambridge, Mass.
24. BLAKEMORE, C. (1974) Developmental factors in the formation of feature extracting neurons, in *The Neurosciences: Third Study Program* (Schmitt, F. O. & Worden, F. G., eds.), pp. 105–114, MIT Press, Cambridge, Mass.

25. EVANS, E. F. (1974) Neural processes for the detection of acoustic patterns and for sound localization, in *The Neurosciences: Third Study Program* (Schmitt, F. O. & Worden, F. G., eds.), pp. 121–144, MIT Press, Cambridge, Mass.
26. PRIBRAM, K. (1974) How is it that sensing so much we can do so little?, in *The Neurosciences: Third Study Program* (Schmitt, F. O. & Worden, F. G., eds.), pp. 249–261, MIT Press, Cambridge, Mass.

Discussion: Triunism

Medawar: This is a completely epigenetic theory of development of the brain and the mind. To complete an epigenetic theory you have to try and explain what, in material terms, is the nature of the potentialities in the brain which are brought out by environmental stimuli, sensory inputs and so forth.

Searle: Could we have a definition of epigenetic?

Towers: Epigenesis is a process in which one thing is developed after, and sometimes as a result of, another, rather than everything being preformed in miniature, so to speak, i.e. the alternative 'preformation hypothesis'. There was much debate about these rival theories in the 18th century.

Medawar: It is normally classed as preformation but it is the evocation by the environment of what was formerly thought to be innate.

Delgado: Consciousness requires a temporal and spatial association between two or more sets of information coming from the outside and combined through established and acquired brain processes. In this way one element is related to others stored inside the brain. Understanding of reality depends on previously learnt frames of reference. Does that answer your question?

Medawar: No, but this is exactly where the meeting started, by talking about John Locke who was a *tabula rasa* man.

Delgado: I don't believe in a *tabula rasa*.

Putnam: I don't think that there is a mind–body problem or mind–brain problem in the usual sense. Everybody says there is this big mind–brain problem and Mario Bunge has a list of possible solutions. When we have said that, we go on to talk about the brain, except that occasionally we wring our hands and say 'are both hemispheres aware or aren't they?' I think that is no accident and that we have here a case of two languages. In fact there are many languages of mind. There isn't just one language in which we describe consciousness. There isn't even *one* language in which we describe what used to be called 'sense data'. The old argument about whether the mental image of the cartwheel is elliptical or circular is an example of confusion on this point. There is always a tendency to try to fit two or more languages for discourses into one. Asking where in the brain the mind is seems to me like asking how many miles from physical facts are legal facts. I argued in an earlier session that empirical facts are relevant to philosophy, but that does not mean that every question one can pose must have a determinate answer and that all we have to do is keep investigating empirically to find it out. Conceptual issues have been badly slighted in our discussion.

Bunge: I don't think that you are postulating the existence of three separate substances, Professor Delgado. Rather you insist on the need to study three different aspects. If anything, as a property pluralist I would quarrel with the number three, which seems too small.

Secondly, your diffidence towards the concept of emergence may be just a question of terminology. 'Emergence' is a name for the appearance of novelty. When you speak of the *appearance* of different functions at different levels of development in a child you might just as well refer to the *emergence* of those functions.

I agree of course that propositions and theories and so on are important. The only question is, are there propositions which are independent of any brains that are capable of thinking them up? Books are materializations of ideas, but will they be read by anyone if we succeed in annihilating ourselves with atomic bombs? I say no ideas will be left. A real dualist would say that there is a realm of ideas that cannot be touched, even by the most powerful atomic bomb.

Delgado: I agree that you could say either emergence or appearance but I am trying to stress that consciousness is not something that will appear only by development of the brain itself. There are other basic elements.

Bunge: I agree.

The neuroscientist's summary

J. Z. YOUNG

The Wellcome Institute for the History of Medicine, London

Before coming to this meeting I put down a note of two considerations that it is essential to remember in any discussion of this problem. The first is that we are limited by the history and current use of language. The second is that this language compels us to refer particularly and constantly to ourselves. It was therefore very satisfactory to find that many contributors also felt that these apparently trite considerations in fact contain important clues.

Searle began by trying to show us that the essence of the definition of a human mind has to do with the concept of intentionality, by which he seemed to mean the direction of interest towards or about happenings. If I understood him right the problem of the nature of this directedness cannot be decided *a priori* and is a matter for observation and experiment, for which he advocated the cooperation of scientists and philosophers. However the observations he quoted by Weiskrantz and Penfield on humans and Lettvin and colleagues on frogs did not seem to me to illuminate the nature of intentionality. I pressed him to define the word but he declined and seemed to say that it was not to be derived from intent or intension.* In a paper that John Searle kindly showed me in manuscript form he proposes to use Intentionality, with a capital I, to distinguish it from ordinary intention. This seems to me a very poor sort of philosophizing and the intrusion of Intension, with an 's', makes it worse still. Surely something should be done swiftly about this. In any case, is the philosophers' Intentionality really so different from intention? It is defined (in Searle's manuscript) as 'this feature of directedness of our mental states'.

---

*A strange feature of the day was the repudiation by some people of the need for definitions, which was repeated by Putnam and Medawar. Others in the group thought that we should not make much progress unless we agreed on the use of words. Delgado repeated the need for this at the end of the meeting.

If it is restricted to 'us' it can only be used as a criterion of mentality if we deny that capacity to animals *ab initio*. But every living process shows directedness.[1] When the cat whines at the window it shows an intention to be let in. The question of the origin and nature of directedness is a question of the origin and nature of life, no less. The discussion surely shows that others besides myself found the concept of Intentionality unclear and unhelpful. I very much hope that Searle and other philosophers may be able to find some better way of explaining their intentions to us.

Molly Brazier's account of the history of the problem of Brain and Mind emphasized early attention to the ventricles and to the persistence of vitalistic concepts. I wondered whether she had sufficiently considered the question of *why* workers directed their interest in this way. It is sometimes possible to get an insight from historical studies into characteristic features of human brain operation. The prevalence of emphasis on 'spirits' of one sort or another may spring from an innate tendency of our brain to use concepts related to humans and therefore to assume that natural events are the product of the operations of some human-like entity. The evidence from the behaviour of young children strongly suggests that we are preprogrammed to give attention to human features when we are young. Indeed we build our whole cerebral model around them and so cannot avoid thinking largely in anthropocentric terms.[2] In short the ghost is in the brain from the start. How far does this limit the way in which we think? It is 'natural' for us to think animistically and indeed, as Piaget shows, only quite late does the child reach the ability to think otherwise (i.e. in terms of natural causes). So the concept of a little person in the head, the mind or soul, came fairly readily to be used as enquiry and language developed. Of course it is not really a primitive concept. Apes do not function with concepts of spirits. One wonders if palaeoliths did.

The big advance was the recognition that what resides in the head is not an actual little man but the essence of one. Having refined the man in the head to his essence (by analogy with vapours), it was very reasonable to suppose that the spirits flowed along the nerves and were produced in the ventricles. The various concepts of spirits and humans formed quite a refined system of thought, as Sherrington showed in his study of 16th century medicine, *The Endeavour of Jean Fernel*.[3]

Dr Brazier emphasized that the strange thing was that people were so obsessed by the ventricles that they neglected the convoluted cortex. A paradigm always has this effect of attracting attention to features that seem to be relevant and neglecting others. Today we pay millions of pounds to study synapses but few people examine the programs of the whole brain, the whole activity of it, because we have no good way of speaking about the actions of the cortex and brain as a whole. So we spend our time and money on the details. Let us not be too proud and think that this is the only way of going about it. I hope perhaps the concept of Programs of the Brain may help us on the way.

I was not impressed by Towers' attempt to show how consciously learnt responses become, in the course of evolution, converted to unconscious reflexes. At one point he distinctly said *Amoeba* has awareness, and implied it even in macrophages. Later he repudiated the charge of panpsychism, but the meeting seemed not convinced.

We had fascinating information about the neurology of speech from Ploog and Bellugi, which I shall not try to summarize. Especially important for our general theme is the evidence about how cells of the auditory cortex that respond to a monkey's calls are inhibited when the animal itself vocalizes. That gives us some interesting thoughts about the possibility that self-awareness depends upon recognizing the difference between our own productions and those of others. It is striking that the higher (cingulate) level of the control system is not involved in cats and dogs. Perhaps they have awareness but not self-awareness. Hints of this sort may be a great help in solving these basic problems. Some such ideas may help with the problem of the emergence of consciousness.

Dr Bellugi's contribution fascinated and instructed us all. The way in which iconic signs become modified to allow indication of more abstract concepts is surely a lesson to those who look for the origin of language. I draw the conclusion that, unusual as our linguistic powers are, we shall one day realize their bases in animal language.

Bennett seemed to me to support rather than refute this possibility. He also emphasized that we really must try to define and refine our terminology, especially for concepts such as awareness that cover multiple situations. His idea that a baby's signs are not received by the mother was repudiated by Crown and later by Trevarthen.

On the second day of the symposium we addressed ourselves more directly to the problem than before. It seemed at times that we were even approaching the point where an answer might be found to the question asked several times by Medawar: 'What sort of answer are we looking for'. Blakemore put us on the right path with his remark that Perception is Constructive Action, and when he emphasized that each sort of animal is born with the capacity to learn the sort of information that is needed for its life. Surely this fact has profound implications for human knowledge. We are not all-purpose creatures capable of knowing anything, but limited to certain types of awareness and knowledge. Blakemore stood firmly on the ground that reality for each species is what is necessary and useful for it to know about. Bunge and others challenging this implied that there is a 'physicists' reality' over and above that of the senses. The point that even physicists are human gained assent but was not followed up. Indeed reality is a baffling subject, for the very truth of this thesis means that we cannot conceive any way in which it could be refuted.

Trevarthen carried the study of innateness further with his emphasis that the early responses of children are especially to human features. The evidence of very early intentional responses is very strong. If this is to be a criterion of mentality we must surely say that a baby already has a mind at birth. I should prefer to say that both intentionality and mentality can be detected also in animals but that human infants show from birth the human type of mentality.

Elizabeth Warrington besides describing the several sorts of human memory brought us to the critical question of what is to be the criterion of consciousness. Subjects with impaired event memory may say that they cannot recall what they have seen, but given some hints they then perform almost normally while still insisting that they are guessing.

At this point I wrote in my notes that 'it is the brain not the mind that carries the information'. After all, the patients are not conscious of the correct answers and deny that they know them. From here on I found myself increasingly insistent that whatever meaning we give to the word 'mind' it must not be considered as a continuing repository of information. It is the *brain* that continues to store our knowledge while we are asleep or when we do not require it. The information store is extremely stable. Much of what is learnt in our first year can still be used a hundred years later if we live that long. This information is not in such a vague entity as the mind. It is written in some material script in the brain. One day we shall understand how it is done.

The states that we refer to the mind, mental states, are conditions in which certain features of brain activity are in evidence to the individual concerned and, sometimes, to outside observers. These states only occur in the condition that we call consciousness but the concepts of mind and consciousness are not identical. We can say 'he has a good mind', but not 'he has a good consciousness'. Mind refers to the organization of the activities of the brain, hence the opposite of mental (which is a mode of functioning) is physical (which is that which functions). The opposite of consciousness (which is presence of a particular form of activity) is unconsciousness (absence of that form).

Susan Khin Zaw seemed to be trying to persuade us that empirical discovery is not likely to influence philosophy and that all that is necessary for philosophy is that perception be due to external objects. I probably misrepresent her views, because I really felt unable to follow them. We need to examine carefully the points of view and objectives with which we start before genuine cooperation can take place between the subtler treatments by philosophers and scientists. Perhaps there should be a conference about what each hopes to achieve—a question that surfaced several times but was never really attacked. As Medawar put it—no one envisages a draft solution. Why not?

Creutzfeldt in his talk (as at various times throughout the meeting) directed our attention squarely to the problems. As he said 'We have a sort of idea of mind and by inference that there is one in a cat or dog'. We are trying to find out what sort of idea this is. He gave us a list of the conditions of consciousness. His analysis of cortical functioning, full of facts and insights, showed how in each cortical area the world is represented in a different aspect in relation to the individual. I liked his brave speculation that the social relations of the individual are represented in the frontal cortex.

Another of Creutzfeldt's insights is that the whole system makes a synthesis by integrating into action. 'Consciousness *is* the continual change in cortical activity'. Unfortunately from this I did not get what he means by *is* and this is the epistemological problem at the core of the whole subject of our conference. Should we not go back to the basic grammar to discover what sort of attribution we wish to make when we say that something *is* something else? Surely this is a problem for philosophers and scientists together. Creutzfeldt believes that we are faced by a dualism that is unexplainable because it is of the nature of consciousness.

Armstrong gave us further definitions of what consciousness might be at various levels. He hopes to demystify the concept by comparing it with proprioception. There is a difficulty here in that we really know very little in detail about the relation of either muscle and joint proprioception or visceral enteroception to consciousness. Curiously enough we know far more about vision and its relation to consciousness than we do about the senses that tell us what is going on within our own bodies. However, Armstrong brought up again the importance of human self-consciousness with the idea that introspection occurs only in human beings.

I have been increasingly impressed over the years by the contribution that clinicians, including psychiatrists, have brought and are bringing to neurology and philosophy. Few people realize how much we owe to clinical science for knowledge of ourselves. We had excellent examples of that here. Cooper's ideas about disinhibition as a basis for revealing suppressed sensory capacities has enormous possibilities. In any multichannel system there must be a part that suppresses the unwanted responses so that only certain parts of the system control behaviour at any one time. Indeed in octopuses we have been able to identify the lobes that are involved in this task.[4] Our own species has an enormous repertoire of possible actions and to exploit them properly needs a very powerful suppressive device. We don't know where it is—perhaps the frontal cortex, perhaps the cerebellum; probably both of these and other sites too. Acting to excess these inhibition areas may well produce many symptoms including those that Cooper described. I hope he will follow the leads that they produce.

Dr Plum made us face further problems of the nature of consciousness in a very dramatic way by showing the difficulty of identifying signs of it when a person is in coma. This gives yet again warning that our intuitive feeling that we can recognize states of consciousness or mentality is not reliable. Where common sense does not give answers it may be that exact scientific observation and description can help. Philosophers can take part by showing where the ambiguities lie. Unfortunately discussion often proceeds on the assumption that the 'ordinary language' meaning is good enough as a basis.

Pat Wall brought out essentially the same point in showing the unreliability of our understanding even of the simple phenomenon of pain, and Marsden emphasized that even consciousness of pain is an obscure and variable phenomenon. Wikler carried the point further, showing us the doubts that philosophers raise not only about pain but other sensations as well. We might find that a major conclusion of our discussions is the rather obvious point that intuitive ideas and everyday language about apparently simple concepts are unreliable and may hinder attempts to solve fundamental problems. We need further exact observation and new linguistic and logical refinements if we are to make any real advance.

Wikler also brought us back to the consideration of intentionality. If pain is not intentional how can we use intentionality as a criterion of mentality? Dunstan reminded us that in the middle ages Pain was a Penance and what we now call pain was a hurt. Ploog reinforced this with the differences between English and German, where emotion is *Gefühl*, *Empfindung* is sensation and *Schmerzgefühl* a pain.

Above all, the pain discussion again brought out how deeply all of our concepts are social. The picture [not reproduced here] of a man in terminal cancer pained us all.

Dr Delgado's triunism introduced new problems and reinforced much of what had already been said. It is very helpful to consider the mind as a heterogeneous entity. Emphasis on the transmateriality of information avoids many of the traps in this subject. Finally Delgado drew our attention back to the fact that our knowledge is written in codes imprinted in the neuronal flesh. He showed us how it is possible to speak intelligently of the material and transmaterial or spiritual aspects of the brain. There is hope for a synthesis in his phrase that 'Mind appears when symbols by material means shape the neurons'.

These themes had recurred earlier in the last session. Crow showed us how for a patient anything is better than to be out of the social world. This is surely what we have been saying all along, that our whole thinking is social. Crow again emphasized how aberrant our perceptions can become. The common-sense view of the world is only one view. So is the view of physicists: it is the world as seen in their particular way. Are we sure they are more right than schizophrenic patients? We all hope so, but people in the future may be very different, perhaps in some ways more like schizophrenic people. It is not impossible—there are signs of that sort! In any case, people in the future will almost certainly be very different from Aristotle, Kant, Locke and us. They will have their own ideas about the relations of body and mind, depending upon the constraints of their technology and language. Their beliefs and intentions will presumably still be motivated by the urge to survive. Crow finally brought us right back to this theme, indeed to where John Searle started us, with the suggestion that dopamine pathways provide directional activation towards rewarding situations. What is that except intentionality?

References

1. YOUNG, J. Z. (1976) Choice, determinism and value in the light of biological knowledge. *J. Theor. Biol. 62*, 459–465
2. YOUNG, J. Z. (1978) *Programs of the Brain*, Oxford University Press, Oxford
3. SHERRINGTON, C. S. (1946) *The Endeavour of Jean Fernel*, Cambridge University Press, Cambridge
4. YOUNG, J. Z. (1965) The Croonian Lecture, 1965. The organization of a memory system. *Proc. R. Soc. Lond. B. Biol. Sci. 163*, 285–320

Chairman's closing remarks

JOHN R. SEARLE

Department of Philosophy, University of California, Berkeley

J. Z. Young is a hard act to follow, and anything I say will be hopelessly inadequate to the challenges that he has presented. On the other hand I have been sitting here in what is for me the uncomfortable role of listening to other people talk without saying a great deal myself. And I am not going to be able to hear myself talk in a feedback mechanism of the type brilliantly described here by Detlev Ploog. I am going to sound more dogmatic than I feel simply because there isn't time to develop the arguments.

First of all I should say that I don't find traditional disputes between dualism and monism at all helpful, for reasons which Hilary Putnam stated very clearly. What I am really interested in is a series of overlapping phenomena—beliefs, desires, pains, tickles and itches, perceptions, actions, intentions, knowledge and information and so on. If we really knew how all this was wired into the plumbing, we wouldn't be worried about how many substances we should count. What we want are detailed answers to quite specific questions, and here I am following what Dr Delgado said.

Secondly, I am very suspicious of the computer analogy. It is useful up to a point, obviously, and I think John Young is right in saying that the brain is preprogrammed for all sorts of things, but it is an empirical question exactly how far it is preprogrammed. But his position is quite different from that of many workers in artificial intelligence and cognitive psychology. What many of those people are saying is that mental operations consist *entirely* of computational operations on purely formally defined elements. That is a very strong empirical hypothesis and I don't know the slightest bit of evidence to show that it is true. Although it might be true, I see no evidence to prove, or even support, the view that in addition to a description of the neurophysiology and a description of the intentionality, we also need to postulate a different level of computational operations and say that mental processes consist entirely of formal operations on that level.

405

In one respect I have been very unclear in what I have said about intentionality. I wasn't citing Penfield's cases and Elizabeth Warrington's experiments
with Weiskrantz *in support of* my views of intentionality but rather as *para-*
doxical cases which any account of intentionality should be able to deal with.
This is characteristic not only of the history of science but also of the history
of philosophy: it is the paradoxical case that forces us to examine what our
hypothesis is and what sort of evidence would bear on it.

A short definition of intentionality is that it is that property of the mind
by which it is directed at objects and states of affairs in the world, including
of course its own operations and including the body in which it is located
and the actions of the agent of which it is a part. But that definition is unhelpful
because it doesn't explain directedness, which is the heart of intentionality,
and which I would like to see as more a part of the research programmes
of neuroscientific investigation than it is now. At present I think it is studied
in an *ad hoc* and disorganized way.

The simplest way to understand intentionality is to see its most obvious form
of expression in behaviour, and that is through speech behaviour. The unit
of human communication is the speech act. With very few exceptions all
speech acts are externalized forms of intentionality: when we make a statement
we are characteristically expressing a belief; when we give an order we are
characteristically expressing a desire; when we make a promise we express
an intention; and so on through a large number of other cases. Speech acts
have a certain kind of structure that is reasonably well understood. To
summarize it briefly, when we describe speech acts such as statements, questions,
commands, orders, apologies, promises, vows, threats and so on, we find it
useful to make a distinction between the content of the speech act and what
has been called the illocutionary force or type of the speech act. For example,
consider the order 'leave the room', the prediction 'you will leave the room',
the optative 'would that you left the room!', the hypothetical 'if you will
leave the room such and such will occur'. All of those speech acts in some
way contain the same propositional content, namely *that you will leave the*
room, but they contain it in different illocutionary acts, one an order, one a
prediction, etc. This is a very useful distinction to make and it is a striking
fact that it seems to carry over exactly to our mental states. Just as we can
order or predict that you will leave the room, so we can believe, hope, fear
or desire that you will leave the room. So the first thing to say about intentionality is that for a large class of cases we can make a distinction between the
representational content of the intentional state and its psychological mode,
whether belief, desire, fear, hope, etc.

There is another striking parallel between the structure of speech acts and the structure of mental states. Speech acts relate to reality in different ways. For example, we might say that it is the responsibility of our statements to match an independently existing reality. If I say it is raining then my statement will be true or false according to whether or not it is really raining. On the other hand if I make a promise that utterance has a different relation to reality, the responsibility for relating the utterance to reality then rests with me; for it is my obligation to keep the promise, i.e. to act in such a way that my behaviour fits the propositional content of my promise. Speech acts such as statements, assertions, descriptions, characterizations and explanations have what I call the word-to-world direction of fit: in these cases it is the responsibility of the words to match the world. We can represent this word-to-world direction with a downward arrow thus: ↓. Speech acts such as orders, commands and promises have what I call the world-to-word direction of fit, and we can represent this direction of fit with an upward-directed arrow, thus: ↑. In these cases it is the responsibility of people to match their behaviour to the words. Characteristically utterances with the word-to-world direction of fit can be assessed as true or false. Orders, commands and promises, however, aren't true or false: orders and commands are said to be obeyed or disobeyed, while promises are kept or broken. Certain other speech acts have no direction of fit. For example if I apologize for stepping on your toe there is no direction of fit, because although we have a propositional content—that I stepped on your toe, in apologizing I am not trying to tell you that your toe has been stepped on, nor am I trying to get it stepped on. Now, these distinctions apply exactly to intentional states. Beliefs, opinions and convictions, like statements and descriptions, have what we could call the mind-to-world direction of fit; but desires and intentions, like orders and promises, have the world-to-mind direction of fit. If my beliefs turn out to be false I can patch things up by changing my beliefs, but if my desire or intention isn't satisfied I can't in that way fix things up by saying I was mistaken in my desire or my intention. Similarly some mental states don't seem to have a direction of fit. Sorrow and pride, unlike belief and desire, have no direction of fit. However, those states contain beliefs and desires and the beliefs and desires have a direction of fit.

It is tempting to think that perhaps we could define all intentional states in terms of beliefs and desires (construed very broadly) together with logical constants, and modal operators. If for example I am afraid that something will occur, it is tempting to say that my fear equals the belief that it is possible that it will occur together with the desire that it should not occur. Thus fear $(p) = $ df. $Bel(\Diamond p)$ and $Des(\sim p)$. That is not a bad start on a definition but it doesn't quite work. For example I believe that it is possible that there will be a San Francisco earthquake and I very much desire, for all sorts of self-interested reasons, that there not be a San Francisco earthquake, but I am not in any genuine sense afraid of a San Francisco earthquake—maybe I ought to be but I am not. And this is even more obvious in the case of terror; I believe very strongly that it is possible, and I do desire very strongly that it not occur but I am not in fact terrified of a San Francisco earthquake. Nonetheless, a fear contains a belief and a desire as part of its structure, even though the fear is not equivalent to belief and desire. What I am inclined to say about the few pieces of data I have had time to present is that they indicate that the analogy between language and the mind, between the structure of speech acts and the structure of the intentional states, is really quite striking. Furthermore it looks as if we can make a kind of map of the mind in terms of these relationships, that is in terms of a rather small number of primitive notions, such as belief and desire, direction of fit, conditions of satisfaction, etc. The analysis will not be reductionist but rather a kind of diagram of interrelations. I doubt if we will be able to reduce everything to these two, *Bel* and *Des*, although they will certainly figure very prominently in the analysis. And you will recognize them as rough analogues to the traditional notions of cognition and volition—the jargon has been discredited but I think there is something in it, at least in the sense that there are two basic ways by which the mind is related to reality, that is the two basic forms of intentionality, mind-to-world and world-to-mind.

It seems to me that we have started to get an answer to the question of what is directedness. I might summarize it by saying that intentional states represent objects and states of affairs in exactly the same sense of 'represent' that speech acts do. And just as speech acts can be true or false, kept or broken, so in general can intentional states that have a direction of fit be satisfied or unsatisfied. The key to understanding intentionality is representation and the key to understanding representation is conditions of satisfaction. Every intentional state with a propositional content and a direction of fit represents its conditions of satisfaction.

Now I want to explain how some of the things that have been said at this meeting have been helpful to me in understanding how intentionality is wired into the neural circuitry and also show how it gets a little more complicated if we try to develop the theory of intentionality to any degree.

First, we never have an intentional state by itself. Such states come in great big networks, with sub-networks that are quite tightly constructed. There are very tight constraints on being proud of something, for example. If I say I am feeling very proud today and you ask me what I am proud of, I can't say 'I am just proud. I've just got this feeling in the hypothalamus and it's called pride'. Pride is intentional; I have to give you a representative content of my pride, and furthermore not just any content will do. I can't say, for example, 'I am immensely proud of the elliptical orbit of the planets' (unless I am Johannes Kepler). In order to be proud of a certain state, p, one must believe it to be the case that p, one must want p and furthermore one must believe that one is in some way connected with p. What one gets then with pride (or sorrow or blame or remorse) is a rather tight network. And there are bigger networks. For example if I believe that Heath is no longer Prime Minister and that Callaghan is now Prime Minister, in order to have those beliefs I would have to have a huge battery of intentional states: I have to believe that England is a country, that it is on this earth, that it is a monarchy but has a constitutional government, and so on. All those intentional states affect each other. The elements in the network are not independent of each other.

I said that these things are all representations but there are some forms of intentionality for which that account doesn't sit comfortably at all. Take perception. If I see this piece of chalk I am inclined to say that there isn't any *representation* of the piece of chalk; I just see it; and in seeing it I have a certain visual experience. Notice that visual experience has intentionality; and there is a very simple argument for that: even if I am hallucinating the piece of chalk, and there is no chalk there, still my visual experience is such as to tell me what the hallucination is a hallucination of. That is, I know what must be the case in order that it *not* be a hallucination, and to say that is to say I know the conditions of satisfaction as part of this intentional state. Perception (and action) involve major variations on our earlier structure. That is, when it comes to perception and voluntary action the intentional states are not representations but presentations that are direct causal and intentional transactions with the real world. This is true not only of perception but also of voluntary action: if I raise my arm I have a certain experience. That experience has intentionality. And again, I know that because the experience has conditions of satisfaction. If I have exactly this experience and the arm doesn't go up, I am having something analogous to a hallucination. The main difference between perception and action is that whereas visual perception has one direction of fit ($\downarrow$), the case of action has the other ($\uparrow$). My perceptions and my intentional actions have another feature, a causal feature built into the conditions of satisfaction. Because, for this visual experience to be satisfied, not only must a piece of chalk be present, but the piece of chalk must also cause the visual experience. So the conditions of satisfaction of the visual experience are self-referential. It refers to itself because its content requires that there must be a piece of chalk which is causing this very visual experience.

Similarly with the intentional action. When I raise my arm the form of intentionality is also self-referential: not only must my arm go up, but the going up must be caused by that particular intentional state. If I am right about this, all of it has to be realized in the neurophysiological mechanisms.

Now I am going to sound very much like a traditional philosopher and say that if we extend this notion of self-referentiality to cover both *presentations* such as visual experiences and experiences of acting on the one hand, and *representations* such as event memories and prior intentions to do something in the future on the other hand, we get a surprising formal symmetry between the structure of cognition and the structure of volition. Let's think of it this way: the relation of a memory to a visual perception is analogous to the relation between a prior intention and an intention in action. The distinction between prior intention and intention in action is for example the distinction between my intention now to drink beer in a few minutes and the intention I have when I am actually raising the glass during the actual experience. In the case of memory and visual perception we get the mind-to-world direction of fit ↓, because the memory and the perception are supposed to match the world; but we get the world-to-mind direction of causation ↑, because events in the world cause the memory and the perception. And the event memory is a representation of a total experience which includes both the visual perception and the object seen, that is, the object that causes the visual perception. But in the case of the prior intentions and the intentions in action the directions of fit and causation go the other way. These cases have the world-to-mind direction of fit ↑, because the world, i.e. the behaviour of the agent, is supposed to match the intentions; but they have the mind-to-world direction of causation ↓, because the intentions cause the behaviour that constitutes their conditions of satisfaction. Unless my intentions cause my behaviour, the behaviour is not a case of carrying out the intentions. Furthermore the prior intention—in a formal analogy to the event memory—is a representation of a total experience which includes both the experience of acting, i.e. the intention in action, and the bodily movement of the agent. These various relations can be seen in Table 1.

Thus there seem to be striking formal similarities between the structure of the intentionality that enables us to find out about the world, namely perceptual awareness and memory, and the structure of intentionality that enables us to act in the world, namely prior intention and voluntary action.

If I am right about this, it must be realized in the neurophysiology. It can't be an accident that the arrows come out like that, and there is a simple explanation for it. If the world comes to be the way I want it to be, that is if I achieve the upward direction of fit, it is because my action makes it be the way

TABLE 1

A comparison of the formal structures of 'cognition' and 'volition'

	Memory (of perceptual events)	Perception	Prior intention	Intention in action
Presentation or representation	Representation	Presentation	Representation	Presentation
Direction of fit	↓	↓	↑	↑
Direction of causation	↑	↑	↓	↓

↓ = mind-to-world; ↑ = world-to-mind

I want it to be, that is the downward arrow direction of causation. Similarly if I see the world the way it really is (mind-to-world direction of fit), it is because the way it really is is what causes me to see it that way (world-to-mind direction of causation). That is a rather simple epistemological explanation of the formal symmetry.

I have been helped in several ways by our discussions. First, pain is a very interesting case where the forms of intentionality which we get in representations, both mind-to-world and world-to-mind, actually affect a mental event. They help to structure the shape, working causally on mental phenomena that from this point of view are not intentional. Concerning the question of how we should categorize pain, I want to say that it does not fit comfortably into either of these categories, simply because it does not have a direction of fit. Originally Professor Wall suggested that it was wrong to regard pain as having an analogy with visual perception, and I think that is correct. But equally it is wrong to classify pain with thirst and hunger because those two are satisfied only if the world changes to satisfy the representation, that is only if I eat or drink, as the case may be. Although I think pain is associated with both beliefs and desires, the pain itself isn't identical with either the belief or the desire. My suggestion is that pain isn't intentional but lies in the middle somewhere.

Elizabeth Warrington's paper was also immensely helpful to me. Blind-sight is a challenge to the intentionalists' model because blind-sight clearly is in some ways like vision yet it doesn't have the form of realization in consciousness that vision has. Blind-sight does not have a self-referential content, because a man with blind-sight doesn't necessarily know that he has it; and amnesiac memory is a similar phenomenon.

Elizabeth Warrington also gave evidence to suggest that we localize various bits of intentionality in the brain. What is especially fascinating about her subjects is that the knowledge is apparently localized in ways that are counter-intuitive. It is counter-intuitive because our natural inclination is to say that the first things to be lost would be the abstract words and that the concrete words would remain. But patient AB lost the concrete words and kept the abstract ones. So his general intelligence apparently can't be involved there. One of the most fascinating questions as this subject develops is, how do you get from the kind of circuitry or synapses that Drs Ploog, Creutzfeldt and others described to intentional states? How do you, for example, get the unity of networks? There are obvious split-brain problems here because it looks as if there may be two partially connected networks of intentionality in the split-brain subjects, but how do you get to the unity of the network in the normal brain? Various answers were suggested to that and I hope to see more work on those lines. One suggested answer was that the explanation is essentially symbolic action. Another answer that seems to be completely independent, and maybe even inconsistent, was that it is morphogenetic, that somehow or other the explanation will come developmentally.

I would like to answer Peter Medawar by saying that the only way we'll know what will count as an explanation of our phenomena is to be able to point to some explanation that seems to satisfy our intellectual needs. One explanation that seems to get part of the way there is the feedback mechanism described by Dr Ploog as a neurophysiological explanation of self-awareness. The organism seems to have a mechanical structure that is somewhat like the formal structure. The reason that is unsatisfying as it stands is that we have no criteria for connecting our intuitive idea of self-awareness to the machinery that he described. There is a gulf between the machinery Dr Ploog described and self-awareness. Wherever we get the phenomenon of self-awareness we find this machinery, but how do we get them together to prove that the machinery realizes the self-awareness?

One of the things that might put them together would be something like the following. If we had behaviour that we were confident was a manifestation of self-awareness—and that is a large claim—and if we could show that that behaviour was tied to that mechanism, we would be a long way towards satisfying ourselves that the mechanism was explanatory in the right way.

I do not think we shall get an answer to the question of what general form of explanation will suit our needs until we start to get some good explanations. One possible form of explanation would involve getting behaviour criteria that manifest the underlying mental phenomena and then showing that those phenomena are correlated with corresponding phenomena in the neurophysio-logical wiring. That is as good a form of causal explanation as we are likely to get in the near future.

Index of contributors

*Entries in **bold** type indicate papers; other entries refer to discussion comments*

Armstrong, D.M. 33, 35, 36, 177, 181, **235,** 325, 330, 366

Bellugi, U. **99,** 129, 130, 132, 133, 134, 136
Bennett, J. 31, 40, 65, 75, **119,** 129, 130, 186, 243, 286, 325, 330
Blakemore, C. 37, 75, 131, **139,** 175, 176, 179, 181, 183, 184, 250, 325, 328, 329, 331
Brazier, M. **5,** 31, 32, 33, 34, 35, 36, 38, 42, 65, 177, 329
Bunge, M.A. 31, 32, 33, 34, 36, 38, 41, 42, **53,** 65, 72, 73, 77, 130, 131, 177, 179, 248, 250, 252, 330, 364, 366, 396

Cooper, I.S. 69, 133, 136, 246, **255,** 285, 290, 325, 332
Creutzfeldt, O.D. 32, 34, 36, 37, 67, 73, 74, 134, 180, 183, **217,** 249, 250, 252, 285, 289, 331
Crow, T.J. 69, 135, 327, 329, **335,** 361, 367
Crown, S. 132, 133, 136, 181, 328, **345,** 361, 362, 363, 366

Delgado, J.M.R. 251, **369,** 396
Dunstan, G. 289, 290, 326

Fried, C. 38, 71, 245, **279,** 285, 287, 288, 290, 292, 323, 362, 364

Khin Zaw, S. **167,** 181, 185, 361, 362
Klima, E.S. **99**

Levy, D.E. **267**

Marsden, C.D. 68, 137, 246, 287, **305,** 329 330, 332, 333
Medawar, Sir Peter 31, 35, 37, 39, 40, 65, 69, 72, 186, 285, 286, 395

Ploog, D. 31, **79,** 130, 131, 133, 134, 135, 136, 137, 179, 181, 327, 328, 363
Plum, F. 34, 66, 69, 74, 76, 133, 136, 246, **267,** 286, 287, 288, 289, 331, 365, 366
Putnam, H.W. 31, 32, 37, 40, 65, 66, 76, 129, 178, 182, 247, 325, 329, **355,** 365, 366, 367, 395

Searle, J.R. **1,** 35, 39, 40, 41, 42, 67, 69, 72, 73, 74, 75, 129, 130, 131, 176, 177, 179, 186, 244, 249, 251, 289, 323, 331, 362, 364, 395, **405**

Towers, B. **45,** 67, 68, 70, 71, 74, 75, 77, 133, 134, 180, 331, 398
Trevarthen, C. 37, 70, 71, 72, 176, **187,** 242, 244, 245, 246, 247, 250, 251, 252, 286, 287, 325, 362, 363, 365

Wall, P.D. 179, 250, 287, 290, **293,** 323, 326, 330, 331, 332, 364
Warrington, E. 134, **153,** 181, 183, 184
Wikler, D.I. 68, 182, 244, 287, 288, **315,** 323, 324, 325, 333

Young, J.Z. 31, 37, 40, 42, 66, 67, 68, 69, 70, 71, 75, 130, 134, 177, 179, 251, 288, 327, 328, 364, 366, 367, **397**

Indexes compiled by William Hill

Subject index

action
2, 247, 409
awareness and 192
centres of 244
control of 190
perception synthesis into
222
unity of 224
affective disorders
337
agnosic syndromes
157
aggression
injury and 299
programming of 57
altruism
57
American Sign Language
100–117, 125–127
cerebral specialization
for signs 114
dimensions of movement
109
grammatical processes
108, 126
hand slips 104
hemispheric dominance
and 126, 133
hierarchies of form and
meaning 112
historical changes in 105
iconicity of 107, 131
inhibition in 132
internal structure of 108
intrusion errors 103

lexical units 114, 126
morphological devices
108, 109
new signs 108
phonology 129
semantic distinctions 109
sublexical coding units
102
syntax 108
wit and poetry in 106
amines
opiates and 311
pain and 310
amnesia syndrome
161, 180
anatomical basis of 164
anterograde 161
retrograde 161
short-term memory and
164
amoebae
75
awareness in 47, 48, 399
analgesia, congenital
300
angina pectoris
303
anima, the
18
animals
awareness in 46, 180
response to injury 294
spatial localization 175
thinking by 56

animal spirits
8, 9, 11, 18
animism
36
anxiety, pain and
301
anxiety-defence mechanism
347
apallic syndrome
219
apes, artificial language in
56
aphasia
3, 291, 374
aphonia
pyramidal tract and 136
Aristotle
6, 74, 359
auditory cortex
94, 131, 133
auditory–vocal feedback
89, 91, 92
awareness
33, 37, 66, 243, 386, 399
action and 192
as property of living
matter 50
commissurotomy and 243
community in 190
conscious 189
consciousness and 188
culture and 212
definition of 72
double 245
environmental 46

417

awareness, *continued*
expressed in play 70
function of 49
in animals 46, 180
in infants 210
levels of 67, 70
of spatial relations 201
realms of 244
self 34, 412

babbling
86, 88, 91, 121
conditioning of 87
role of 90
babies
battered 286
communication with 132,
208
development of
consciousness in 70
discrimination in 120
interest in actions 250
interest in toys 250
sensory inputs 392
signals 121
Bacon, Francis
11
Baglivi
14
basal ganglia
consciousness and 225
pathways 256
role of 290
surgery of 285
behaviour
345
consciousness and 193
environment and 140
evolution and 59
importance of 59
pain and 323
behaviour, abnormal
361–368
communication and 345
deviance 348
humanist-existentialism
347
institutionalism and
compliance 349
behaviourism
54
Berkeley
10

Bichat, Xavier
19
biological elements of mind
369
biological solipsism
150
blindness
172
hysterical 181, 350
blind-sight
142, 411
body image
132
bradykinesia
226
bradyphrenia
226
brain
embryogenesis 251
brain death
267, 281, 289
brain development
382
brain function
23
brain growth
56
brain injury
care of 268
consciousness and 204
effect on vocalization 85
localization and 146
memory in 157
prognosis 281
brain lateralization
57
brain–self identity
267
brain surgery
285–292
implications of 155–166
legal and ethical
implications 279, 289
Broca's area
134, 230
Burton, Robert
11

Cabanis
14
cardinal cells
149

category mistake
40
cerebellum
function of 20
cerebral cortex
as site of psychic spirits 9
auditory 131, 133
chronic stimulation of 265
controlling voice 123
electrical stimulation 21
language and 229
larynx area 84
localization of function
17, 19, 21
memory and 220
pain and 310
retinal pathways to 171
role of 398
size of 197
stimulation of 290
visual 142, 149, 178, 205
cerebral dominance
American Sign Language
and 115
cerebral hemispheres
function of 20
cerebral neocortex
anatomy of 220
consciousness and 219
diversity of functional
representations in 219
hierarchical synthesis in
221
cerebral palsy
266
cerveau isolé
227
children
development of vocal
repertoire 120
reared among animals 378
Chomsky's hypothesis
31, 124, 129, 130
chorea
258
chromosomes
379
cingulate area
in vocalization 83, 93
cognition
79, 411
coma
402

clinical signs and outcome
of 270
definition 271
eye movements in 273
prognosis 269, 281
recovery from 271, 274
commissurotomy
effects of 198, 199, 201,
243, 245, 246
communication
80, 372
see also language
abnormal behaviour and
345
among primates 47
and the individual 346
by chimpanzees 373
in social interactions 350
in social situations 345
interpretation and 358
language in 373
medical care and 287
pain for 364
perception and 351
psychiatric treatment and
352
voice 373
without speech 99
computer
brain as 32, 356, 364,
367, 405
computer science
38
Condillac, Abbé de
12
conditioned reflexes
24
conscious intentionality
189, 199
consciousness
46, 184, 243–253, 278,
387, 395
aspects of 188
awareness and 188, 189
basal ganglia and 225
basis of 251
behaviour and 193
biological function of 367
brain anatomy and 195
commissurotomy and
198, 199, 201
cultural habitat and
212

definitions 76, 188, 217,
367, 401
description of 249
development of 70, 92
dualistic aspect 217, 229
environment and 192
evolutionary aspects
45–52, 192, 197, 238
fitness of world for 192
hemispheric dominance
and 292
images for movement in
190
information uptake and
191
in infancy 208
inner motivations and 206
in split-brain subjects 198
introspective 237, 252
levels of 218
mechanism of 187
midbrain systems and 226
minimal 235
neocortex and 219
neurophysiological
mechanisms 217–233
of self 240, 241
perception and 237
prognostic aspects of 269
reflex 239
self-reflective 46, 71
speech indicating 249
tasks of 187–215
types of 235–241
unification 189
wakefulness and 66
cooing
86, 87
core self
358
corpus callosum
absence of 199, 203
cortico-fugal output
223
creativity
132
crying
86, 87
cultural evolution
72

Darwin, Charles
53, 65, 70, 187

deafness
philosophical discussion
and 130
death
brain 267, 281, 289
definition of 281, 289, 291
decerebrate rigidity
21
decussation of nerve tracts
48
demons
11
depression
pain and 302, 310
Descartes
8, 9, 33, 34, 35, 38, 39, 42,
147, 176, 218, 219, 230
De Stutt de Tracy
14
deviance
348
Diderot
13, 36
diminished force
13
discrimination
120
Down syndrome
135
dreaming
237, 356
dualism
32, 33, 55, 56, 65, 73, 326,
330, 363, 370, 383, 396,
401, 405
Cartesian 37
materialistic 36
nature of 38, 39
religious context of 37,
38, 42
Sherrington's 35
substance 39
Du Bois-Reymond
23
dystonia musculorum
deformans
258
dystonic-spastic syndrome
262

Eccles, J.C.
35, 59, 65

emergence
396
emergentist materialism
46
emotion
79, 181, 328
speech and 85
encephalitis epidemica
226
enkephalins
311, 321
and pain 307
distribution of 308
functional control of 309
environment
awareness of 46
behaviour and 140
consciousness and 192
effect of actions on 90
knowledge of 168
manipulation of 91
relation to organism 252
response to 68
epigenesis
395
epilepsy
246, 266, 310
epiphenomenalism
72
epistemology
140
event memory
see under memory, event
event perception
191
event recognition
131
events research
181
evolution
53
behaviour and 59
brain growth during 56
consciousness and 45–52,
192, 197, 238
continuity of 55
cultural 72
development 69
genetic variation and 58
nature of 67
of brain 377
of intelligence 60, 66
of language 95

pain and 323, 325
qualitative novelties 54
social 73
evolutionary perspectives
53–77
evolutionary psychology
53
eye movements in coma
273

face
cortical control of 123
facial expression
88, 90
Flourens
20
functional localization
17
fun of living
49

Galen
9, 17
Gall, Franz Josef
19
Ganser state
132
genetic codes
379, 380
global agnosia
219
God
51
Goltz
21

Hall, Marshall
23, 24, 32
hands
manipulation with 244
neural control of 204
Hartley, David
14, 32
Hebb's principle
57
Helmholtz
23
hemiballismus
258
hemiplegic dystonia
262
hemispheric development
247

hemispheric dominance
201, 374
in American Sign
Language 128, 133
language and 125
hemispheric functional
specialization
247
historical background
5–43
Hobbes
32, 33
Homer
8
hominids
60
homunculus in the head
176, 177, 181, 249, 378,
398
Hoyle, F.
67
humanization
process of 378
Hume
10
humours
11
hunger
300
Husserl, E.
40
hypoxic ischaemia of brain
272, 274
hysteria
181, 350

ideas
12
identification
143, 194
identity
348, 358
identity theories
248
image problem
182
inductivism
32
infants
awareness in 210
consciousness in 208
infectious hepatitis 303

information
    363
    molecular carriage of 381
    receipt and storage 390
    transmaterial 387
injury
    326
    acute 299
    animal response to 294
    detection fibres 332
    human response to 296
    pain and 319, 331
    pain-free 297
    phases of response to 297,
        319
    recognition of 306
    recovery phase 323
    relation to pain 293–304
    sensory behavioural
        response to 294
institutionalization
    349
integration in brain
    179
intelligence
    artificial 55, 182
    evolution of 60, 66
intensive care units
    287
intentionality
    2, 33, 34, 40, 74, 130, 229,
        397, 402, 406, 409
    centre of 244
    commissurotomy and 245
    conscious 189, 199
    definitions 40, 406
    localization of 412
    realization of 41
interactionism
    36
internal feedback loops
    223, 224
isomorphism
    perception and 176, 179
itches
    324, 325

justification
    65

Kant, Immanuel
    23, 31, 34, 169, 228, 238,
        240

knowledge
    391
    sharing of 189
    theory of 66, 73, 139

Lamarckism
    69, 72, 74
Lamy, Guillaume
    9
language
    38, 79, 99–117, 124, 372,
        391
    among primates 47
    brain and 88
    cerebral control of 125
    cortex and 229
    effect of commissurotomy
        on 201
    evolution of 95, 381
    grammatical structure 124
    in communication 373
    nature of 3
    neurons and 130
    of mind 395
    origin of 57, 399
    relationship with reality 1
    role of 12, 42
    sound and 129
    understanding of 200
    use of 373, 397
    without speech 99
language organ
    129
larynx
    cortical control of 123
    position of 134
laughter
    57
Laycock, Thomas
    23
learning
    122, 376, 382
    brain structure and 381
    transmission of 71
Leibniz
    34, 218, 219
Leonardo da Vinci
    7, 8, 10
life
    value of 286
limbic area
    in phonation 85
    in vocalization 87

lipotropin
    308
living
    fun of 49
localization
    145, 171, 173
    in space 171, 173, 175
    of function 17, 21
Locke, John
    10, 12, 54, 238, 380
locked-in state
    271, 275, 282, 291
locomotion
    193
Luciani
    21
Ludwig
    23

Magendie
    19, 21
materialism
    18, 24, 53, 73
    emergentist 46
mathematics
    42
matter
    behaviour of 68
meaning
    recognition of 390
mechanistic concept of brain
    23
memory
    13, 175, 236, 382, 400, 411
    cortex and 220
    immediate processing 102
    pain and 329
    quantification of 181
    selective 206
    visual perception 410
memory, event
    157, 160–164, 165, 240
    central representation of
        163
    impairment of 161
memory, semantic
    156–160, 164, 181, 183
    impairment of 157
    relationships 164
memory, short-term
    103, 153–156, 367
    American Sign Language
        and 134

memory, short-term,
continued
among deaf people 134
central representation of
154
iconicity in sign language
and 104
impairment of 155
interrelationships 164
memory systems
183
interrelationships of 164
multiple 153–166
mental activity
377
midbrain
consciousness and 226
mind
existence of 371
ownership of 375
molecules carrying
information
381
monadology
34
monism
72, 363, 383, 388, 405
psychoneural 57
mood
201
pain and 310, 315, 323
morality
57
morphine
307
motor development
90
movement disorders
291
surgery for 255–266
Munchausen syndrome
132
mutation
59

naloxone
308, 309
natural spirits
11
nature and nurture
379
Naturphilosophie of Schelling
18

nerve impulse
147
nerve tracts
great decussation of 48
neurological illness
legal and ethical
implications 279
outcome influencing
decisions 267–277
prognosis of 269, 281
neurology, clinical
285–292
neuronal activity
dynamic complexity 376
neuronal processes of
behaviour
24
neurons
language and 130
pattern detection 389
Newton, Isaac
10

opiates
307, 311
orienting
193

pain
315–321, 411
acute 299
amines and 310
as penalty 324, 325, 326
as perception 315, 317,
325, 329, 333
as social response 331
behaviour and 323
chemistry of 305
chronic 302
classification 300, 316
cortex and 310
depression and 302, 310
emotion of 305–313
enkephalins and 307
evolutionary implications
323, 325
feelings of 306
for communication 364
function of 318, 320, 323,
324, 330
gate control theory of 307
in acute injury 299
injury and 319, 331

interaction of nervous
functions in 306
measurement of 330
mechanisms of 293, 327
memory and 329
mood and 310, 315, 323
private nature of 316
psychological aspects of
329
recognition of injury and
306
relation to injury 293–304
social aspects of 402
stimulation and 328
pain-controlling region of
brain
309
panpsychism
67, 74, 75
paranoia
350
parental behaviour
57
Parkinsonism
226
effects on mental state 285
treatment of 257, 285, 291
partial-orienting systems
195, 197
Pavlov
7, 24
perceived events
150
perception
3, 131, 168, 169, 170, 175,
188, 409, 411
action and 177, 399
ambiguity of signals 147
communication and 351
consciousness and 237
delusional 339, 340, 356
gating mechanisms 226
in plants 176
isomorphism and 176, 179
localization 145
logical problems 145
measurements 191
memory and 410
neuronal time factor 372
neurons and 171
pain as 315, 325, 329, 333
psychology of 191
reality and 139–152

schizophrenia and 339,
340
synthesis into action 222
unity of 222, 224
validity of 168
variations in sensitivity
149
perceptual categorization
184, 185
Perrault, Claude
12
petit mal
3
Pfluger
17
philosophy
1
as conceptual analysis
39
relation to science 167
research and 3
phonation
79
brain structures in 95
development of 87
limbic area in 85
phrenology
179
pineal gland
38
placebo reaction
299
plants
perception in 176
talking to 70
Platonic universals
170
play
70, 210, 250, 252
pontifical neuron
222
Popper, K.R.
35, 59, 65, 72
posture
193
Pourfour de Petit
17
presentation
410
pride
409
primates
language in 47

Prochaska
15
prognosis
269, 281, 288
proprioception
238, 330, 401
protein S100
376
protolanguage
247
psychiatric treatment
352, 358, 361, 366
psychology, evolutionary
53
psychoneural identity theory
58
psychoneural monism
57
psychoneurotic symptoms
346
psychosis
361–368
psychosurgery
279
pulvinar lesions
262, 291
pyramidal tract
136, 251

Radishchev
15
rational thought
32
reality
168, 178, 181
absolute 178
in animals 181, 184
logical problems 145
of external world 169
perception and 182
perceptual representation
of 139–152
validity of 169
receptive fields
143
recognition
143, 184
reflexes, conditioned
24
reflexes of brain
23
reliability
65

religion
37, 38, 42
representation
410
reserpine
311
reticular substance, lesions of
227
retina
direction selective
ganglion cells in 148
inhibition in 145
pathway to cortex 171
representation in brain
146
robots
76
Ryle, G.
39

Schelling's Naturphilosophie
18
schizophrenia
132, 266, 335–343, 355
auditory hallucinations
340
concept of 335
definition of 336
delusions in 356, 363
delusions of control in 339
diagnosis of 336, 365
genetics of 366
meaning of symptoms 340
neurochemical basis of
341
perception and 339, 340
psychotherapy of 366
symptoms of 337, 338,
340, 363
thought insertion in 338,
364
Schrödinger
69
science
and values 370
relation to philosophy 167
Sechenov, Ivan
23
seeing
149
self
267, 358
consciousness of 240, 241

self-awareness
    34, 92, 119, 132, 412
    definition of 119
    in infants 120
self-destruction
    361
self-expression
    362
self-representation through
    reflective loop
    229
semantic category mistake
    40
sense organs
    behaviour-environment
        interaction and 140
sensitivity
    149
sensory information pathways
    256
sensus communis
    8, 9, 16
Sherrington, C.S.
    7, 21, 23, 24, 25, 35
signals
    ambiguity of 147
    from babies 121
sign language
    100
    see also American Sign
        Language
    configuration and
        movement 102
    iconicity 100, 101
sleep
    288
sleep–wakefulness cycle
    226
smiling
    57
social communication
    345
social evolution
    73
social interaction
    350
social signalling
    101n
soul
    6, 9, 389
    disturbance of 11
    sensory action of 14
    site of 8, 16, 17

sound
    language and 129
spatial localization
    171, 173, 175
spatial relations
    awareness of 201
    interpretations of 147
speech
    399, 406
    articulation 86
    emotion and 85
    hemispheric dominance
        and 201
    indicating consciousness
        249
    in Parkinsonism 285
    vocal signalling and 123
speech act theory
    190
speech areas
    381
speech disorders
    85
split-brain phenomenon
    243, 246, 386, 412
Stahl, Georg
    18
strokes
    272, 275
Stuart, Alexander
    15, 16
subarachnoid haemorrhage
    272
substance dualism
    39
suicide
    361
surgery
    legal and ethical
        implications 279
Sylvius
    9
symbols
    391

tabula rasa
    10, 31, 395
terror
    408
thalamus
    257
thoughts
    among animals 56

brain area responsible
    for 136
    in Parkinsonism 285
thought insertion in
    schizophrenia
    338, 364
tongue
    123
transmaterial information
    387
tricyclic antidepressants
    311
trigeminal nerve
    332
trigeminal neuralgia
    303
triunism
    369–396, 402
truth
    66, 178

unconsciousness
    236

values
    370, 386
vegetative state
    268, 275
    definitions of 271
    legal and ethical
        implications 282
    prognosis 288
Vellansky
    18
verbal span tasks
    155
vision
    205
    cortical 205
    cortical lesions and 142
    function of 141
    intentionality and 409
    two system theory 142
visual cortex
    142
visual input
    371
visual world
    analysis of 141, 145
vitalism
    14, 15, 398
vital spirits
    11

vocal behaviour
  brain control of 122
vocalization
  anatomical aspects of 135
  brain structures
    responsible for 81
  cingulate area and 83, 93
  development of 87
  effect of brain lesions 85
  limbic area in 87
  preprogramming of 89
  species differences 121
vocal responses
  123
vocal signals
  role of brain in 80
voice
  373

  control of 92, 95
  development of 120
  instrumental use of 122
volition
  411
Voltaire
  10, 12

Wada test
  136
wakefulness
  288
  consciousness and 66
walking
  49
Whewell
  10, 32
Whytt, Robert
  16

Willis, Thomas
  9
Wilson's disease
  258
words
  comprehension of
    meaning 157
  concrete and abstract
    159
  selective preservation of
    159
world
  symbolic representation
    of 230
world of mind
  231
World 3 concept
  37, 59, 72